HERBAL MEDICATION FOR THE PEOPLE

The MEDICAL HERBALIST

Edited by

J. R. YEMM, F.N.A., D.O., N.D.

Published by
Melvin Powers
WILSHIRE BOOK COMPANY
12015 Sherman Road
No. Hollywood, California 91605
Telephone: (213) 875-1711

Printed by

HAL LEIGHTON PRINTING COMPANY
P.O. Box 3952
North Hollywood, California 91605
Telephone: (213) 983-1105

ISBN 0-87980-309-6
Printed in the United States of America

CONTENTS

THE MEDICAL HERBALIST

Incorporating "The Herb Doctor and Home Physician"

EDITORIAL

*". . . . . hills and dales,
thistles as well as daffodils."*

And so it is in life. Recently in a contemporary journal we read: "A legal M.P. in a recent public speech declared that he read the *Medical Herbalist* regularly, and it is indeed in many respects funnier than *Punch.*" That may have been meant for a thistle, but if our Journal affords the legal gentleman a good hearty laugh, then it fulfils a useful mission.

Just think of the numerous muscles called into activity by a good hearty laugh; notice the transfiguration of the physiognomy. The frowning brow, cold, hard eyes, and tight lips of the unemotional legal luminary is transformed, apart from the beneficial action on the abdominal viscera.

Laughter is internal gymnastics, and calculated to do far more good than a bottle of medicine dispensed out under the N.H.I. Scheme, and may be as good as a dose of herb tea.

Laughter is essential to life; it is the spice of life, although it is not given to all to appreciate the same kind of fun. We view life from various angles, and what may seem to be a very serious problem to a legal mind, would to another individual appear to be funny—"funnier than *Punch.*"

Of course, we have always had respect for the legal profession, not that some of its members have not afforded us some fun. Legal opinions, like doctors' diagnosis, oft-times disagree; but let anyone outside the profession dare voice an opinion, then—it's "funnier than *Punch.*"

We remember an occasion some time ago, whilst travelling up to London, a lady and a gentleman entering our compartment. They seemed just ordinary individuals. At the next stopping place another gentleman came into the carriage, and judging from his deportment and cut of his clothes, he was above the ordinary John Smith. The three entered into conversation; it seemed that they were acquainted. And we, in our corner, "all quiet and unconcerned like," could not help overhearing the conversation.

The lady was rather solicitous about her husband, and as it was nearing lunch time, she took from a bag a bottle of medicine and a glass. Pouring out a dose of medicine, she handed it to her husband. He looked apologetically at us and said: "It's not Scotch." "No, we know the colour; a drop of Scotch may taste better," we replied.

Then the last gentleman to enter came into conversation with the lady. "I see you are going to the City." "Yes; we have an appointment with Dr. ———, Harley Street, at 3 o'clock." "H'm!" "Dr. ——— made arrangements for us; he does not seem satisfied." "Ah, yes, he's a very good man." Then the patient spoke: "I don't know what we are going for. I feel grand for weeks, then an attack of giddiness will come on; it will pass off again in a few minutes. It's she that is worrying. We will hear what this man has to say, but he is not keeping me there."

Then the other gentleman spoke: "I do not suppose there is much wrong. Dr. ——— is very smart. I expect it's just a germ floating about in the brain." Just then he left the compartment, and we said to the lady: "That seems a nice man; he has a very intelligent face." "Oh, yes, he's Mr. ———, the barrister; a very clever man." Then to the gentleman we said: "Ah, so you are going to get some more medicine. It's a bad thing when you are in business if you do not feel up to scratch." The gentleman told us he was a bank manager, and when the train arrived at its destination we wished each other good day and the usual compliments.

Our readers may not see anything in the relating of this incident, but it has afforded us much fun. We make a study of psychology, and inwardly we were laughing when the legal gentleman gave his diagnosis of "a germ floating about in the brain." Had we been the patient, we would have questioned the statement. Undoubtedly the legal gentleman had read of the existence of germs, and probably believed that these little germs remain quiescent for a period, then give you a kick just to show you they are there, and go to repose again; it's—"funnier than *Punch.*"

We would not advise our readers to enter into an argument with a medical or legal man. They have been trained along certain lines, and honestly believe they are the *crême de la crême* of knowledge, the ambassadors of progress. Yet when we review the conflicting theories in medicine, and notice the spikes and loopholes in law, it's—Thistles.

We do ocasionally have a few daffodils. The same morning as we read the report quoted above, we received a letter from French Equatorial Africa, saying how "interesting and instructive" they have found our Magazine. Many M.P.s have written us and stated how much they appreciate our efforts, while from our numerous readers we have received many a bouquet—and a few thistles—to urge us forward in our task.

There is just a bit of the philosopher in us, for as Bacon said: "The eye of the understanding is like the eye of the sense; for as you may see great objects through small crannies, so you may see great axioms of Nature through small and contemptible instances." To us, this little instance opens out a huge vista; we use the political and economic lens to aid us. All great movements are born of the masses; it was ever so. It is so in Nature. The slower the growth, the more sturdy the plant. We believe the system of Herbalism to be founded on Truth, and before it reaches its zenith must go through the same stages as other great truths — indifference — ridicule — persecution.

Personally, we are content to wait, just pushing along slowly, gradually winning converts to our faith. Ultimately they must come, for deep in the minds of all men is the conviction that Nature is supreme. And, when by education and discernment the tinsel will be torn from many of our present-day legally protected systems, they will be exposed, in their nakedness, we venture to say they will present a sorry sight.

That is what we hope for. We desire a revolution, not the kind of revolution where there will be great upheavals and things reduced to chaos. But that gradual process whereby man will realize his duties as a citizen and take a personal interest in his own welfare. Then will he come to realise that, apart from economic factors (which he will be able to control), disease is the result of progressive life, the violation of natural laws. There can be no cure other than the obedience of these laws, and, as man is a product of Nature, so must he go to her for sustenance, be it food or medicine.

Again the philosopher comes uppermost. We cannot but realise our unworthiness to act as an advocate for such a great truth as is expressed in Medical Herbalism. We do our part, and in our simple way endeavor to present the truth as we understand it.

All great truths are simple. Scientific terminology may make them difficult to understand, but, fundamentally, all sciences are simple laws. The intelligent application of these laws will give the same results to prince and beggar.

"The Messiah cometh mounted on an ass." God grant that our Journal shall be the ass to carry health and happiness to His people.

Substitute for Tea and Coffee

To the Editor, "The Medical Herbalist"

Sir,—I have several times noticed in "The Medical Herbalist" references to substitutes for Tea and Coffee. The following formula is what I have used as a beverage for breakfast and tea daily for the larger part of my life. I have now passed my 80th birthday, and enjoy good health; and for this I believe I am largely indebted to the daily use of my formula for breakfast and tea:—

R Fl. Ext. Agrimony
" " Avena Sativa
" " Dandelion Root
" " Raspberry Leaves

Take an equal quantity of each. Mix and filter. Then to the full amount of filtered liquid add an equal amount of Simple Syrup B.P. Mix together. Use one teaspoonful or more to each small teacupful of hot milk or milk and water in suitable proportions. Add sugar if required.

Yours faithfully,
J. WARNER.

Allestree, Derby.

Bulbs

Gardener's Little Son: "My daddy's busy. He's putting plenty of bulbs in our garden."

Electrician's Little Son: "Oh! then what a blaze of electric light you will be able to have there."

ELDER DWARF.—*Sambucus ebulus*

Known also as Ground Elder, of which the leaves only are used medicinally, they are actively diuretic and are suitable for suppression of the urine; the infusion may be used either externally or internally the same as the flowers.

In Field and Garden

PLANTS OF THE FYLDE

Their Medicinal Values

And he spoke of trees from the cedars of Lebanon even unto the Hyssop that springeth out of the wall.

In the fields and ditches and even by the roadside you may have seen someone gathering an odd plant here and there as you have rushed past in car or 'bus. Perhaps you have wondered what he was doing and why.

The gatherer of plants was, in all probability, a botanist acquiring a few specimens for his collection or perhaps in order to subject them to closer scrutiny under the microscope.

If you had known this as you passed him by, you would probably have said to yourself: "Of what use is the botanist, and to what end does he aim? And, when he gets there, of what use will it be to mankind?"

The Answer

In reply, the botanist would point to the orchards, vegetable gardens and the like, and tell you that the vegetables and fruits we eat every day are but highly cultivated forms of wild plants and trees, and that all varieties of roses and garden flowers in general are there as a result of the inquiring minds of the botanists of yesterday.

Further, he would point out that were it not for botanists and herbalists, we should know nothing of the therapeutic or medicinal value of the herbs of the field, and much human suffering would go unrelieved.

There are many who, on their journey through life, see the general colouring of the world, but nothing of the great beauty of even the smallest of Nature's handiwork.

They see a plant in the fields, and can only tell you that it has a yellow flower and that its leaves are green, but of its name, generic order and virtues they know nothing, neither do they care.

If You Can—

Are you one of those? Can you name even a dozen herbs which grow in the Fylde, give the medicinal properties of three of them and say what diseases they are used to alleviate or cure? If you can, you are an exception.

In a day's outing in the Fylde the Herbalist should be able to gather the following herbs without difficulty:—Agrimony, Avens, Burdock, Celandine (lesser), Celandine (great), Coltsfoot, Chervil, Centaury, Comfrey, Chickweed, Dandelion, Elderberry, Eyebright, Fumitory, Figwort, Ground Ivy, Mouse-ear, Nettles, Plaintain, Purple Loosestrife, Pellitory-of-the-Wall, St. John's Wort, Sauce Alone, Scarlet Pimpernel, Yellow Dock, Tansy, Wood Betony, and dozens of others.

He may find one which is almost if not quite extinct. The latter is Sea Holly, which used to grow along the coast, but owing to the extensive building of recent years the land it grew on has been turned from waste land into gardens and building sites.

The botanist, as distinct from the herbalist, would find innumerable plant life to interest him, but to give a complete list of the flora of the Fylde would require several pages of this Journal alone.

M. H.

ANSWERS TO READERS' ENQUIRIES

By MEDICON

Question.—I have suffered from Bronchitis for some time, and am very short of breath. I can't stand tobacco smoke or fog, and even the changing from a warm room into a cold one starts me coughing. I have trouble in clearing my tubes of a nasty sticky phlegm. Of course, I feel ever so much better in the summer, when the weather is warmer. I will feel very grateful if you could give some advice as to treatment. (A. L., Colchester.)

Answer.—You do not give your age; but chronic Bronchitis is at any time a very obstinate complaint, and any treatment must be persevered with. The obvious thing for you to do is to avoid changing temperatures. It will not help you to sit in a stuffy room any more than in a chilly one. So long as the weather is fair you should get plenty of fresh air, but do not over-exert yourself. Here is a prescription which should give you a good deal of relief:—Horehound, Licorice Root, Coltsfoot, Spikenard, and Elecampane, one ounce of each. Boil in 4 pints of water for 30 minutes. Strain, and add when cold 2 drams each Tincture of Lobelia and Tincture of Cayenne. Dose: A wineglass four times daily.

Q.—My father has been troubled with Eczema for two years now. His body is all out in spots, and his legs are very bad, too. The itch is torture. He is 68 years of age, and has been in poor health generally. (B. Jones, Cardiff.)

A.—We have no doubt that the general ill-health from which your father suffers has allowed the toxins (poisons) to get a hold on the system. In order to obtain results, the blood will need to be purified. The skin eruptions are a sign that the organs are unable to deal with the poison in the usual way, and consequently it is being thrown to the surface. First of all, attention must be paid to the diet. Greasy and rich foods must be avoided, and the consumption of meat and sugary foods moderated. Plenty of green vegetables and fresh fruit should be included in the daily menu. If your father is unable to masticate his food, it may be mashed or cut into small pieces; or, better still, grated. The bowels must be kept open, since through this channel the majority of the poison is eliminated. To purify the blood, give the following:—

Yellow Dock Root.....	1 ounce
Burdock Root	1 "
Figwort Herb	1 "
Sarsaparilla Root	1 "

Boil in one quart of water for 20 minutes. Strain when cool, and take a wineglassful three or four times a day. Obtain an ointment from your local Herbalist.

Q.—I have noticed a hard lump about the middle of the abdomen on the right side, which seems to be about the size of a man's fist. There is no pain and no discharge. I went to a Naturopath last July, and he said it might be a cyst or a fibroid. About 8½ years ago, I underwent an operation for a supposed cyst, and perhaps this influenced the mind of the Naturopath. Of late years (four or five) menstruation has been exceedingly profuse except for the last eighteen months, when the periods have become fewer and discharge much less. This year, the only periods of show being January, July, and just a week ago, discharge slight, sometimes continuing for a week, sometimes a day or two, and no pain. I want to know first, what to do to thoroughly clear up the menopause, and then what is the best course for me to take with regards to the lump in the abdomen, always bearing in mind that I want to avoid an operation if possible. (Miss M. H., London.)

A.—First of all I would advise you that no attempt can be made to "clear up" the menopause, that a normal menopause is best managed by hygienic methods without recourse to medicines. During the "change of life" the body is readjusting itself both mentally and physically, and thus it is not surprising that any tendency to ill-health will make its appearance at this time if the system is abused. Any medicine taken must be mild, and even then only if the symptoms are severe. Avoid stimulating foods, condiments, and rich, spicy articles, and get on to fruit, vegetables, salads, and wholemeal bread. Do not drink tea in large quantities, but try to substitute for it Dandelion Coffee. Give the body plenty of freedom, that is to say, do not wear tightly fitting clothes, and get out into the fresh air, and avoid stuffy rooms. Another point is always to remember to keep the bowels regular. If you are prone to nervous symptoms, as a great number of women are at this time, take a course of the following:—

F. E. Motherwort . . . ¼ ounce
" Scullcap . . . . . ¼ "
" Black Haw . . . ¼ "
" Prickly Ash . . ¼ "
" Chamomile . . . ¼ "
Syrup Ginger . . . . . . 2 ounces

Dose: One teaspoonful morning and night.

Regarding the abdominal swelling, I can only say that cysts have a habit of recurring, and I would suggest that you put yourself in the hands of a qualified Herbalist without delay.

Q.—My sister, 44 years, has been told that she is suffering from Gall Stones, and I write for advice from "Medicon." Would a liniment help? (Moore.)

A.—My experience is that internal remedies are most beneficial for Gall Stones, and I would recommend the following herbs:—Agrimony, Clivers, Dandelion, Barberry, Black Root; of each half ounce. Add three pints of water; boil down to two pints. Add 2 drachms Tinct. Lobelia when strained. Dose: A wineglassful four times daily. If there are acute attacks of pain, these are best relieved by poultices of Lobelia seeds. It is necessary for you to avoid all greasy foods and those which are highly spiced. Finally, one of the best things for Gall Stones is a daily dose of Olive Oil.

Q.—Can you give me a cure for Trigeminal Neuralgia without an operation, as at times I suffer terribly with it. I would be very grateful. (A Great Sufferer).

A.—Trigeminal Neuralgia is a very obstinate trouble, as you have probably found, and any treatment must be persevered with. Do not be persuaded to take depressive drugs, since although a certain amount of relief may be obtained, the reaction is always worse. Avoid stimulating foods such as meat and cheese, and be very sparing with condiments, especially salts. I would recommend you to try a course of the following herbs:—Jamaica Dogwood, Scullcap, Valerian, Black Cohosh, Prickly Ash, and Cinchona Bark, of each equal parts. To each ounce put 1½ pints of water. Boil down to 1 pint. Strain, and when cool take a wineglassful thrice daily. If you can obtain tinctures and fluid extracts, you may get quicker effects.

Q.—I have suffered from a very bad taste in my mouth for this last twelve months or more, tongue coated with a yellowish covering every morning. I am 60 years old and 14½ stone in weight. ("Anxious to Know," South Shields).

A.—A yellowish coating on the tongue certainly points to a disordered liver, and this may quite possibly be due to dietetic errors. Take no greasy food, avoid the frying pan, eat no pastry or richly spiced foods. If you are not a teetotaler be strictly moderate, and see that you are not smoking too much. A course of the following herbs should put you right.—

F. E. Black Root ...½ ounce
" Bogbean .....½ "
" Centaury ....½ "
" Clivers ......½ "
" Mandrake ..1 teaspoonful
Syrup Ginger ....3 ounces

Add water to 8 ounces. Take a tablespoonful three times daily before food.

Q.—I have three swellings or lumps, one on top of the breast, hard; another nearer the arm, softer; and a small lump in the armpit. Have noticed, also been treating them for two years. I have never been strong, and am so easily tired. I should be so glad if you could recommend treatment, external and internal, containing something for nerves. What I have used has made no difference to the swellings as yet. Age over 40. There is no pain. (Yours truly B. L. Rotherham).

A.—It is extremely difficult to say what the lumps are, and I would advise you to consult a qualified Herbalist for an examination. Most probably certain glands are blocked and swollen, thus causing the lumps. This trouble is sometimes due to constitutional hereditary weakness, which may not develop until later in life. Plenty of fresh air is needed, and if you are well protected, I would advise you to spend as much time in the open air (and sunshine) as possible. The nervousness of which you complain may be a sign of general debility, and therefore you will be helping to overcome this difficulty by treating and strengthening the whole glandular system. Here is a prescription which will help you:—

F. E. Tag Elder ....½ ounce
" Queen's Delight ....½ "
" Blue Flag ....½ "
" Echinacea ....½ "
" Yellow Dock ..½ "

Add water to 8 ounces. Take two teaspoonsful in water four times daily. Apply externally Marshmallow Ointment.

Q.—I suffer from an enlarged spleen, caused by having Malaria during the war. I do not have the fever, only my left side troubles me, and this mostly when I have been standing in one position for some time, or when I feel cold; thus dull pain is always there. I might add that I took a great deal of Quinine during the war. If you would say if this could be cured, or what would give relief, I would be most grateful. (D. C., Malton.)

A.—After all this time, I would not be so rash as to promise a cure, but if you would give the following prescription a fair trial, it should certainly help you:—

Tr. Ginger........ 2 drachms
Tinct. Hydrastis...½ ounce
F. E. Dandelion....½ "
F. E. Blue Flag....½ "
Add Water to..... 6 ounces

Dose: Two teaspoonsful in water before meals. Always keep the bowels well open, and avoid greasy foods, which tend to upset the liver.

Q.—Ever since my periods commenced I suffer untold agony each time. I am 37 years of age, of small build, married and have one child, a boy of five years. I thought that after having a child, things would improve; they have not done so. For days before they come I have to go to bed; otherwise I am in good health. Please help if you can, as my doctor can do nothing for me. (Periods, Workington.)

A.—It is extremely difficult to tell the cause of the trouble, since it may be brought about in many ways. It is quite possible that it is due to the way in which you are made; and if this is the case, you will unfortunately have to wait until the change of life. However, there is no harm in trying the following prescription:—

F. E. Helonias ....3 drams
F. E. Black Haw......3 "
F. E. Avena ....3 "
F. E. Wild Yam......3 "
F. E. Raspberry Leaves.3 "
F. E. Black Cohosh....3 "
Add Water to.........8 ounces

Dose: Take one tablespoonful in water three times a day before meals.

CASE IN PRACTICE

STUDENT 608

An interesting case came my way some twelve months ago. I was requested to call upon a lady who had been subject to epileptic fits for nearly twenty years, during which period she had been consistently treated without much success, and for the first few weeks I confess to little progress, until we noticed accentuation of each menstrual period. Enquiry revealed an incident associated with the beginning of the trouble and overlooked by the medical attendant at the time, since when the following agents have proved completely effective:—

No. 1.

Stinking Arrach,
Blue Cohosh,
Pennyroyal, equal parts,

just prior to menstrual period to bring about a natural determination to the uterus, following with the combination below upon cessation of above:—

No. 2.

Vervain,
Scullcap,
Cramp Bark, equal parts.

These have apparently eliminated the sources of irritation set up at each uterine cycle via the sympathetic nervous system, with the happy result of freedom from the above thraldom of twenty years.

Q.—I am the victim of chronic nasal catarrh. I have been suffering for about three years, and as a result my general health is very much undermined. There is a persistent mucoid discharge from nasal passages, and the membranes are rather inflamed. I have a tendency also to have an intermittent cold in the head. I have used some nasal douches without effect, and have tried various mineral drugs internally, obtaining only little relief. I would be most thankful if you could help me. I promise to adhere to your remedies and advice. I am 26 years of age and unmarried. (J. P. S., Ireland.)

A.—Chronic nasal catarrh will not, unfortunately, stop at that point, but will gradually spread throughout the system. The stomach may be affected by the swallowing of mucus during sleep. Catarrh is caused by a relaxed state of the mucus membranes. Normally there should be just sufficient mucus present to moisten the membranes, but when an irritation is set up either by dust or certain odours, there is an increase in the amount of mucus secreted, this being an effort by Nature to remove the irritating matter or to protect the membrane. The object, when treating catarrh, is to tone up the membranes, and for this purpose astringents are necessary. I do not entirely believe in douches, and would rather rely on internal treatment. For this complaint I would prescribe a simple but effective remedy, namely, Composition Essence. Regular doses of this in hot water will bring about excellent improvement. Do not despise this remedy because it is so well known, for I can assure you that it cannot be surpassed.

Q.—Male, 54 years old. For some time now I have suffered the inconvenience of my discharging water. When I go to make water I have a fair flow for a time, then it just dribbles at the finishing part; have to make an effort time and again to empty the bladder. I rise twice through the night to make water. (Moriti, Cumberland.)

A.—Were you a little older I should put your trouble down to the prostate gland, but in the circumstances it may just be one sign of nervous debility. This would cause an irritability of the muscle which guards the entrance to the bladder, and as soon as the urine irritates it, it will relax and let the urine through. However, being irritable, it will tend to close spasmodically near the end of urination, thus causing the symptons of which you complain. I would advise the use of the following herbs:— Black Willow, Uva Ursi, Damiana, and Golden Seal. Use equal quantities of each. Add to each ounce one pint of boiling water. When cool, strain, and take a wineglassful four times daily.

THREE DOCTORS FINED

"Two doctors were each fined £25 by the Middlesex Insurance Committee yesteday for failing to return a number of medical record envelopes. It was stated that one doctor had previously been fined for a similar offense, and that the second had been fined three times for failing to keep his medical records properly.

"A third doctor was fined £5. It was alleged against him that he treated a young school teacher for indigestion. There was no improvement in her condition, so she consulted another doctor, a woman, who, she said, found a very large cyst, and sent her to a hospital specialist, who advised an operation.

"At the hospital she was told that the cyst had been forming for five years."

"The Daily Telegraph," Dec. 3, 1935.

"FOLK MEDICINES" RETURN TO FASHION

"The years since the war have seen a remarkable revival of interest in folk-songs, folk-lore, and even folk cookery. It is not surprising that even learned medical men, tired of the knife and disappointed with this gland or that, are turning to 'folk medicine.' No branch of study of the past is more interesting than that of the medicine of our forefathers, who lived naturally, and when they wanted physic returned to Nature herself for it. Now ancient tomes are being re-read and old men and women, some of whom can neither read nor write, are being interviewed in an endeavour to recall and record priceless gems of information before they are lost for ever.

"More than one surgeon has won success and fame by reviving the Seton, re-introducing 'blood letting,' and again employing the leech. But it is the physician to whom the medical literature and practices of the past appeal with greater force. Generally he is faced with two difficulties—where can he find the Nature remedy he desires and how can he get it properly administered and prepared?

"Yeast as Blood Purifier

" 'Miracles' can be worked with yeast as a blood purifier. Some say that in its freshest state, yeast will beat every vaccine and synthetic preparation the chemist can produce. It is not easy to get and few understand its administration. The doctor and patient who take the trouble to get it fresh from its source will be rewarded with surprising results such as never followed the administration of a medicine or the injection from a syringe.

"Medicinal herbs were used in the past not only to cure but also to prevent disease. As a precaution against contagion, Rue and Rosemary were sprinkled in the Old Bailey. Even to-day Lavender and Camphor are used for the same purpose. Modern research has proved that our grandmothers used herbs without our present-day knowledge of what they contained, but they were wise in their generation in doing so. We know now that many herbs contain essential oils superior to anything the chemical laboratory can offer us.

"The plants and seeds used in 'folk medicine' are easily and cheaply procured. They are hardy, and well repay the little trouble required to cultivate them. They sometimes afford relief when all else has failed.

"Value of the Dandelion

"Among the most famous remedies of the past is the Chamomile poultice which is still popular, whilst the tea made from the flower has much to be said in its favour and is extensively used in France. The Dandelion taken in the form of a decoction has become famous for its liver, kidneys and stomach complaints. Celery in the form of tea has been long known as a remedy for neuralgia and sciatica, and its active principle is sold at a high price under another name.

"Chestnut leaves made into a fresh infusion are almost a specific for certain types of spasmodic cough. Kidney trouble may be relieved by a fresh infusion of Broom tops, and Stinging Nettles are not only a novel vegetable, resembling Spinach, but also in the form of a strong decoction, a remedy for the miseries of feverish gout. Another good remedy for winter coughs and colds is a Thistle infusian.

"These are but a few examples of rustic remedies which suggest that spare ground in the garden might be put to profitable use. It opens up a new hobby which is not without profit to both body and pocket. With the ever increasing demand, it is possible that supplies may give out, while our modern knowledge of vitamins makes it almost essential that to get the best results, the infusion or decoction must be freshly made from freshly collected herbs. To have the herbs growing as it were, at one's doorstep is almost equivalent, for ordinary complaints, to having the doctor and chemist under one's own roof."
—Press cutting.

Simplified Directions for compounding the Prescriptions in this book that are to be used internally only.

Most of the prescriptions in this book which are made up of Fluid Extracts and Tinctures may be made at home in tea form.

In place of the fluid extract, use the same quantity, by weight, of the dried herb. Mix the herbs and place three teaspoonfuls in a cup of boiling water. Allow to stand for thirty minutes and strain. Add as much honey as you have liquid and keep in the refrigerator.

Dose two or three tablespoonfuls three times a day.

Answers to Readers' Enquiries—Cont.

Q.—My wife, 43 years old, is now having all the signs and symptoms of an ulcer on the stomach, so the doctor says. Six months ago she fell off a ladder, and her left leg went into a boiler of nearly boiling water, and, he says, no doubt shock has been one of the causes. Bitterness and sourness after food gives her much trouble, and pains in the stomach for some months have been bad; also pains in the back are in evidence. She is in bed, and has been for a week with her periods; they have been missing five months, and came on the 30th December, 1935, for one day and one night, and lost very little. This was brought on by shock a week after she saw a motorcycle accident. (Box, Cumberland.)

A.—The series of shocks have undoubtedly upset the nervous system, and the stomach has, apparently, suffered. Another result of the nervous derangement may be that the change of life may come on sooner than usual, so do not be surprised if there are menstrual disturbances. The symptoms of the stomach trouble certainly point to a threatened ulcer, even if one has not already developed, so I am going to give you a treatment for gastric ulcer.

Now, first and foremost, a diet is essential, and even more important than medicine, I would suggest that for a fortnight your wife follows out the following plan.

Take a teaspoonful (or more) of Olive Oil before each meal. Let each meal consist of Slippery Elm Food, Slippery Elm Cocoa, and white bread and butter. Three or four meals may be taken daily, but only of those things mentioned. This will give the stomach a rest, and allow the ulcer to heal. After a fortnight, if all goes well, light articles of food, such as boiled eggs, boiled fish, and baked custards may be added to the diet. When the pains have gone, add vegetables gradually until the patient is back on normal rations. Remember, however, that the process must be slow.

As a medicine, the best thing to take is Tincture of Golden Seal in small but frequent doses. This will soothe the inflamed tissues, heal the ulcer, and tone up the stomach membrane and muscle.

Finally, I want to impress upon you that the medicine is of no use unless the diet is adhered to.

Q.—I am 64 years of age, and have been troubled with Piles for over 20 years. For the last 10 or 12 years I have rarely missed a day without being troubled with them. They come down like a fleshy protuberance about the size of a half-grown tomato, and when down for several hours, often discharge a mucus, and at other times bleed. They usually come down when I have been at work an hour or two, and have to be pushed back. Also, they have to be pushed back when the bowels are emptied. The stools are kept just short of a watery condition. I have tried Sulphur, Confection of Senna, Liquid Paraffin, Cascara, also many advertised remedies, without receiving benefit. (Hopeful, Grimethrope.)

A.—After having suffered for 20 years, the lower bowel will be in a chronic state of relaxation, which is shown by the mucous discharge and the watery stools. Therefore, the only successful method of treatment will be the one which aims at astringing and toning up the mucous membranes. For this purpose I will give you the following prescription, which must be persevered with for months if necessary:—

F. E. Prickly Ash...3 drachms
F. E. Stone Root....3 "
F. E. Witch Hazel...3 "
F. E. Black Root....3 "
F. E. Burr Marigold.3 "
Add water to.......6 ounces

Take two teaspoonsful in water before meals. If you prefer to use the crude herbs instead of extracts, obtain an ounce of each. Put one ounce of the mixed herbs into one and a half pints of water. Boil down to one pint. Strain, and bottle. Take a wineglassful three times daily. In addition, obtain Green Pilewort Ointment from your herbalist and apply after every motion. Regarding your diet: Avoid all greasy and spicy foods. Be sparing with meat, cheese, and eggs, and cut down the consumption of salt.

Q.—My wife suffers from the cramp in both her legs, and has done so for some time. Doctor's medicine has done her no good. It comes on every night when she is in bed. She is 57 years of age. (Have Suffered, South Shields.)

A.—The cramps from which your wife suffers show that the blood circulation is feeble. Consequently, I am going to give you a prescription which will improve this condition. Take one ounce each of Prickly Ash Bark, Black Cohosh, Vervain, Bogbean, and Guaiacum Rasps. Add six pints of water and boil for half-an-hour. Strain, and add two ounces of Composition Essence. Take a wineglassful four times daily. You need not make all of this quantity at once. Half the amount of herbs can be used to make up half of the medicine. The treatment must be persevered with, since it cannot be cured in a short time.

Q.—What are the best herbs to take for a fatty heart, and hardened arteries of the heart? Also, the best herbs for appendicitis. I know another man with a slight pain at bottom of right ribs, on towards his navel. (W. Herbert, Tredegar.)

A.—If there is fatty degeneration of the heart, there cannot also be hardened arteries. However, here is a prescription which will help the arteries:—Valerian, Lime Flowers, Wood Betony, Motherwort, equal quantities of each. To one ounce of the mixed herbs and roots add one pint of boiling water. Simmer for three minutes. Let stand for half an hour. Strain and bottle. A wineglassful is to be taken three times daily. The diet is quite right if it contains a lot of vegetables, since these contain a substance called chlorophyl, which is good for the heart. The best herbs for appendicitis are Elder Flowers and Peppermint. This is a very simple remedy, but effective. A pain around the navel is sometimes a sign of colic, but it is difficult to say without knowing more detail. It may be, again, a sign of trouble in the gall bladder, or ulcerated duodenum. I would advise a visit to the nearest qualified herbalist.

Q.—One of the family has gradually become in a run-down condition, and is also nervy. Wrinkles have formed on the forehead, her hair has become dull and thin. Her eyes have been dull, and recently they have become large and prominent. What should be done to overcome this condition. As she is about to take Cocoa and Slippery Elm, what proportions do you recommend of each, and if fine sugars should be added. (T. Yorks, Ossett.)

A.—All the symptoms point to severe nervous debility, which will have to be checked before a breakdown occurs. Here is a prescription for the nerves which will tone and stimulate:—

F. E. Scullcap .....3 drachms
F. E. Valerian .....3 "
F. E. Mistletoe ....3 "
F. E. Hops ....3 "
F. E. Gentian .....3 "

Add water to 8 ounces. Take two teaspoonsful in water before meals. Regarding the Cocoa and Slippery Elm, why go to the trouble of mixing when you can obtain Slippery Elm Cocoa which is already prepared?

Q.—I have read with interest the copy of "Medical Herbalist" you have been sending me, and I am wondering whether you could help me. I have attacks of Migraine with the usual symptoms: sight distorted and severe pain over left eye and temple. At these times my motions are very pale in color, and I get constipated. For years I have taken Calomel or blue pills, and this seems to clear me, and my motions then become dark. I take very little fat; eggs and onions, I cannot digest. I am 66 years of age. The attacks are more frequent since I left the footplate to come to Parliament. If you would advise me on the above, I should be grateful. (M.P., House of Commons.)

A.—You do not say whether the attacks end with vomiting or not. This is usually the case with Migraine. The pains in the head become more and more intense until an attack of nausea and emesis relieves it. Migraine is, as a rule, classed under nervous affections, but I am inclined to think from experience that in your case the whole trouble lies in the liver and gall bladder. The dark color of a normal motion is due to the bile pigments it contains. Clay colored stools point to a deficiency of the pigments, showing that the liver and gall bladder are obstructed in some way. Calomel is a strong liver stimulant which will relieve the obstruction, but the objection I have to its use is that it exhausts the liver and leaves it in a worse condition than it was before. In other words, it can never cure, only relieve. Now in the treatment of Migraine by herbal remedies I have found that a combination of gentle liver and nerve herbs has proved very effective. Here is a prescription which I have known to give definitely good results:—

Tinct. Gelsemium .. 2 drachms
F. E. Wahoo Bark. .½ ounce
F. E. Black Root . .½ "
Tinct. Pas. Flower. 2 drachms
F. E. Scullcap ..... 2 "
F.E. Am. Mandrake. 30 drops

Add water to 8 ozs. Take one

tablespoonful in water night and morning.

I would advise you to continue with the medicine between the attacks, as the object of it is to cure, and not only to relieve.

Regarding your diet, the following facts may help you. Soups made with vegetables are good, but meat broths, fatty soups and cabbage soup are forbidden. Meat is permitted in small quantities only two or three times per week. White meat and poultry, fresh lean ham, and cold pork are well tolerated, but veal, hot pork, liver, kidneys, brains, sweetbreads, fats, stews, preserved meat, game, and sauces made with acid condiments, are forbidden. Fresh lean fish such as turbot, halibut, sole, whiting and trout may be taken, but avoid all shell fish and oysters.

Eggs are forbidden, even when used in sauces. Milk should be skimmed, and butter taken only in small quantities. Cream and fermented cheeses are bad.

Cereals and semolinas are quite good.

Bread in any form is not good, so cut it down to a minimum.

Green vegetables and plain boiled potatoes are permitted, as are also salads without seasoning. The following are forbidden:—Cabbage, spinach, sorrel, tomatoes, turnips, and radishes.

Heavy pastry and cakes, containing eggs must not be taken. Chocolate and cocoa should be cut out.

Salt, vinegar, and lemon may be used in strict moderation, but spices, pepper, mustard and pickles must not be taken.

If you will give both the medicine and diet a fair trial, you should get excellent results. I shall be only too pleased to enlighten you further if there is any point upon which I have not touched.

Q.—The change of life is now established twelve months, and my headaches are terrible at times. I have also "whites," some days I am free of the discharge, other days quite the opposite. My age is 43 years. The mouth and tongue of a morning are very foul indeed. I am a poor eater, troubled with wind in the stomach, but the bowels are nice. Some days I am listless, other days I can work well, but tire about 3 p. m., and have to rest. The heart beats very fast and heavy at times. (Cumbria, Cleaton Moor.)

A.—At the change of life the whole nervous system is disturbed, and it is very easy for a woman to become very run-down at this time. This is why you have the "whites," which is a sign of debility. It may be difficult for you to realize that all the symptoms you have are the outcome of the nervous trouble, but I can assure you that this is so, and I will therefore give you a prescription which will get to the root of the trouble. Take an ounce each of Scullcap, Wood Betony, Valerian, and Hops. Boil in 2½ pints of water down to 2 pints. Strain, and when cool take a wineglassful three times daily. Make an infusion of Chickweed, and use it as a douche regularly.

Q.—I have had a three months' miscarriage recently, a great disappointment to us. My doctor was unable to tell me the reason for this miscarriage, but I myself think there is some weakness of the womb and it just wants toning up. There is no displacement, I have been examined for that, and the periods are regular and normal. Can you suggest any herbs I could take to strengthen the womb, and also a herb that prevents miscarriages. (Mrs. G. W. Folkestone.)

A.—There is a remedy for strengthening the womb and preventing miscarriages which is very effective, but often over-looked becaused of its simplicity. I refer to Raspberry Leaf Tea. This is made in the following way:—To one ounce of Raspberry Leaves add one pint of boiling water. Allow this to stand for twenty minutes, then strain. Take from half-a-pint to one pint daily, sweetened if desired with sugar or honey. This should be continued throughout pregnancy, and not only will it prevent a miscarriage, but it will ensure an easy confinement.

Q.—Please would you advise me on the following, as I have tried several kinds of ointment, etc., and all of them no use. Occasionally, there grows on my ear very hard small lumps just like a very big corn, and it is very painful and sore to the touch. I had three of those cut off by my Panel doctor, but they come on again. There is no discharge from them, just solid flesh. (Troubled, South Shields.)

A.—There are such a variety of growths that it is impossible for me to diagnose through correspondence, and I should advise you to pay a visit, to a qualified Herbalist. However, in the meantime, I should like you to try Chickweed Ointment, which has a good reputation for removing all kinds of growths.

Q.—Would you please give me advice and tell me what you could do for my wife. She is 61 years old and is suffering from Blood Pressure, and it has affected her sight very badly and she cannot see to read. She suffers with terrific pains in the head, all at the right side, and her hands are always very cold. There is also a great deal of Asthma. (Robert James Stewart, Southwich-on-Wear.)

A.—In this case I have come to the conclusion that your wife is of the nervous type. Blood Pressure is not a disease, it is only a symptom, and can be caused by several conditions. Nerve tension is one of these, because there are nerves which, if they get out of hand, will cause contraction of the blood vessels and thus cause the blood pressure to rise. The Asthma can also be of nervous origin, but in this case, instead of the blood vessels being contracted, it is the lung tubes which are compressed, thus preventing the air from flowing in and out freely. However, the first thing to do is to bring the blood pressure back to normal, and so here is a prescription which will help. Take of Lime Flowers Valerian Root, Black Cohosh Root, Motherwort, and Scullcap, one ounce of each. Mix the whole together, and then take half of the quantity and put in 2½ pints of water. Boil down to 2 pints. Strain and bottle, and take a wineglassful four times daily before meals. If your wife persevere with this, she will obtain great benefit.

Q.—Will you please advise me in the following cases? (Maolmhurie, Fermanagh.)

Q.—(1) Girl, aged 24 years, has eczema of four years' standing. General health very good.

A.—(1) Take of Queen's Delight, Yellow Dock, Blue Flag, and Clivers, equal parts. Infuse one ounce to one pint. Dose: a wineglassful four times daily.

Q.—(2) Man, aged 55 to 60 years. Numbness, coldness and creeping in legs from waist down, also in hands.

A.—(2) Obviously a nerve condition, so prescribe this: Scullcap, Valerian, Black Cohosh, Mistletoe, equal parts. Make infusion as before.

Q.—(3) Kidney trouble, frequent passing of urine, constipation. Pain in back of neck and head, with headaches. General tired feeling. Excitable, irritable, etc.

A.—(3) I would give Wood Betony, Hops, Motherwort, Scullcap and Gentian.

Q.—(4) Married woman, several family, cough and spittle and generally run down.

A.—(4) Give Comfrey, Hyssop, Vervain and Iceland Moss.

Q.—(5) Man. 50 years. Pain in knee and stiff at joints.

A.—(5) A good prescription for rheumatism is the following: Bogbean, Agrimony and Centaury. Equal parts, made into an infusion. An infusion of Celery Seed should be made separately and then the two liquids mixed. This treatment will be a long one.

Q.—(6) Man, 45 to 50 years. Kidney trouble with pains passing urine.

A.—(6) Prescribe Wintergreen Herb, Clivers, Juniper, Hydrangea and Pellitory.

Q.—My age is 63. I suffer a great deal with soreness in the stomach. I have been like this for three years, more or less. I take a little Cascara at night; is that right? (Hopeful.)

A.—A continued soreness of this kind is probably due to a mild inflammation of the digestive tract. Here is a prescription which should help you. Take of Cranesbill Root, Raspberry Leaves and Centuary, 1 ounce, and of Clivers and Agrimony, ½ ounce. Boil the whole in three pints of water down to two pints, strain, and take a wineglassful four times daily. Whilst the trouble continues, your diet should be confined to light foods such as eggs, fish, tripe, and milk puddings. Vegetables can only be taken in small quantities. Malted Slippery Elm Food is a good standby in your case, as it is both soothing and nourishing. It is quite safe for you to take Cascara, as this is one of the best herbal laxatives.

Q.—For about a year I have had trouble with my left eye. A dark spot appeared in it, which looks like a fly. It is not a fixed spot, as it floats around as though it were flying. What would you advise me to do? A member of our family is a sufferer from Piles. If you could help me, I should be grateful. (A. D. Longman, Somerset.)

A.—The black spot is certainly due to a part of the eye having ceased to function, and my best advice to you is not to worry over this, but to employ a means to strengthen the muscles of the organ. For this purpose I would recommend the following: Take one ounce of Eyebright herb and pour on it one pint of boiling water. Strain and bottle, and use this as a lotion regularly.

It is quite possible to cure piles if the patient will persevere with this prescription:—Take 1 ounce each of Shepherd's Purse, Pilewort Herb, and Stone Root. Boil in three pints of water down to two pints. Strain, and take a wineglassful four times daily. An ointment made from the Pilewort can be obtained at your nearest herbal store, and this should be applied externally.

Q.—Will you advise me what to get for my daughter. She is 18 years of age, well built, strong, good appetite, etc., but when she moves her arms, the shoulder bones make a grating noise, and the ankles and fingers the same. There is practically no pain. Her hands are blue at times when she is cold. (Mrs. Badham, Birmingham.)

A.—I am of the opinion that the trouble is a form of rheumatism which has caused the ends of the bones to become roughened. At the same time, the circulation is not so good as it might be, and, therefore, the treatment should be directed to improving this.

Here is a prescription which will prove effective if persevered with.

Take equal quantities of Black Cohosh Root, Prickly Ash, Bogbean Herb, Centaury Herb and Agrimony Herb. To one ounce of the mixture put one and a half pints of water. Boil down to one pint, strain, and take a wineglassful four times daily.

Finally, I would stress the importance of avoiding dampness, since this will certainly aggravate the trouble and perhaps cause the bones to enlarge.

A pain in the small of the back may be present with kidney trouble, but it is also found in a number of cases in which the womb is undergoing changes, and by this, I do not mean there is any disease. Personally, I do not think that you have anything to worry about, but if doubt still lingers, take a sample of urine to your nearest Herbalist, and ask him to test it for you. He will be able to tell you definitely if the kidneys are affected or not.

Fireside Talks on Health

J. MAXWELL, N.D.

IS YOUR HEART IN TROUBLE?

Muscular tissues and the blood vessels become encumbered by the retention of toxins which are the undigested and putrefying end products of certain foods. The heart is a bunch of muscles, and in the blood vessels we have also to think of the muscular walls of those tubes. The health, the elasticity, the pliability, of these muscles depends upon the chemistry of our foods. These muscles as well as all other muscular tissues in the body, must be kept supple and pliable if the body is to function well as a whole.

If poisonous wastes are retained in the system, particularly where there is constipation, gases are given off from those putrefying wastes of sedimentary matter, and as this is sent through the blood vessels during the circulatory processes, it begins to line the arteries and veins with a sticky, mucoid material, which decreases the diameter of those blood vessels and interferes with the proper functioning of the heart. Its action may be to change the structure of the heart muscles, to decrease their elasticity, to cause a slight shrinkage or otherwise slightly change the valves between the auricles and ventricles.

Instead of contending that heart disease proceeds either from rheumatism, fever or infections, let us consider that the heart is poisoned by the toxins that caused the rheumatism, etc.; that heart trouble is always the result of a toxic condition of the blood stream. Instead of whipping up the heart's action or depressing it under other conditions, which in all cases produces enervation, it were far better to seek the removal, from the blood stream and muscular tissues, of the poisonous toxins, by natural methods through the various eliminatory organs. Strychnine, digitalis, and various coal-tar derivatives which are so freely used in various heart affections are all paralyzers, and do much harm. Cleansing, not stimulation, is the course to pursue.

"Stimulants," said Dr. Henry Lindlahr, "precipitate the fatigue products from the circulation into the tissues of the body. They do this by paralyzing the power of the blood to dissolve and carry in solution uric acid and other acids and alkaloids that should be eliminated from the organism—stimulants benumb and paralyze the inhibitory nervous system, and allow the driving powers to run wild when Nature wanted them to slow up or stop." It is rest, not depression, rest and cleansing of the blood vessels by means of the natural juices in alkaline foods, that Nature calls for in such cases. The muscles of the blood vessels as well as all other muscular tissues, must be kept supple and pliable if the body is to function well as a whole.

When the system is loaded with an increasing quantity of uric acid (the end products from meat, fish, poultry or other high protein foods), when this acid accumulates in the blood, beyond the power of the eliminatory organs to clear it out of the system; sedimentary matter, lining the arteries and capillaries, throws an extra burden upon the heart, increases the blood pressure in the main arteries, and clogs the blood vessels in the extremities of the body.

All disease is caused by the excessive accumulation of morbid waste in the body, which clogs and obstructs the capillary circulation, interfering with cell nutrition and drainage. The question is: How can this sticky, mucoid material be removed from the blood stream and tissues? It is evident that we must relieve the heart from any strain that is unnecessary. Respiration must also be made easy.

The blood, on a low protein diet and when green leafy vegetables are freely used in salad form, will be high in hemoglobin, and red blood cells; therefore, respiration can be carried on with the least exertion on the part of the heart. Further, a low protein diet is richer in alkaline elements, which will neutralize the uric acid and other acids, and thus tend to bring the blood back to its normal alkaline condition.

To check hardening of the arteries and stiffening of the muscular tissues of the heart, the diet should be rich in organic potassium and sodium. Both these minerals are of an alkaline nature. Heart disease is generally preceded by gluttony. To bring about suppleness of the muscular tissues of the heart and other organs, use the following foods: tomatoes, cabbage, lettuce, turnips, rutabages, celery, Swiss chard, watercress, cucumbers, cauliflower, radishes, beets, spinach, Brussels sprouts, Jerusalem artichokes, green kidney beans. Among fruits take lemons, oranges, peaches, apricots, grapes, prunes, watermelon, cherries, blackberries, raspberries, plums, strawberries, pineapple, grapefruit, apples, figs, dates, bananas. These foods will also help clear the blood stream of those mucoid obstructions, make the heart muscles more supple, and thus relieve distress in that organ.

The respiratory organs should be eased as much as possible, for when they are in distress there is interference with the heart's normal action. There is trouble after eating more carbohydrates than the amount of oxygen inhaled can oxidize, so that a residue is left behind. As the bronchial tubes are the exhaust pipes carrying such residues out of the body in the shape of carbonic acid gas, if overwork is thrown upon them by gluttonous consumption of starchy foods and sugars, this brings about obstruction in the lung area, a lessened intake of oxygen and lessened elimination. That brings further burden upon the heart.

Great is the power of fine fresh fruits, nuts and green crispy vegetables, to relieve distress, to bring the body into balance. These can be served up in many enticing ways, but there will always be better and surer action when they are taken in an absolutely natural condition, uncooked, just as they come to us from the hand of Nature.

FATS AND BATHS

The pleasures of the bath are fully shared by many of the lower animals, and all those qualities which make the perfect human swimmer may be seen in an exaggerated form amongst the inmates of the Zoo.

All animals can swim in some fashion instinctively; many habitually do so in the pursuit of a livelihood, whilst others, like ourselves, indulge in it for the sheer pleasure of the exercise.

Fat is a vital portion of the animal "wet bob's" make-up. With the exception of the whale, no other animal can compare with the hippopotamus or seal in the matter of adipose tissue, which not only fortifies the swimmer against cold but also materially augments his buoyancy.

The hippo, though so unwieldy upon land, is extraordinarily active in the water, and at certain times of the year these animals at the Zoo spend all the day and half the night submerged.

Most people not unnaturally regard most aquatic animals as taking to the water from birth, but this is often far from being so. The infant hippopotamus is carried into the water.

VOMITING

By J. MAXWELL, N.D.

The Roman architects, when they built a banqueting hall, always erected a room alongside, which they called a vomitorium, the name clearly indicating its use.

Vomiting is often a healing process of Nature, to rid the stomach or other organs of morbid accumulations.

Possibly, the first time you took a sea voyage you fed the fishes. In trying to fathom the reason why, think of the previous abuse of your stomach, overloading on improper combinations of food, demineralised, denatured victuals.

Such vomiting that simply relieves does not prove that the stomach is diseased. It just discharges what Nature considers should not have an abode within your system.

If one is suffering with indigestion, the vomited material is usually acid, sour. In cases of catarrh it may be alkaline. If the liver is gorged and large quantities of bile are thrown into the intestines, it may regurgitate into the stomach, causing vomiting, which will be streaked with bile. If there is strangulated hernia, fecal matter will be vomited—a serious condition if the strangulation is not soon corrected.

Hæmorrhage of the stomach, if the blood is bright red, indicates ulceration. If dark, resembling coffee grounds, it may mean malignant ulceration.

During fasts people will sometimes vomit. If they have taken calomel or some other form of mercury, Nature, during the cleansing brought about during a fast, may produce violent vomiting as the body makes an effort to rid the liver and stomach of this metallic poison. In case the vomiting continues daily and is too severe, it may be advisable to break the fast for several days and give the white of egg to soothe the inflamed lining of the stomach.

There may be vomiting where there is inflammation of the brain, scarlet fever, bowel complaints, etc., indicating that the system is loaded with toxins and has no desire, at that time, to be burdened with more food. Hot weak lemonade or water will be grateful and comforting, but abstain entirely from food until the system is quite easy and free from pain.

Disturbance of certain nerve centres may cause vomiting—for instance, if there is a migraine headache, or accumulation of uric acid in the blood, or through the use of various drugs.

Vomiting in infancy generally denotes over-feeding. If the child is being fed from the mother's breast, the mother's milk may have been more or less disorganised by improper feeding, or emotional excitement, anger, grief, worry, etc. If the child is bottle-fed, the food may be too strong and should be diluted with water, or the child may have been overfed. In any case of continued vomiting, cease feeding until the child is perfectly at ease and calls for food, and place hot applications over the stomach. Never refuse water when thirst calls for it.

Belching may result from gas in the stomach, produced by fermentation, generally incompatible foods having been eaten together, as starches with acids, or there has been gluttony, overfeeding.

The accumulation of old fecal matter in the colon has been known to cause vomiting; a reverse movement of the intestine has been brought about.

Sometimes the intestinal tract gets rid of unwelcome material by purging, sometimes by vomiting. Neither should be suppressed, but helped, by the drinking of tepid water, until the intestinal tract has been cleansed. Then a little warm peppermint tea will be found grateful and comforting.

Vomiting in pregnancy is brought about by wrong feeding, incorrect habits, and is not a normal diet. With a leaning towards the daily use of fresh fruits, nuts and crisp green vegetables, with sufficient daily outdoor exercise, with rest periods, and uninterrupted sleep at night, there should be no abnormal disturbances, vomitings, etc.

Of course, I advocate a non-flesh diet, having practised that for more than thirty years and seen many hundreds of people benefited by its adoption. One should be able to see that man is not intended to be a carnivorous animal. His teeth are so different from those of the lion, tiger, dog, etc. No canine tusks. It would be impossible for him to tear another animal limb from limb. His teeth are too soft to crunch bones, and his gastric juice could not digest crushed bone. He cannot live on blood. The muscular tissues of another animal give a very acid reaction when eaten.

There is not likely to be any vomiting when one eats moderately of fresh fruits, or nuts, or fresh vegetables. There will be no putrefying residues left in the colon; and if plenty of vigorous exercise is taken daily, there is not likely to be constipation.

If, through indiscreet living, one is attacked by vomiting, accompanied by acute pains, take an enema, juice of a lemon in two quarts of lukewarm water injected into the bowels. Then drink several cupfuls of lukewarm water, which will help bring about a more complete vomit of the offensive matter in the stomach; and, as before stated, a drink of peppermint tea will afterwards help to settle the stomach. A hot moist compress can also be placed over the stomach region.

We must look upon vomiting as a warning signal, directing us to stop, look and listen to the voice of Nature. It is a rebellion against our former habits, evidence that the body has been mistreated. Better an empty house than a bad tenant.

Samuel Thompson, the founder of the Thompsonian System of herbal medicine, advocated and practised vomiting as an aid to Nature Cure. He poured a cupful of boiling water on a teaspoonful of powdered Lobelia herb or seed, and a very small portion of Cayenne Pepper, then used the warm tea as an emetic. This would generally dislodge a lot of mucus which had lined the stomach. That was usually followed by a vapour bath. These simple remedies were the sheet anchors of his practice.

I would prefer using one ounce of powdered Lobelia, one ounce powdered Boneset herb, and a quarter teaspoonful of cayenne pepper. Pour on this a pint and a half of boiling water. Let it settle off the clear liquid and give one ounce of the tea, warm, every twenty minutes until vomiting takes place.

Nearly fifty years ago, I had a case of a young blacksmith, who for a long time had been inhaling the smoke and fumes from his smithy fire, until he came down with an acute attack of indigestion, had to quit work, and could not eat. A single dose of Lobelia emetic caused him to vomit a lot of dark, stringy mucus which had been lining his stomach. Then his recovery was rapid; in a few hours his vigour returned.

There are doubtless many cases where such a vomiting would do much to clear the intestinal tract of accumulated mucus and waste material. If this were followed by a fast of a day or two, take nothing but water, and then confine the diet to fresh fruits for a few days, it would work wonders.

Note the heavy coating on the tongue as evidence that the whole intestinal tract is foul. This, accompanied by offensive breath, shows the urgent need of internal cleansing. If that is neglected, presently Nature will take away all desire for food, and produce nausea; her remedy may be some acute attack of disease to clear out of the body, by more or less forcible means, morbid matter that has accumulated there. Vomiting and diarrhœa and heavy sweats are often the agencies that she uses.

But under all circumstances, avoid inorganic mineral drugs or any suppressive agencies, any opiates or narcotics that tend to drive toxic material back into the tissues. Let Nature purge out the old leaven. Then, if all the eliminatory organs work freely, cleansing will take place, the body take on a new lease of life, and if in future one chooses a rational diet and otherwise lives sanely, a measure of health, far superior to anything experienced in the past, should be within reach.

[Dr. Maxwell is a well-known Lecturer and Dietician; writer of Daily Health Column in the "Milwaukee Leader"; Radio daily broadcaster over WCFL, Chicago, U.S.A. An Englishman by birth, brought up in the County of Kent, is over 70 years of age and still young.—Editor, "M.H."]

Diseases of the Kidneys and Bladder

J. R. YEMM, F.N.A., D.O.

Undoubtedly the most painful of kidney and bladder troubles are caused by gravel and stones. Most people have noticed, at some time or other, that their urine, after it has stood for some time, deposits a brick red or brownish dust, and that the quantity of urine passed is smaller than usual, and the colour higher or deeper.

Many people are apt to get alarmed when they first notice these symptoms, and think they are threatened with some serious illness. In most cases, however, these deposits do not indicate kidney disease, but some slight digestive derangement or probably a cold. For instance, the urine will show a heavy deposit (when the patient is recovering from a fever) and which should be looked upon as a favourable sign.

The deposits in urine may consist of urates, oxalates, or phosphates, and sometimes the particular colour of the dust aids in determining its particular variety. Oxalates are dark brown, urates, reddish brown, phosphates a greyish white. Sometimes other substances are present, but the exact composition of the deposit can only be ascertained by chemical analysis.

It is the excess of particular elements in the system that forms a starting point or nucleus for gravel or stone. Some of the solids, instead of being held in solution in the urine and carried away from the system, deposit in the kidneys or bladder, where they gradually accumulate and form gravel, which may, before it has become large in size, pass out of the body with very little pain or trouble. But when it has become large in size, the passage down the ureters is attended with agonizing pains, the rough edges of the gravel cutting and tearing the delicate lining membrane of the ureters, thus causing much suffering. Should particles of gravel remain in the kidneys or bladder, they gradually accumulate there, and form stones of a larger size. When these stones are in the bladder they are called Vesical Calculi, if in the kidneys, Renal Calculi.

The symptoms of gravel are well known to many people, especially to those who have experienced an attack. The pains may come on suddenly, beginning in the region of the kidneys and shooting down towards the bladder. Vomiting may set in, with alternate chills and perspirations. There is a constant desire to urinate, although very little urine is passed, which burns and scalds. Blood may be present in the urine, together with small shreds of mucous membrane. During the whole time the stone or gravel is passing down the ureters, the patient experiences severe pain, which may suddenly cease when the stones reach the bladder, to be renewed again when the contents of the bladder are discharged.

Stone in the kidneys or bladder presents different symptoms, although there is much in common in all kidney and bladder cases. A renal calculi may be suspected when there is a dull, aching pain in the loins, aggravated into sharper twinges after exercise, retraction, and possibly pain in the testicle, on the side affected. The urine again contains blood and epithelium from the kidneys. If the stones gain a large size suppuration is exercised, and pus will be found in the urine. The chief indications of a vesical calculi is severe pain in the bladder, perineum, and urethra; and frequent micturition, the act being frequently stopped by the stone being forced against the neck of the bladder. The urine often thick, ropy, tenacious, and brings, as the stone excites inflammation of the bladder, a muco-purulent discharge, and in many cases blood will be voided.

Although these symptoms are prominent and present in the majority of cases, a person should not think he has a vesical calculus until he has been assured so by a competent practitioner. Many a case has passed through my hands, in which the patient was supposed to be suffering from a calculus and contemplating an operation, but after going carefully over such a case, I have diagnosed a chronic cystitis and enlarged prostate gland. Eventually the patient has responded to suitable treatment.

Treatment.—During the passing of gravel from the kidneys the first object should be to give relief to the sufferer. The patient should be placed in a warm bath as hot as he can bear it, and the region of the kidneys bathed with hot water. Copious draughts of Marshmallow or Linseed Tea, with about 20 drops of the Fluid Ext. of Lobelia, should be given, but the Lobelia may be given every quarter of an hour, until sickness is felt; it should then be stopped. This treatment is relaxing, and will do more to get "gravel down" than the use of opiates and the usual "drugs," which are generally administered. The Lobelia acts as a relaxant and antispasmodic; it causes a relaxation of the ureters, so that they expand and the spasmodic contractions are abated. The Marshmallow or Linseed acts as a demulcent and soothes the passages, and also heals the membranes which may have been cut by the rough edges of the gravel. If no Marshmallow or Linseed is at hand, use Slippery Elm, Hollyhock, or Gum Arabic—in fact any demulcent. After an attack of gravel I have found the following bring about a wonderful result:—

℞ Gravel Root, ½ ounce.
Uva Ursi, ½ ounce.
Parsley Piert, ½ ounce.
Comfrey Root, ½ ounce.

Boil these in 2½ pints of water down to 2 pints, and strain. When cold, take a wineglassful 3 times a day. To get rid of the trouble altogether, one should place oneself in the hands of a competent Botanic practitioner, who will be able to prescribe for the alterative treatment his system requires. In nine cases out of ten faulty digestion lies at the bottom of the whole thing. When a stone has formed and has gained a large size, it requires active medical treatment to get rid of it, although I have been told of many cases which have been cured by drinking an infusion of Parsley Piert and Clivers. There are many people under the impression that "stones" can be dissolved by strong acids and alkalines. Theoretically they can, but when we come to carry this theory into practice it falls short of our expectations, inasmuch as it is very, very rare that we find a stone formed of one particular substance. We may, as an illustration, have a stone formed with a calcium oxalate nucleus, and then coated with urates. Now the stones cause irritation, which results in phosphates being given then the stone gets a coating of these, and so on. The best advice I can offer to any sufferer is to consult a Botanic practitioner. There are many remedies which have a solvent action on these calculi, and the remedies can be taken for any length of time without fear of damaging the system, as mineral acids and alkalines will do. Of course, one should see that his drinking water is pure; a filter would be a good investment—in fact, it is a necessity. Pure water alone would help in breaking up these troublesome intruders.

NATURE CURE TREATMENT FOR NERVE DISORDERS

By J. MAXWELL, N.D.

Originally a nervous person meant one who had strong robust nerves. To-day, it generally represents one whose nerves are pained and weakened by disease. The highest development of the body is in the brain and nervous system.

Representing telegraph wires which not only convey messages, but have feelings, the nervous system is divided into two circuits, each with own switchboard. One is called the Voluntary, and the other the Involuntary or Sympathetic nervous system. The first is directed by the will. The other is under the better direction of the abdominal brain, centering in the solar plexus. The brain directs the Voluntary muscles in carrying out mechanical work, directs the organs of speech, etc. The brain is to a large extent under the control of the mind, and constantly receives reports from all over the body.

The mind influences the health and activities of the whole body through the nervous system, which regulates and controls the secretions of the cells and glands, but food is first necessary out of which those secretions can be manufactured. Food must be of good quality, undenatured, not demineralised if normal nourishment is to be given to every cell in the body.

Equally important is the fact that the mind has a great influence upon the entire nutrition and metabolism of the body. A disturbed mind may make good food of little value in nutrition, by interfering with digestion. A tranquil mind and undisturbed nervous system assists in making good food thoroughly acceptable.

Disease is either a disturbance of the function of the cells of the body, or of the substance of the cell, primarily caused by faulty foods or the retention of the end-products of those foods. If we had retained natural instincts, as do other animals, we would intuitively choose foods suitable for our upkeep, and choose them in their prime, natural condition. But the instincts of civilised humans have been lost, or they are only faintly conscious of them.

Food deficiencies affect the mind, the temperament, the whole substance of the body. We are also affected by environment.

Food is unquestionably fundamental. Without it there will be no bodily life in which mind can function. Therefore, we should take an inventory of our foods and banish all that are not above suspicion. Condiments may generally be classed as irritants, not foods. This applies to salt, vinegar, pepper, mustard, etc.

Nerve balance is interfered with when the blood loses its normal alkalinity, when one suffers with hyperacidity. All nervous people, all who lack nerve control, are better without meat, fish, poultry, eggs, denatured cereals, white flour or any thing made therefrom, refined white sugar, coffee and tea.

When potatoes, apples, pears, peaches, are peeled, these foods are robbed of a good portion of their minerals, and the nerves and whole being suffer from mineral starvation, if a liberal supply is not obtainable from other foods. The frying pan spoils many foods. The albumen, the white of an egg, is toughened and made almost as indigestible as leather by frying.

The nervous system is strengthened most by foods which give an alkaline reaction—foods rich in potassium, sodium, calcium, magnesium and iron. Most of the digestive juices are mainly mineral elements in solution. Poisonous so-called "preservatives" in foods, metallic or coal-tar extracts, salpetre, aniline dyes and other foreign substances, often partly neutralises the potency of the different digestive juices and interfere with nutrition.

Eternal vigilance is the price of safety. It needs a watchful eye and good food sense to detect all the food faking that is prevalent today. To keep strong nerves we must be well nourished on natural foods in all their naturalness. Refinement of food generally brings calamity in its train. Many cooks, many diseases. Study not how many more dishes and how much greater variety you can place on your table than your neighbor can. Don't be stirred by emulation in that way.

Women flock by the thousands to note some new cookery demonstration, to learn how to compound the 57 varieties, as one pickle manufacturer puts it. And when they later practise on poor husband, he might as well be measured for his coffin, for he will surely die before his time, if the foods used are demineralised, denatured, or otherwise damaged, by processing.

Tranquility of nerves will generally follow a natural simple repast. Few ever felt distress from a fresh fruit breakfast taken daily. On starting out with such a regime distress may be felt for a day or two, not caused by the fruit, but its great cleansing properties have stirred up toxins that have been stored in the system, to throw them out by the eliminatory channels. Cleanse the body internally; then all the works will function smoothly. Start the day with fruit, all your appetite calls for. Fresh fruit and two tablespoonfuls of nuts. How many of you suffer needlessly!

Your body is a piece of machinery which should function smoothly day by day, without ache or pain. The strong nerves should feel no distress. A well-fed body has courage, endurance, and leaves little room for fear and worry.

Feed largely on natural alkaline foods and the heart will beat stronger, the brain think clearer, breathing will be deeper, digestion more active, eyes brighter, cheeks ruddier, skin will take on a finer texture, and you will feel at peace with the world. Primarily, nervousness is the call of the nerves for real food. Of course, the food may be good, but lack of exercise will lead to the imperfect elimination of wastes, leaving in the system poisonous toxic residues which, being acid, irritate the nerves.

Then one may fly to stimulants to tone up the jaded nerves. At first this may take the form of tea or coffee. As the effects of these, by constant use, become weaker, my lady nicotine is then called up to narcotize the poor, weak nerves. Later, many form a habit of taking still more dangerous substances, as quinine, digitalis, arsenic, strychnine, aspirin, acetanilid, phenacitin; or bromides, and their condition becomes piteous in the extreme.

These nerve paralysers get a terrible grip upon many people. They interfere with certain brain centres, act as permanent depressants, and their continued use may soon bring one down to the grave. With all the persuasion at my command I urge you to quit the use of all such medication.

The Hop

By JOHN BARLEYCORN

Doctor: "Does your husband take his medicine religiously—four times a day?"

Wife: "No, certainly not; he always swears!"

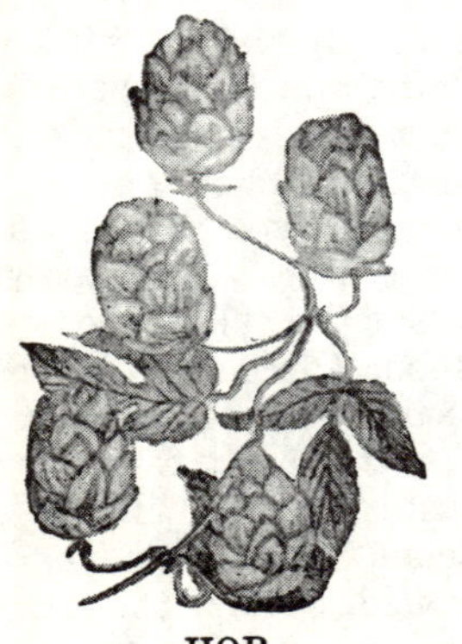

HOP

Reading the above in a daily newspaper raised a smile, set me thinking, and decided an attempt to make a little contribution to the columns of "The Medical Herbalist," a Journal much appreciated from its inception.

The patient caricatured above must have been passing through a "bitter" experience — sickness and physick, as the ancients used to describe their bitter yet healing potions. It is the bitters, particularly of the botanic system of medicine that give tone and stimulation to the vital organs of the human body. To apply the same theory to daily life, we find that it is the bitter experiences thereof which stimulate us to overcome and conquer. A simple yet wonderful analogy—the bitters of life spur us on to achievement; the bitter herbs, provided by a Bountiful Creator, invigorate the physical system to overcome disease.

Having refreshed myself with a decoction of one of the "bitters," I am inspired to write of its history and virtues, not recollecting any record of such having earlier appeared in this Journal. I refer to the Hop **(Humulus lupulus)**, the French **Houblon,** German **Hopfen**. The modern word "Hop" is derived from the Anglo-Saxon **hoppan,** signifying to climb. Etymology is a very interesting study, and regarding our subject we find the generic name to be derived from **humus,** moist earth, as hops flourish best in rich moist soil. The word **Lupulus** is a diminutive of **Lupus salictarius,** the Willow Wolf because, as recorded by Pliny, the plants suffered to grow among osiers strangle and destroy them, as wolves do the shepherd's flock. From the latter it is readily apparent that the Hop was originally, and even still is, of wild growth, valued by people of the country-side. Yet cultivation has progressed over many centuries.

In "The British Flora Medica," a very valuable work by Benjamin H. Barton, F.L.S., and Thomas Castle, M.D., F.L.S. (1837), revised in 1877 by John R. Jackson, A.L.S., Curator of the Museums of Economic Botany Royal Gardens, Kew, we read: "The first mention of Hops occurs in a letter of donation by King Pepin (King of the Franks. d. 768), which speaks of **humulariæ**, meaning probably Hop-gardens. Beckman does not find the word **Lupulus** to occur earlier than the 11th century. About the beginning of the following century Hops were introduced into the breweries of the Netherlands. They seem to have been unknown in England—for brewing purposes—till brought from Artois about the year 1524."

Mentioning the use of Hops in brewing tempts me to give historical records; yet fear that so to do may bring criticism from temperance friends upon the Editor for passing the matter. Then let him take a quaff with me and thereby fortify his courage. Why scruple? I believe the Editor delights in honest, straightforward criticism. Truth is that it is not the presence of hops in beer or ale that produces the staggering gait or the temporary mental unbalance; rather is it the other ingredients combined with the process of manufacture. We can now have delivered at our door a sparkling "Hop Bitters," "Hop and Burdock Bitters," etc., which certainly would quench the thirst, without raising the slightest qualm of conscience, of such stalwart temperance advocates as Lady Astor, Mr. Isaac Foot, and other Members of Parliament we hold in high esteem. Such preparations from the Hop and other herbs are satisfying to the palate of abstainer and non-abstainer alike; appetising, stimulating, and costing little for the reason that the Customs and Excise Authorities can make no duty demand.

The original use of hops in the manufacture of beer was as a preservative, and at the present day severe penalties are inflicted on brewers who use any other bitters for the purpose. 'Twas not ever thus! Synonyms of botanical plants render a clue. **Alehoof** and **Tunhoof** have, for long ages, been applied as common names for Ground Ivy which, prior to the introduction of Hops and Parliamentary sanction for the use thereof, was used to clarify and preserve the beverage prepared from malt alone. The latter was a drink to quench the thirst in similar manner to our own use of simple barley water with perhaps lemon juice added for piquancy. Ground Ivy—**Glechoma hederacea**—having definite diuretic and tonic property exhibits that, knowingly or otherwise, the brewers of five centuries ago thereby added therapeutic value to their malt beverage.

Medicinally, the **flowers** of the Hop are used, properties attributed thereto being stomachic, diuretic, tonic, more or less narcotic, anthelmintic, and antiseptic. When required as a stomachic, it is better taken as a beverage at meals than in the character of medicine. It promotes digestion, and is particularly useful to obviate the lassitude and debility felt by persons of relaxed habits. A simple infusion may be employed for that purpose.

As a stimulating and relaxing nervine **Humulus lupulus** is indicated as a remedy for all nervous conditions, being invaluable by producing sleep and allaying pain. Insomnia is a terrible complication, physical condition thereby weakening and the power of disease resistance seriously impaired. Dr. Maton records: "Besides allaying pain and procuring sleep, the preparations of Hops are capable of reducing the frequency of the pulse, and increasing its firmness in a direct manner."

A gentleman I met recently, and who appeared to be in robust health, informed me that for three years he had been continuously under varied doctors for nervous debility and insomnia. Treatment which included bromides and other narcotic drugs had been of no avail. Being induced to try natural medicine, he prepared infusion from Hops, half-ounce; Gentian Root, crushed, half-ounce; Scullcap, one ounce. After only one week of the herbal treatment he was sleeping well; at the end of two months fully recovered. Such a revelation was interesting, the simplicity of the formula agreeing essentially with my own method of prescribing for such conditions:—

℞ Tinct. Lupuli
" Avenda Sativa a.a. ʒ iv
" Gentian Co....... ʒ vi
Aq. Menth pip p.s..... ℥ viii

Dose.—Tablespoonful in water 4 times a day after food. Add suitable hepatics if indicated.

The fragrance or aroma has a soothing influence upon the nerves, and long since originated the now famous Hop Pillow. Probably this came from observation of the **cradeled infants of Hop pickers,** who, arriving fretful, soon enjoyed sound sleep and thrived wonderfully during sojourn in the Hop gardens. We are told that pillows stuffed with Hops were first prescribed in 1787 to George III, and it is further recorded that similar was used with great effect about 1879 in the Prince of Wales' severe illness. So the Hop pillow may be ascribed as under Royal Patronage, and further, as prescribed by the King's Physicians. Oh, ye Herbalists! Hold high the banner of "Nature's healing power."

A word of warning in conclusion. The active principle of Hops resides in the yellow translucent glands sprinkled on the scales of the cones (flowers) near the base. This active principle **(Lupulin)** is about 14 per cent of the whole, and it may be readily conceived how by beating and sifting this may be to a great extent separated. I am informed that lupulin is valuable to the brewer. Therefore, for whatever purpose required, secure only Hops of guaranteed quality, and you will be amply repaid by results for the extra cost.

Herbal Aids to Beauty

To Cure Gnat Bites

When bitten by gnats, immediately obtain some Liquid Ammonia dilute with half part water, and apply to the part bitten every fifteen minutes until the inflammation disappears. A little green Marshmallows Ointment may be applied, after for a day or two.

FOR THE CHILDREN

By "AUNTIE JENNIE"

"Hello! Children." How familiar is that greeting, which opens the wireless broadcast of the "Children's Hour." We older ones even take it as a call to shed our years and gather with the youngsters to enjoy the pleasures provided. We hear the Zoo man tell of animal life, star-gazer describe the wonders of the night sky, and Chief Os-ke-non-ton tell his stories of child life in North America.

That thought leads me to endeavour to institute a "Hello! Children" in "The Medical Herbalist." We might name it "The Children's Corner," "The Children's Page," or head it with the B.B.C. phrase, "Hello! Children." But I am sure the Editor would like his young friends to decide (1) whether they decide a page of the Magazine all to themselves, and (2) the title you would like to see at the head of the special children's item. Will you all write with either pen or pencil your answers to above? You may also say what particular subjects you would like to appear on the page. Then address the envelope to "Auntie Jennie, % The Editor, 41, High Street, Ammanford, Carm."

We shall get together a band of interested Uncles and Aunts. Uncle Dick, of Lancashire, is bubbling over with a keen desire to entertain you. We shall have Uncle Alfred to relate some of the botany stories told to Alan, Margaret and other wee bairns during country rambles. Then we hope to have the help of Aunt Rebecca, who can draw from a well of knowledge, County Durham abounding in botanical wealth.

Some years ago I was accompanying two little boys through fields green with flourishing herbage. As is usual with children, they scampered ahead thrilled with the venture. Suddenly one came racing back, his face radiant with apparent joy. "Look, Auntie," he exclaimed, holding up a spray, "Yarrow for Colds!" And true it was; he had secured a beautiful specimen. That small boy of many years ago is now a doctor in one of the largest cities of England. We are told that early impressions are lasting, and with me you will hope that doctor has never forgotten the early intuition.

How distinct is the above affectionate recognition of God's handiwork and intention when compared with the indifference of the wayfarer portrayed by Agnes Strickland in her poetry:—

"Green Yarrow, Nature's simplest child,
  Thy leaves of emerald dye,
And silvery blossoms undefiled,
On rugged path, or barren wild,
  The traveller passes by
With reckless glance and careless tread,
Nor marks the kindly carpet spread
  Beneath his thankless feet;
So poor a meed of sympathy
Do generous herbs of low degree
  From haughty mortals meet."

In reference to the beauty and grace of the plant, with its erect stem bearing a dense tight cluster of flowers, sometimes white, other times more or less tinged with a pinkish or purple hue, a wealth of leaves peculiarly sessile and bipinnate, so often to be found in our churchyards. Miss Strickland continues:—

"But thou a meeting place has found
Which none disputes with thee:—
The silent churchyard's lowly bound,
Where sweetly on the hallow'd ground
Thou growest wildly free;
Aye mantling o'er each nameless mound
Thy graceful foliage creeps around,
And thy pale blossoms wave,
Wet with the dew's descending shower,
Beneath the yew's funereal bower,
And mourners in the autumn hour,
Behold and bless the gentle flower,
That decks the peasant's grave."

The Editor has kindly placed at our disposal one page for educational entertainment of our young friends. Due to necessary introduction, I may have overstepped the allotment, yet would ask his generous indulgence for a few more lines of information, and, further, that he will favour us with a drawing of the plant we have before us.

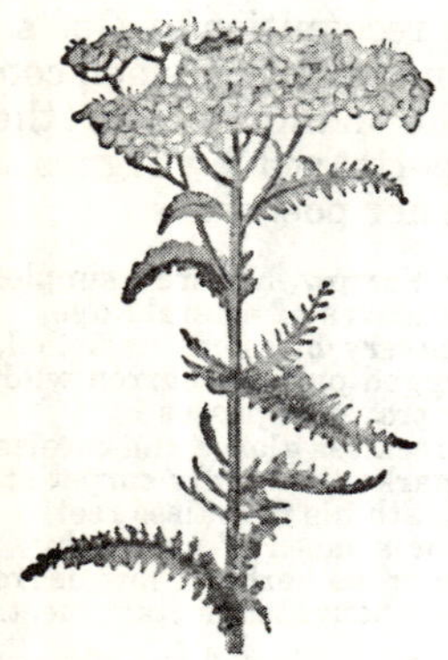

YARROW

You will all know that it was Linnæus, a Swedish naturalist (1707-78), who by his system of classification and naming of plants produced order from chaos and made the study of Botany more easy and entertaining. **Achillea millefolium** is the name given to the common Yarrow, and clearly demonstrates how Linnæus frequently combined historical association with peculiar characteristics of plant formation in fixing definite names.

Achilles, King of the Myrmidons in Thessaly, is said to have been the first to use the herb for staying hæmorrhage and healing wounds. One of our old names — **Soldier's Wound-wort**—is significant of its former use. In addition to "Yarrow," there is yet another common name much used in some parts of the country. This is "Milfoil," which you will readily notice is an abbreviation or corruption of the specie name **Millefolium,** signifying that thousands of minute leaves compose the beautiful foliage. The principal present-day use of Yarrow is by infusion for obstructed perspiration frequently brought about by a chill and which, if neglected, results in a fevered condition. That should always cause us to remember "Yarrow for Colds."

Herbal Aids to Beauty

To Prevent Gnat Bites

Purchase from the Herbalist ½ or one oz. of Quassia Chips, make these into a strong infusion by allowing ½ oz. to stand in cold water (about a large cupful or more) for 8 or 9 hours overnight. Wash the skin that will be exposed before you go into the country, this may tinge the skin but it will wash off, can be made weaker for the ladies if desired.

NATURE CURE TREATMENT FOR GAS PAINS, INTESTINAL GASES, INDIGESTION

By J. MAXWELL, N. D.

Aim to remove causes of these troubles and not be content to deal only with symptoms.

Sometimes through over-eating, gas pains are developed. The body can only assimilate a certain quantity at one time. The surplus has to be disposed of, and the easiest way for the body to do that is to ferment it. That fermentation produces carbonic acid gas and alcohol. The former causes acute pain as it moves about in the intestines. The alcohol makes one heavy, dopey, sleepy, and generally slows up the body. At other times the gas may originate from the introduction into the stomach of incompatible or indigestible foods. Starches and acid foods eaten together produce trouble. An excess of sweets upsets the stomach, particularly when there is at the same time an excess of cereal foods.

The use of tobacco has a very harmful effect upon the nervous system, and thus interferes with digestion, therefore, when the body is under the influence of tobacco, food that is in the stomach will ferment, instead of being digested; hence the production of gas.

Those who suffer from indigestion and subsequent gas pains would do well to avoid all acid fruits in combination with starches —refrain from refined sugar, all condiments, coffee and tea, cream, fatty foods, gravies, pastries, stimulating and intoxicating beverages, tobacco, white bread and anything made from white flour, also meats, fish and poultry. The last-named animal foods produce a very acid condition in the body. Do not be tempted to go back to these foods. The colon should be kept clean with nightly enemas. The preliminary treatment should be the elimination diet. Take a glass of warm lemonade first thing in the morning. Another glass later in the day, before noon, and another at night, sweetened with honey.

First meal of the day should be fresh ripe fruit—nothing else save two ounces of shelled nuts flaked or well masticated, and sometimes a glass of certified (raw, not pasteurised) milk. Always sip the milk, never gulp it. At noon, and for supper, a large plateful of raw green vegetable salad, with dressing, and a baked potato, the jacket of which should also be eaten, well masticated. Take time over these meals, thoroughly chew every particle before swallowing. Drink water, sip it, if thirsty, or take a glass of water after the meal.

If there is disturbance after eating, and the food has been well masticated and eaten slowly, the cause is probably some old obstructions, undigested residues in the system, which the fruit juices or the salads are trying to dislodge or chemically disintegrate. In such cases persevere with the above diet, and the disturbance is likely to disappear in a day or two.

Symptoms in the form of irritability, nervousness, abnormal appetite, and sometimes mental depression are evidences of a highly acid condition, and the alkaline elements in the above-mentioned diet will neutralise that; the potassium, sodium, calcium, magnesium and iron will help to bring the blood back to its normal alkaline condition.

Do not eat when overtired or emotionally excited.

Be guarded against over-eating; always leave the table when you would like a little more. Not too many varieties of food at the same meal.

Keep to natural unsophisticated foods. Avoid cakes, dainties, candies, pancakes, waffles, mushy foods, tapioca, all fried foods.

Do not eat the heavy meal of the day between working hours.

Keep optimism uppermost in the mind. A merry heart doeth good like a medicine. It has a good deal to do with perfect digestion.

Guard against constipation. Use enemas until bowels act freely. Correct diet, sufficient exercise and right mental attitude will in time bring about normal action of the bowels without other aid. Salads and fresh ripe, raw fruits will help much towards that end.

Dried beans and dried peas sometimes causes gas formation when eaten cooked. Certain cooks add a teaspoonful of bicarbonate of soda to the water when cooking beans. It is not a good practice. Rather get the Sodium in an organic form by taking some green vegetables whenever using dried beans or peas as a part of the meal.

In some cases baths, massage, deep breathing exercises, air and sun baths do a great deal in bringing back the body to a condition where it can readily assimulate food.

When the system has been well cleansed by the aforementioned eliminating diet, take a simple meal, after the following order:—A baked potato with sweet butter, a large baked or steamed onion, sip a glass of certified milk whilst eating other foods. Still continue to take one vegetable salad meal a day—every day—and with it a glass of raw milk or a bowl of vegetable soup. Sometimes add a medium-sized baked potato.

Gradually introduce a few starchy foods into your diet, but always take breakfasts of fresh fruits whenever obtainable. Glass of raw milk and a few nuts can be added when desired. Also always have some raw green vegetable salad during the day.

Shredded wheat biscuit or rye crisp, or whole wheat crisp are good forms of bread, because they compel mastication. Take one or other, with a little honey, sweet fruit such as dates or figs, with a glass of raw milk, and you have a very good meal.

Another time a small vegetable salad, one or two steamed or baked vegetables, two ounces of cottage cheese, and a bowl of vegetable soup.

Or take a salad, including grated carrot and grated raw cauliflower, green peas, steamed unpeeled potato, cottage cheese. Glass of raw milk or cereal coffee sweetened with honey.

Or celery salad, steamed spinach and green beans, nut roast with brown gravy. Bowl of vegetable soup.

Or half head of lettuce. Vegetable stew—composed of carrots, turnips, onions, celery, flavoured with a little Sativa; butter added after stew is cooked. Baked potato. Glass of water or milk.

Sometimes take two or three fruit meals a day, with a few nuts and certified milk.

Take any two fresh vegetables as they come into season, with a little butter and corn bread. Glass of water or bowl of vegetable soup.

Simple meals like these will be easily digested, and there should be no distress after eating. Get your protein supply mainly from nuts, cottage cheese or a poached egg occasionally.

RHUBARB (Rheum)

Turkey Rhubarb—The Root

Properties.—Astringent and cathartic.

In small doses it exhibits stomachic and tonic properties, assisting digestion and creating a healthy action of the digestive organs when in a condition of torpor and debility. In large doses it produces a brisk, healthy purge, without clogging the bowels and producing the constipation too consequent upon the use of some of the more active purgatives.

Propagation of Herbs

J. PASKE

The vegetable kingdom includes a great variety of forms, some simple in structure and exceedingly small, while others attain a great size.

The simpler forms of plant life includes the Seaweeds, Toadstools, and Mosses, while the higher forms being the Trees, Flowering Plants, and Ferns.

Observations clearly show that there are several distinct methods of propagation of wild plants, which include dispersal of the seeds or fruits: (1) By wind; (2) Explosion of the seed vessels; (3) Seeds which adhere to the clothing or passing animals; (4) Fruits carried by birds. Some plants shed their seeds around the parent, and by the action of summer's heat and winter's frost, the soil becomes broken up, and into the cracks the seeds find their way.

Burrowing animals, especially earth-worms, contribute to this process of disintegration, whilst fallen leaves add protection to the seeds below. It is nearly always essential for the transference of pollen from the stamens to the stigma for the production of the seeds or fruits. Pollen can be conveyed by various agencies one of the commonest being insects and wind. Wind pollinated herbs are usually green, and inconspicuous, such as the Dog's Mercury and Stinging Nettle. These lack the attractive features of the insect pollinated flowers. The chief pollinating insects are bees, moths, flies, beetles, and butterflies, which possess a special sucking organ (except the beetle), which is curled up when not in use.

Some herbs produce seeds without fertilisation, such as Dandelion, Hawkweed and Lady's Mantle. It will be noticed that almost all herbs produce far more seeds than can survive, the bulk being killed as the result of competition with the more successful ones. Again a large percentage of seeds are carried to places unsuitable for their development, and will not germinate.

The wind dispersal seeds consist of minute and very light seeds, such as all the Thistles, Dandelion, Mouse-ear, Golden Rod, Ragwort, Coltsfoot, Fleabane, Elecampane, and Valerian; also many grasses.

These wind-carrying seeds are covered with fine hairs, or pappus, which form a kind of parachute, which drift through the air; thus the seeds only get dispersed under favourable conditions, when they fall to the ground, being worked into the soil by the rain.

Herbs whose seed vessels explode include such plants as the Shepherd's Purse, Broom, Cranesbill, Fumitory, and Violet. Some will have heard, when out on a ramble, the Broom exploding, shedding its seeds everywhere.

A number of herbs develop hooks on their fruits, which are usually distributed by hairy animals, as in the case of the Cleavers, Enchanter's Nightshade, Herb Bennett, Bur Marigold, Agrimony, and Burdock. These fruits adhere to the clothing or passing animals, and often carried many miles; and crop up in unexpected places.

The last method is seeds of fruits carried by birds. These include all plants that produce berries, such as the Black Currant, Blackberry, Bryonia, Bittersweet, Juniper Berries, and Strawberry. These fruits, after being eaten by birds and passing through the digestive tract, are deposited in all parts of the country.

Some seeds only germinate after being subjected to the action of the digestive juices within the animal's body.

In the case of the Mistletoe, the fruit is very sticky, so that it adhere to the bill of the bird, which rubs it off on to a branch of a tree. Other herbs drop their seeds where they are to grow, being so heavy that they cannot be carried away, such as the Foxglove, Primrose, Daffodil, and Bluebell. These plants, when found, are usually found in great profusion owing to this reason.

FOR ECZEMA AND OTHER SKIN DISORDERS

Fl. Ext. Yellow Dock .. 1 ounce
Fl. Ext. Mountain Grape 1 "
Fl. Ext. Burdock Seed.. ½ "
Simple Syrup to....... 8 ounces

Two tablespoonfuls three times a day, half an hour before meals.

Herbal Aids to Beauty

Dry or Scurfy Skin

If your skin happens to be dry or scurfy do not despair, try this: —take two teaspoonfuls of fine oatmeal and mix it into a very soft paste with cold water, or if your skin is very bad, mix it together with Olive Oil in the same manner, then add to this, half a cupful of very hot water and let it cool, then separate the liquid from the ingredients and it is then ready for use. Dab or pat the skin with this two or three times a day and allow it to soak in. Do not keep this preparation too long but make it fresh every other day.

SOME BRITISH WILD PLANTS AND THEIR USES

By W. COMPTON, N.A.M.H.

Tormentil

Potentilla Tormentilla (Sib.). N.O. Rosaceæ.

Synonyms.—Ewe Daisy, English Sarsaparilla, Septfoil.

Habitat.—Grows commonly on hilly districts and dry pastures in Britain, Europe, Western Siberia, and the Azores. Flowers June to September.

Description. — Root perennial, thick, roundish, irregular, knobbed, woody, fibrous. Color dark brown on the outside, reddish inside. Stems numerous, somewhat trailing on the ground or prostrate, roundish, wiry, hairy-like branched and in pairs; height, 6 to 10 inches. Leaves occur in regular succession, or alternate, surrounding the stem nearly, without foot stalk, leaflets 3, shape lance-oval, saw-like edge — serrated— slightly hairy; color, bright green above, pale beneath. Flower erect. Calyx 8 cleft, segments ovate or egg-shaped. Petals usually 4, golden yellow, like miniature buttercups in color. Time of flowering, June to September.

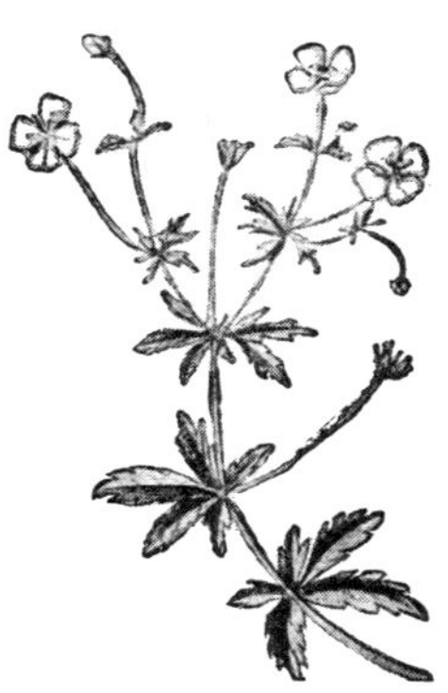

TORMENTIL

Part Used.—Root, herb.

Chemical Composition. — Tormentil contains about 30 per cent of tormentil-tannic acid, and nearly 20 per cent, tormentil red, equal to that of horse chestnut, similar to rhatany-red; also small quantities of kinovic, and ellagic acids, with resin and mucilage.

Medical Properties.—Persistently astringent, alterative, antiseptic. It imparts its strength to the digestive processes. Is a specific in diarrhœa and other discharges. Is non-stimulating, and alkaline in decoction. The foliage is sometimes eaten by cows, goats, sheep, and pigs; horses will not touch it. Removes the corruption which tends to form on the walls of the bowels. Has been proved in many cases to clear the skin from eruptions, and lumps in the neck, in combination with other herbs as follows.

Preparation and Uses. — This plant has been employed as a gargle in ulcerated throat and mouth. The gargle being made from the decoction of 1 ounce to 1½ pints water; boil 10 minutes. In Leucorrhœa, Spermatorrhœa, etc., one of the most useful remedies will be found as follows:—

Tormentil (Tormentilla Potentilla) . . ½ ounce
Willow Bark (Salix Nigra) . . . . ½ "
Vervain (Verbena Officinalis) . . . . . . ½ "

Steep in 2 pints of water a few hours, then simmer half-hour; towards the end add:—

Red Sage (Salvia Officinalis) . . . . . ½ ounce
Ginger (Zingiber) . . . . ¼ "
Strain.

Dose.—One small wineglassful three times daily for an adult.

The above has been used successfully in such diseases as spitting of blood, and passing blood with urine. A ¼ ounce of Cinnamon added to the above will usually allay vomiting; it is also a certain cure for dysentery, inflammation and ulceration of the bladder. Also it quickly reduces fever.

In nocturnal emissions it would be necessary, whilst taking the above, to inject into the uretha an infusion of:—

Yarrow Achillia Millifolium) . . . . .1 ounce
Water . . . . .1 pint

Or:

Elder Flowers (Sambucus Nigra) . . . . .1 ounce
Water . . . . .1 pint

infusion. Inject as above.

Should it constipate, omit the Cinnamon and substitute:—

Comfrey Rt. (Symphitum Officinalis) . . . . . .1 ounce

It need hardly be stated one should seek the advice and guidance of a qualified Medical Herbalist in all cases. Dr. Cullen recommended it either alone or combined with Gentian in intermittent fevers. A piece of line soaked in a strong decoction and constantly applied to warts is said to remove them. Make as follows: Tormentil Root, 2 ounces; water, 1 pint; boil 10 minutes; then strain. When taken internally, the infusion is taken in doses of 1½ ounces three times daily. The above has been used as a wash for piles.

In Fluxes, Dr. Thornton gave 1 dram of the root in an infusion of Hops four times daily.

Thornton also states that an old man made some remarkable cures of ague, small-pox, and whooping cough from an infusion of 1 ounce of the powdered root to 1 pint boiling water. The old man became so celebrated that Lord William Russell gave him a piece of ground on which to cultivate the plant; this he did, keeping it secret for a long time. A good compound powder of Tormentil is made as follows:

Powd. Tormentil Rt. (Tormentilla Potentilla) . . . . ½ ounce
Powd. Galangal Rt. (Alpina Galanga) . . . . .½ "
Powd. Comfrey Rt. (Symphitum Officinalis) . . . . .½ "
Powd. Ginger Rt. (Zingiber) . . . . 2 drams

Infusion.—Pour on the compound 3 gills boiling water, cool, strain.

Dose.—One to two dessertspoonfuls every half-hour until relieved, then take it three or four times daily.

FOR THE CHILDREN

By "UNCLE DICK"
(*Fro' Lancashire*).

Dear Children,—Do you want to become strong in Mind and Body? Of course you do; and your mother and father and your Herbalist friends also want you and all the children of the world to grow up better and stronger in every way than we have been.

Of course, Children, we adults have many faults, as well as good points; so we admit it at once.

We know of your difficulties and your joys. Let us try to help you avoid many mistakes we have made. Then we may expect you to carry on our work and carry a message to other Children and adults, to help them understand what must be done by you and others: to make people healthy, happy, and more intelligent.

Study the flowers, plants and trees when you can, by the aid of books, and our Medical Herbalist Magazine. If you are eager to know anything, ask the Editor. He is one of the best Herbal Teachers in our ranks. He loves the Cause and the "Medical Herbalist" and tells us when he thinks we are wrong, and he helps us to do right. He wants to help you and all children, so please rely on the Editor to assist you any time you write to him.

If you join a Botanical Class, or go on a ramble with Herbalists, you will learn the names of herbs; where they grow, and their use. You will find some lovely flowers and berries, and will learn that some are called poison; so don't put them to your mouth, because poisons do harm to body and mind.

Perhaps you are poor, but even so, you should keep on trying to buy a few books to read. Also try to obtain other books from a lending library to help you study more. Take care of all books you may borrow, and be sure to return them without delay.

We know a man who worked in a cotton mill, and later became a Cabinet Minister. Every day, he wrote several words and sentences in a foreign language, then placed the cards over his looms. By that means he learned more words each day, and became an expert speaker in six languages whilst working as a weaver. The last time we saw him he could speak and write ten languages.

It takes a long time to learn a subject, but you will succeed if you try to learn a little more every day. To become a Herbalist, you will need to learn about herbs, roots, barks, flowers, berries; also about the human body; deep breathing; exercise; cleanliness; the value of foods, and many other subjects.

You may perhaps learn more about herbs and their uses, about the body and other subjects, than we have done if you try. So please try your best, Children, to learn all you can.

Many people do not know the value of herbs, or they would demand herbal treatment to keep them well, or to cure their ills. Nature provides all we need, and if you rely on Nature, she will supply all your needs.

Uncle Dick wants to talk to you about books, physical training, and other subjects; and sometime will add a little fun because we believe laughter is good medicine for everyone.

We have a few books on our shelves, bought 40 years ago as a boy. There are many more books now; and some are costly; but we love to keep those penny, threepenny, and sixpenny books which help us so much in our youthful days. They are old and trusted friends; always reminding us of our early struggles.

You must never spurn books or human friends who help you to learn; or to grow strong and healthy. Simple books are good friends. Your mother and father are your best friends; and your uncles and aunts in the herbal cause, led by the Editor, hope to guide you into the paths, along which you may travel to spread the Herbal Message of Hope.

How the Self-Heal Got Its Name

There is a plant occupying our short-grassed meadows from July into autumn which is commonly distributed and as commonly ignored. Since children have taken to field work, it has perhaps gained more attention than at any other time. Usually we receive plants of it under the impression it is the Bugle, which is an earlier plant and does not hold its own as long. On the other hand, the Self-Heal is given the name of Bugle. Self-Heal was not always a plant cast aside, being held to be a specific in so many ailments that the name of Self-Heal was at once evident in its appropriateness.

It is a labiate or lip plant, and this group of plants is one giving great pleasure in discrimination. The calyx tubes in most of them are quaint and of differing build, so that it is capital work to try and name the plants from these tubes. I am afraid we too often take a plant at face value, and I am sure that Self-Heal has become so frequent we pass it over in a cursory

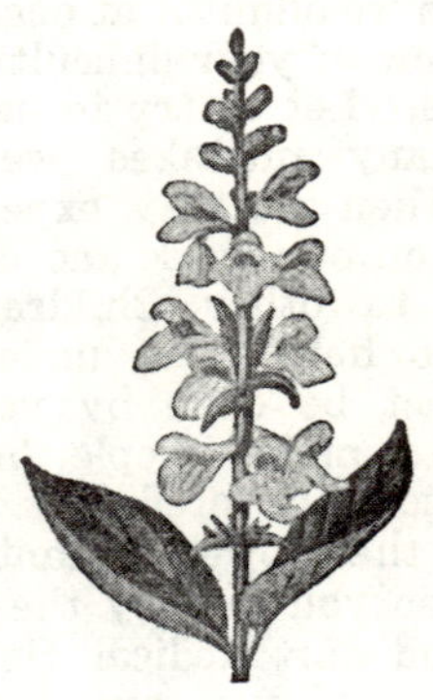

SELF-HEAL

fashion, ignoring the structural interest it might have.

The other day a piece of a plant was submitted to me which had only the steam and calyx tubes present. The flower parts had gone, the inflorescene was shrivelling up, and the freshest part was the base of the flower head. Not much to identify a plant by. The calyx tubes were, however, peculiar enough, and those soon settled the name.

Self-Heal and Bugle

A glance with the naked eye provided little information, but the use of a field lens revealed those minute parts and features which mark out a plant so well. By calyx we mean the outer part of a flower, the holding cup as it were. In the order to which this plant belongs this is always tubular, and usually a complete tube. In this instance the calyx is composed of two parts, the upper lip having seven ribs behind it, and notched. The lower lip is composed of two spear-shaped segments, each marked with three lines, and serrated, with short, stiff hairs. The flowers are densely whorled, forming a solitary oblong spike. This is how this dry specimen of the plant looked, with its flowers gone.

Let me say a word or two as to the full plant. It is variable in height. In some situations it may not be more than an inch, as was this one examined. In woods and shady places it may approach a foot. So height is no guide. Purple may be given as the general colour of the flower, this tint extending also to other parts. It may, however, be found white and even blue, though the plants sent to me to discriminate have been the usual purple colour, the resemblance to Bugle being merely in the habit. Looked at casually, the plant appears smooth, but Self-Heal is hairy enough when examined. The calyx tube of the Bugle is divided into five equal sections, which is sufficient in itself to distinguish the plant from Self-Heal.

The Position of Bracken

One thing which came to my mind while traversing a wood was the position of Bracken in the past, its distribution and its quantity. I will tell you why. I passed on the way places where there used to be delightful gullies, to judge by photographs taken for me in years past. Now these gullies are choked with Bracken. It is the same in the case of the edges of woods where Brambles used to hold sway. These are now hidden by the ever-climbing Bracken. I know there used to be tall Bracken. I have been in woods where they have completely hidden one from other people's view. But they were so over a long period of years. They did not spread.

In the case of one wood, taking this as an example, the trees have only been planted these 35 years. Before there were great gaps, and Bracken was but a mere trifle. Now it is a man's height and crowding out everything else. Is it that its use in times past in many ways for utilitarian purposes served to keep it in check? We know it is even now conveyed down from some hill-sides and used for bedding by farmers. Yet acres of it are ignored. Had the increase noted been kept up down the ages, we should have had no other vegetation left to us.

A Remarkable Instance

On an occasion during the war when lights were obscured, I was unfortunate enough to get out at Withnell Station instead of Feniscowles, and in the dark it was not easy to estimate exactly how the country could be crossed to home. It was done in an incredibly short space of time. I was over the ground again last week when dusk had fallen. There were lights on the hills and in the valleys. Yet it gave me then cause for wonder however I had estimated and traversed the shortest way home on the other trip. It was difficult enough with lights to aid. One of the changes which time had brought about was in the walk, where I had to stop and consider in which direction the true path lay, so mystifying were the Bracken-covered sides.

Butterflies Sunning on Stones

That butterflies should like to sun themselves on the sides of stones in warm weather one can well understand. I have seen them in numbers so disporting on the banks of the Ribble, only being disturbed by passing shadows. They are very susceptible to shadows. It is one of the things a new beginner in insect stalking has to learn—the way in which to approach an insect at rest. As I say, it is not difficult to understand an insect's attitude on a warm day. But I have amended my own opinions as to the reason for this sunning. So often recently have I seen them gyrating in strange places it has left my opinion very open and quite altered preconceived notions. I saw one some days ago—a fine small tortoise-shell. It alighted on a large pebble in the midst of a garden path. When my shadow crossed it it flew away, only to return, and once again to the same pebble.

There were other pebbles quite as conspicuous, but they were ignored. Only this one pebble was the attraction. I puzzled over the circumstance, but am still left in wonder as to what the attraction of this pebble could be. It was not the warmest of days either, and there was nothing in the colour of the stone to suggest any sort of protection.—(Press cutting),

HERBS YOU CAN GROW

Herbs often used as remedies can be grown in your garden. Here are hints on some ofthem:—

Thyme.—Sow seeds in April and afterwards thin seedlings to an inch apart. A sunny position is best.

Lemon Thyme is the most aromatic, but it is less hardy than common Thyme and cannot be raised from seed. For drying it should be picked in July.

Sage.—Seeds can be obtained, but propagation by "slips" is a better method. It should be grown in a light dry soil in a warm corner, and picked during August and September for drying.

Sage has been known for centuries to assist digestion.

It will make a good gargle, and Sage tea is considered to allay irritability of the stomach.

Marjoram is little used nowadays, but it is a very aromatic herb and gives flavour to soups, broths, stuffings, etc. It likes a warm, dry soil. Seeds should be sown in April.

Gather herbs to be dried on a fine day. Wash them immediately and dry in a cool oven on trays.

When dry, either hang them up in paper bags in a place where there is a good draught, or pound the leaves in a mortar, pass them through a sieve, and put the powder into bottles, which must be kept closely corked.

In the United States the Indiana Botanic Gardens of Hammond, Ind., are headquarters for Medicinal Roots and Herbs.

Some British Wild Plants and Their Uses—Cont.

WILD CARROT

Daucus Carota. N.O. Umbelliferae.

Synonyms.—Bird's Nest, Bee's Nest.

Habitat.—The plant is indigenous to Britain, growing most abundantly near the sea, in the fields, and in many of the waste places of Europe, Northern Asia, West Asia, America, and so far as India.

Description. — Root perennial, rather woody, slender, firm, yellowish, sinking deeply in the soil, having occasionally small rootlets. Has an erect, round, branched, slightly furrowed hairy stem, 2 to 3 feet high. Lower leaves large, bipinnate; higher ones decrease in size, and are tripinnate, having linear, lanceolate acute segments. Both stem and leaves are more or less covered with stout hairs. The white flowers are clustered together, the stalks of which arise from one point, in rays like an umbrella. The Carrot may be distinguished from other umbels by its having the central flower of the umbel, or sometimes a tiny umbellule brightish red or deep purple in colour, the outer rays white.

Parts Used.—The whole herb, seeds and root.

Composition.—One of the chief constituents is peptic acid. Also a volatile oil is extracted from the seeds, tinged with yellow, or colourless; also "carotine" in red crystals and albumen.

Medicinal Properties.—The seeds are a mild, persistent positive aromatic, diffusive, stimulating, diuretic, deobstruent. For chronic diseases of the kidneys, the whole herb is given in an infusion of 1 ounce herb to 1 pint boiling water, taken in wineglassful doses three times daily. The same infusion is used in gravel and stone. The seeds relieve wind, chronic coughs, dysentery and hiccough. They have been considered beneficial in jaundice. The herb clears the bladder. Removes lithic aid, or gouty condition, with the deposit of brick dust sediment in the urine after standing.

Preparation.—In cases of cloudy urine and lumbago, use the following:—

Parsley Piert (Alchemilla Arvensis)	½	ounce
Wild Carrot (Daucus Carota)	½	"
Motherwort (Leonurus Cardiaca)	½	"
Juniper Berries (Juniperus Communis)...	¼	"
Wormwood (Artemisa Absinthium)	¼	"
Cayenne of Ginger....	1	dram

Let the above simmer 10 minutes, closely covered in 2 pints of water. Strain. Dose: One wineglassful three times daily.

In dropsy of the subcutaneous cellular tissue, the following has been of great service:—

Parsley Piert (Alchemilla Arvensis)	½	ounce
Broom (Cytisus Scoparius)	½	"
Pellitory-of-the-Wall (Parietaria Officinalis) ...	1	"
Wild Carrot (Daucus Carota)	½	"
Senna Leaves (Cassia Acutifolia)	½	"

Juniper (Juniperus Communis) .... ½ ounce

Simmer for 10 minutes in 3½ pints of water, closely covered. Strain. Dose: One wineglassful three times daily.

When the urine contains blood, use the following:—

Wild Carrot (Daucus Carota) .... ½ ounce
Dandelion Rt. Crushed (Taraxacum Off.) .... 1 "
Burdock Rt. Crushed (Arctuim Lappa) ..... 1 "

Simmer in 5 gills of water 15 minutes; filter. Dose: One wineglassful three times daily. The above has given useful service, particularly in relieving elderly gentlemen, or an effective substitute may be found as under:—

Wild Carrot (Daucus Carota) .... 1 ounce
Parsley Piert (Alchemilla Arvensis) .... 1 "
Parsley Rt. (Petroselinum Sativum) .... 2 "

Add a little Capsicum (Cayenne).

Boil in 2 quarts of water half-hour. Strain. Take half-teacupful three times daily.

Apply stimulants locally and sit over hot water in case of stone or gravel.

It is needless to point out the necessity of seeking the advice of a qualified Medical Herbalist in every case.

THE SCOURGE OF MALARIA

New German Drugs
British Association Meeting

"Norwich, Monday.

"The Chemistry Section of the British Association to-day held an important discussion on the chemistry of drugs for the treatment of malaria, in the course of which Professor R. Robinson, who is generally regarded as the most brilliant living British chemist, said that the British Empire is now in pressing need of an institute for research on the chemistry of drugs for treating malaria and other diseases. The resources necessary for the advance of these researches are now beyond those of any private laboratory. A national institute of chemical therapy should be founded.

"The discussion was started by Colonel S. P. James. He said that the malaria outbreak in Ceylon during November, 1934, and April, 1935, had cost the Government £350,000 in treatment and preventive measures; 14½ tons of quinine had been bought at an expense of £50,000, and £20,000 worth of the German drug atebrin.

"In India, a region twice as big as England, was recently prostrated by malaria. The normal October death-rate of the area rose from 6,048 to 76,250. The small island of Mauritius had spent 3,500,000 rupees since 1909 in combating the disease, and Lagos had spent more. All of the natives in that place over one year of age have malaria.

3,500,000 Deaths a Year

"During the last war the British Army that invaded Macedonia from Salonika was reduced at the rate of 100 a day, and 70,000 soldiers were ultimately put out of action. The French Army at the same place was reduced in strength by 60,000, and in the end only 20,000 troops were left in the line. The German Army suffered equally badly.

"It is estimated that at the present time 3,500,000 persons die of malaria every year. Most of these deaths occur in parts of the British Empire, which spends nearly half a million pounds on buying quinine for malaria treatment every year, yet the British Empire spends less than one two-hundredth part of this sum in its yearly expenditure on research into the solution of the malaria problem.

"In spite of the immense consumption of quinine, its mode of operation is still little understood. It is now known that preliminary doses of quinine will not prevent infection by malaria germs. It is necessary to discover new drugs to supplement the quinine treatment and improve on it. Even doses of three grains, a prodigious amount of quinine, will not kill the germs, nor will quinine prevent relapses.

Two New Drugs

"In the last eleven years two important new anti-malarial drugs have been discovered by German chemists. These are plasmochin and atebrin. In some ways they are superior to quinine and prevent relapses in the treatment of some of the various forms of malaria, but for benign tertiary, malaria quinine is more effective.

"Colonal James concluded his review with a criticism of the backwardness of research in England on the chemistry of anti-malarial drugs, in spite of the outstanding humanitarian, economic, and Imperial importance of these drugs to the Empire.

"The discussion was continued by Professor Schulemann, of Elberfeld, who has contributed so much to the German school which has produced plasmochin and atebrin. He said their success had been largely the result of the invention of new methods of testing the anti-malarial properties of new synthetic substances by biologists. Progress depended on the growth of a sympathetic understanding between chemist and biologist and a proper mixture of intuition and organisation. Without these qualities, the launching of extensive researches by trial and error or empirical methods would not be successful. Plasmochin was the thirty-fifth substance in a certain series to be tried, and since 1924 only one other effective substance had been found. It had been shown that quinine interferred with the malaria germ in the early stages of its development, while the two synthetic drugs interfered in the later stages.

"He said that the mode of their operation was still largely obscure, and was to be found, he surmised, in the phenomena of the chemistry of surfaces—for instance, a joint application of the two drugs might produce abdominal pains, whereas the application of one immediately after the other did not. He remarked that mice could be killed if given drugs on an empty stomach, but if given after a meal they suffered no ill-effects. Yet if some of the juice from the stomachs of these mice was injected into other mice which had not had anything to eat, the latter would be killed. This showed how drugs might be absorbed on the surface of particles of food.

Stimulus Needed

"Professor R. Robinson gave an account of researches carried out under his direction on anti-malarial drugs. He said that 24 synthetic drugs had been discovered, but none of them had the required effectiveness. The research had now reached a stage where further advance was impossible without more funds and adequate laboratories. Chemists needed a certain psychological stimulus in order to find the zest to make all the routine preparations of synthetic substances. The chemical and the biological co-operation could be made satisfactorily only when conducted under one roof, and that was why a national institute for research in chemical therapy should now be founded. They had discovered many interesting lines of research which showed promise, but they could not be continued without more adequate support.

"The anti-malarial properties of drugs are investigated by studying their effects on birds infected with malaria. Bird malaria is, in a considerable degree, parallel in its reactions to human malaria. Canaries are often used for these biological tests. The contribution of the canary to human welfare is becoming considerable, for they have been much used for the detection of poisonous gases in mines, and now they are helping in the malaria problem.

"Canary-breeding is one of the minor industries of Norwich. In former times there was much malaria in Norfolk, and in the spring it was customary to ask people: 'Have you had your spring ague?' This was the spring relapse after the infection contracted in the previous summer."—Press cutting.

WINTER GREEN (Gaultheria Procumbens.)

The Leaves

Properties. — Aromatic, stimulant, astringent.

Wintergreen must **not** be used where fever or inflammation is present, as it aggravates these symptoms by its action.

It has been used with considerable success in diarrhœa, but there are far more suitable astringents in the botanic practice. As a stimulant it has been used in some affections of the skin, principally in combination with alteratives.

Oil of Wintergreen is of very great value for deafness, dropped into the ear.

SHEPHERD'S PURSE

Capsella Bursa Pastoris (Medic).

N.O. Cruciferae.

Synonyms.—Shepherd's Sprout, Mother's Heart, Lady's Purse, Rattle Pouches, Blind Weed, Pick Purse.

Habitat.—The plant is found in all parts of the world, withstanding equally the tropical as Arctic rigour. It grows abundantly in Britain throughout the year.

Description.—The plant is evergreen, slightly rough with hairs. The large leaves spread out, forming a circle at the foot of the stem close to the ground, 2 to 6 inches long, broadish; they may be either pinnatifid, indented at the edges, or entire. The slender stem springs from the centre of the rosette of leaves, reaches from a few inches to 2 feet high according to the richness of the ground, bearing a few arrowshaped leaves at the base; above these are found a large number of small white flowers at the top forming little clusters. Then follows the wedge or nearly heart-shaped seed vessels, these pods being like the shepherd's purse; hence the name.

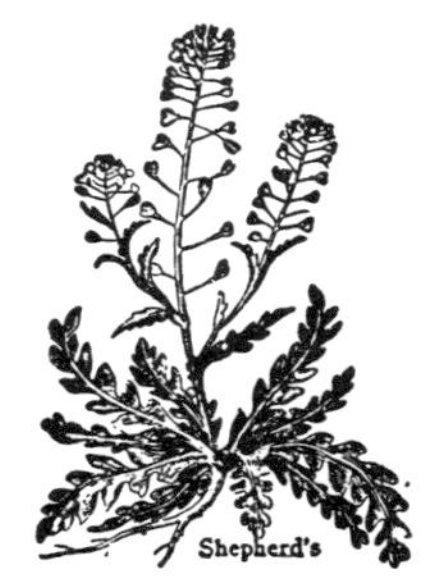

SHEPHERD'S PURSE

Chemical Composition.—Taste, sharp acrid during the summer. Bombelon found an acid which he named bursinic acid, also a tannate, and an alkaloid, Bursine. A volatile oil resembling oil of mustard, a soft resin 6 per cent., and a fixed oil are also present.

Medical Properties.—Anti-scorbutic, stimulant, diuretic, mucilaginous. Its influence is directed towards the renal and vesical organs, soothing irritation, relieves hæmaturia. Gives positive relief in excessive menstruation. In ulcerated condition, catarrh, and abscess of the ureters and bladder it has proved effective; with Couch Grass it is a rare combination as a stimulating diuretic. It is gently stimulating and mildly relaxing to the renal and urinary tract. The flow of urine is relieved and increased. Its results are positive in lumbago. In urethral irritation, in cases of scalding urine, its benefit is soon felt. It alleviates catarrhal conditions of the renal organs and irritable spermatorrhœa. Indeed the whole pelvic viscera is charged with new vigour, either directly or indirectly, it is evidently one of the best agents to be used as stated. Some claim to have cured St. Anthony's fire and several skin diseases. Bleedings and floodings are said to come under its arresting influence; also dropsy. Puerperal hæmorrhage has been known to promptly cease a few minutes after a cupful of the infusion has been taken, and has often been similarly and successfully employed in many forms of hæmorrhages. Make as follows:—Shepherd's Purse, 2 ounces; Water, 3 half-pints; boil down to 1 pint. Dose: One wineglassful four times daily.

Preparation and Uses.—Dr. Ferine states that "The Shepherd's Purse has been announced as the chief remedy of the seven 'Marvellous Medicines' prepared by Count Mattei of Bologna, which are believed by his disciples to be curative of diseases otherwise intractible, such as cancer, aneurism and destructive leprosy." Aneurism is a morbid diltation of an artery. The other six remedies are given as follows:—Knotgrass, Watercress, Water Betony, Cabbage, Stonecrop, and Fever-few.

For bed wetting, use the following:—

Shepherd's Purse (Capsella Bursa Pastoris) . . ½ ounce
Agrimony (Agrimonia Eupatoria) . . . . .½ "
Lady's Slipper (Cypripedium Pubescens) . . ½ "
Corn Silk (Stigmata Maidis) . . . . .½ "
Oak Bark (Quercus Robor) . . . . .½ "
Liquorice Rt. (Crushed) (Glycyrrhiza Glabra) . . 1 "

Steep a few hours in 2 pints boiling water; strain; add 2 ounces Glycerine. Dose: One teaspoonful before each meal and at bedtime.

In case of gritty or gravelly deposit in the urine, make the following:—

Shepherd's Purse (Capsella Bursa Pastoris) . . ½ ounce
Peach Leaves (Prunus Persica) . . . . .½ "
Marshmallow (Althaea Officinalis) . . . . .½ "
Red Sage (Salvia Officinalis) . . . . .½ "

Steep in 2 pints boiling water 30 minutes; strain. Dose: From one teaspoonful to a wineglassful as required.

The following is quite as useful in incontinence of urine:—

Shepherd's Purse (Capsella Bursa Pastoris) . . ½ ounce
Yarrow (Achillia Millefolium . . . . .½ "
Agrimony (Agrimonia Eupatoria) . . . . .½ "
Prepare as above.

In the United States The Indiana Botanic Gardens of Hammond, Ind., are headquarters for medicinal roots and herbs.

BOGBEAN

Menyanthes Trifoliata (Tournef). N.O. Gentianaceæ

Synonyms. — Water Trefoil, Buckbean, Marsh Clover, Marsh Trefoil.

Habit.—Grows throughout Europe, abounding in bogs and marshy and shallow water in the North of England, not so plentiful in the South.

Description.—Main root perennial, white, thick, long creeping, round, jointed, bearing many

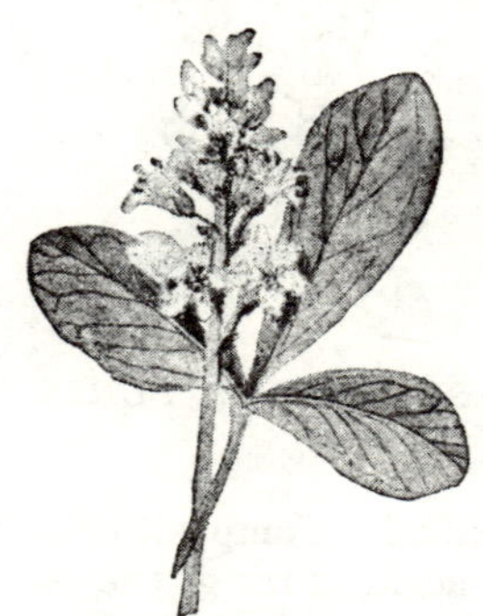

BOGBEAN

fibres. Stem about 1 foot high, being round and procumbent. Leaves, on long fleshy petioles, three partite, leaflets entire, about 2 inches long, 1 inch broad. Flower stems issue from the sheathed base of the leaves on long stalks 6 to 18 inches high, the flowers stand at the top above the leaves in a short thick spike. Corollary funnel shaped, ¾-inch across with 5 ovate, lance shaped, acute segments, with fringed inside with lovely filaments, tinted rose colour. Stamens, 5. It is claimed by many as one of our most beautiful flowers.

Chemical Composition.—A bitter substance imparted to water or alcohol either by infusion or maceration. A gum resin which is bitter, acid, and astringent. A nutritive property.

Medicinal Properties. — Cathartic, deobstruent, febrifuge, tonic.

It exerts its weight of influence chiefly on the glandular system, and the secernent. Large doses cause vomiting, yet they cleanse, and stimulate the liver. The urine is also increased. As an anti-periodic and alterative it is valuable. In scrofula and skin diseases, while there is much impurity of the blood it gives good service. In nervous diseases, such as periodical headache, hypochondriasis, palpitation and paralysis, it is claimed to have proved effective. Its destruction and evacuation of intestinal worms in children has given satisfaction by using ½ to 1 dram doses.

In jaundice, hepatic obstructions, uterine hæmorrhages, it has been well marked. Where ague and low fevers abound, there the Bogbean is most plentiful, consequently it is deemed remedial in those complaints; experience gives us a better reason for its success. Authorities vouch for its efficacy in skin diseases of an apparent cancerous nature, as also the relieving of gout by the application of the fresh leaves to the pain. When sheep and goats suffer from rot, they will quickly recover after feeding on the plant.

Preparation and Uses.—Make as follows:

Bogbean, Dried Leaves..1 ounce
Boiling Water ....1 pint

Dose: One wineglassful frequently.

In cases of dyspepsia, make and use:—

Bogbean (Menyanthes Trifoliata) .... 1 ounce
Wormwood (Artemisa Absinthium) ....½ "
Sage (Salvia Officinalis) 1 "

Pour on the above 1 quart water, simmer closely covered 10 minutes. Strain. Dose: One wineglassful four times daily.

A most useful preparation for worms may be made as follows:—

Bogbean (Menyanthes Trifoliata)...1 ounce
Wormwood (Artemisia Absinthium)...½ "
Tansy (Tanacetum Vulgare)...½ "
Gentian (Gentiana Lutea)...½ "
Indian Pink (Spigelia Marilandica)...¼ "
Male Fern Rt. (Dryopteris Felix Mas)...¼ "
Wormseed (Chenopodium Anthelminticum)...¼ "

Boil in 3 quarts water down to 3½ pints, sweeten with treacle or a little glycerine. Dose: For adults, one small wineglassful four times a day; every other day a good diet drink. Reduce the dose for children to one teaspoonful four times daily.

The above is useful for seat or ascarides, and the teres or round worm.

The following has been tested in spasmodic asthma. Make as here given:—

Bogbean (Menyanthes Trifoliata)...1 ounce
Horehound (Marrubium Vulgare)...1 "

Lobelia (Lobelia Inflata) 1 ounce
Agrimony (Agrimonia Eupatoria)...1 "
Liquorice Rt. (Glycyrrhiza Glabra)...1 "
Comfrey Rt. (Symphytum Officinalis)...1 "
Vervain (Verbena Hastata)...1 "

Boil in 5 pints water down to 2 pints. Strain. Dose: One dessertspoonful four or five times daily, and one in bed if need be.

The above preparations have proved effective in numerous cases.

We always urge the necessity of a qualified Medical Herbalist being consulted in all cases.

YARROW

Achillea Millefolium (Linn).
N.O. Compositæ

Synonyms.—Milfoil. Thousand Weed, Nose Bleed, Staunch Weed, Bloodwort, etc.

Habitat.—Yarrow is found everywhere, on the roadside, pastures, and meadows of this country. In all temperate and colder parts of Northern Asia, and North America.

Description.—Root perennial, round; slender, creeping, white or pinkish, underground shoots being fibrous, stem erect, simple smooth below, towards the top woolly, branched somewhat, with many leaves of a reddish purple tinge, varying from a few inches to a foot or two high. Leaves 4 to 5 inches long, 1 to 1½ inches broad, alternate, sessile, long, bipinnate, segments very finely cut, the leaves thus assuming a feathery appearance. Flowers terminal forming a cluster, each like a minute daisy, with flattened loose heads or cymes. Colour, white or pale lilac. The whole plant is more or less covered with a silky down.

Part Used.—The whole plant.

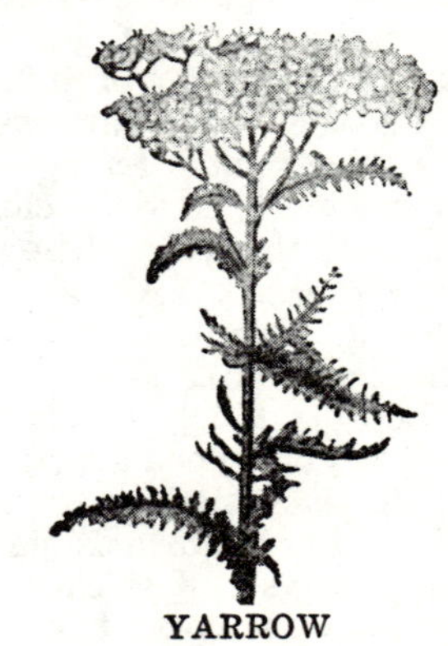

YARROW

Chemical Composition.—Achillein, achilleic acid, supposed to be identical with aconitic acid. A volatile oil, of a dark green colour, with gum, resin, tannin, also earthy ash and composed of phosphates, chlorides, nitrate of potash, and lime.

Medical Properties.—The herb is a mild aromatic, slow stimulating astringent tonic, and diaphoretic. The mucous membrane of the digestive tract comes under its influence. Favourable results are given in chronic diarrhœa, and chronic dysentery. Yarrow tea is unsurpassed in the treatment of colds, as also in early stages of fevers. The infusion taken cold is reliable as a general tonic to the system, both stimulating the appetite and toning the organs of digestion. A hot infusion is specially serviceable in children's colds, measles, and other eruptive diseases. Its influence is directed to the generative organs when used with uterine tonics. It gives good service in piles, gleet, leucorrhœ, hæmorrhages. Its action on the skin is swift and certain, producing sweat. It is claimed by many great herbalists, past and present, that there is not one other herb more gratefully acknowledged to prevent disease and save doctors' bills, especially after drinking a hot infusion and applying a damp cloth round a hot-water bottle to the feet.

Preparation and Uses

Yarrow (Achillea Millefolium)....1 ounce
Boiling Water ....1 pint

Let it stand near the fire half-hour, closely covered. Strain. Dose: One or two wineglassfuls frequently, in bed, with a hot-water bottle as above. This is useful in colds, measles, and other eruptive diseases of children. Cotton wool dipped in it and pressed into the nostrils will stop bleeding. A stronger infusion will halt hæmorrhages of the bowels. A useful combination remedial for piles is as follows:

Yarrow (Achillea Millefolium)...1 ounce
Golden Seal (Hydrastis Canadensis)..1 "
Ginger (Zingiber Officinale)...½ dr.

Simmer in 2 pints water 10 minutes, closely covered. Strain, and while hot add ½ lb. Black Treacle. Dose: Half teacupful three times daily. Apply Chickweed ointment to the piles.

About this time of the year, many suffer from influenza or catarrh; in such cases make up and use the following:—

Yarrow (Achillea Millefolium)..1 ounce
Boneset (Eupatorium Perfoliatum)..1 "
Black Horehound (Ballota Nigra)...1 "
Sage (Salvia Officinalis)..1 "
Balm (Melissa Officinalis)...1 "

Simmer, closely covered, in 5 pints of water, for half-hour, then add Capsicum and Ginger combined half-teaspoonful. Dose: One wineglassful three times daily. A hot bath should be taken immediately symptoms of influenza are felt, and then straight to bed with a hot-water bottle wrapped in a damp cloth placed at the feet; regulate the bowels once or twice daily. Should there be any complications, then the advice of a qualified Medical Herbalist should be sought at once.

VALERIAN

Valerian Officinalis. N.O. Valerinaceae

Synonyms.—Allheal, Phu, Great Wild Valerian, Capon's Tail, etc.

Habitat.—Siberia, Japan, Western Asia, Europe; banks of streams, and most woods of this country.

Description. — Root perennial with longish, slender, dusky brown fibres, which tend to merge into a short, round root-stock or erect rhizome. This often takes a few years to develop before the flowering stem is sent up, though slender horizontal branches terminating in buds appear earlier; from the buds aerial shoots proceed, which after taking root produce new plants. The flowering stalk is upright, smooth grooved, round, branched, and reaches from 3 to 4 feet high. Leaves on stem in pairs upon short broad sheaths. Each leaf being composed of a series of lance shaped segments, nearly opposite each other on each side of the leaf. Leaflets vary in number from

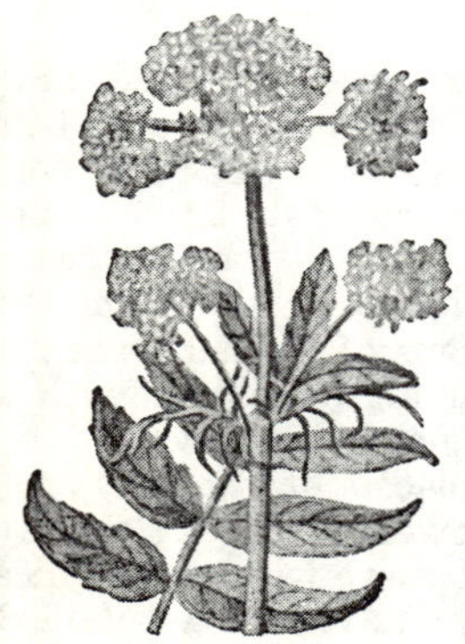

VALERIAN

6 to 10 pairs and vary also in breadth, being broader when few, and narrower when more numerous, length from 2 to 3 inches. The flowers are small, white or purplish in colour and terminate the stem in large bunches. In bloom from June to September.

Part Used.—Root.

Chemical Composition. — The root contains formic, malic, valeranic, and acetic acids; also resin, starch, and some mucilage. The characteristic unpleasant odour is due to an oily liquid isovalerianic acid; this is the normal acid contained in the chief constituent of Valerian, the yellowish-green or brownish-yellow oil, which is claimed to be present in the dried root to the extent of 0.5 per cent.

Medicinal Properties.—Valerian is a powerful, persistent, stimulating, and relaxing nervine. It is soothing and diffusive, gives relief in irritability of the nervous system, insomnia and hysteria, and especially suitable to children's nervousness. It exerts a marked influence on the cerebro-spinal system, acting directly on those parts, thereby causing steadiness in unbalanced conditions. The root eases pain and promotes sleep. Those suffering from overstrained nerves find it specially beneficial. It has a quietening, soothing, and gently relaxing effect on the bowels; with other suitable agents causes a natural evacuation.

Preparation and Uses.—Make the infusion as follows:—Valerian, 1 ounce; Water (boiling), 1 pint. Dose: One or two wineglassfuls four times daily.

The old Herbalists used the root for a cough, boiled with the compound as follows:—

Valerian (Valeriana Officinalis) . . 1 oz.
Aniseed (Pimpinell Anisum) . . ½ "
Raisins . . . . 1 "

Boil in 2 pints of water for 10 minutes; sieve. Dose: One wineglassful four times daily.

Make and use the following in case of chronic constipation, in conjunction with infections of warm water:—

Black Horehound (Ballota Nigra) . . 1 ounce
Life Root (Senecia Aureus) . . 1 "
Valerian (Valeriana Officinalis) . . 1 "

Comfrey Root (Symphytum Officinalis) . . 1 ounce
Centaury (Erythrea Centaurium) . . 1 "

Boil in 5 pints of water half an hours, closely covered; strain. Dose: One to two wineglassfuls four times daily.

The following has given satisfactory results in convulsions, hysterical affections, and epilepsy:—

Powder Comfrey Root (Symphytum Officinalis) . . 1 ounce
Powder Valerian (Valeriana Officinalis) . . 1 "
Powder Scullcap (Scutelaria Lateriflora) . . 1 "
Powder (herb or seed) (Lobelia Inflata) . . 1/8 "
(or 1/2 teaspoonful of each)
Powder Black Cohosh (Cimicifuga Racemose) . . 1/4 "
Powder Cayenne (Capsicum) . . 1/8 "
Powder Ginger (Zingiber Officinalis) . . 1/8 "

Mix thoroughly. Dose: half a teaspoonful of the Powder in half a teacupful of hot water, sweetened or not, as desired. Children half dose or less, according to age.

Another compound which is said to be useful for troublesome bowels follows:—

Valerian (Valeriana Officinalis) . . 1 ounce
Lobelia (Lobelia Inflata) . . 1 "
Wormwood (Artemisia Absinthium) . . 1 "

Simmer in 3 pints of water for 10 minutes. Sieve. Dose: One wineglassful three times daily.

We need hardly point out the importance of asking the advice of a qualified Medical Herbalist in all cases.

FIGWORT

Scrofularia Aquatica. N.O. Scrofulariacaeæ

Synonyms.—Water Betony, Bishop's leaves, Feddlewood, Brownwort.

Habitat.—Europe, North Africa, Western Asia to the Himalayas. Fairly abundant in this Country on the side of ditches, and in moist places.

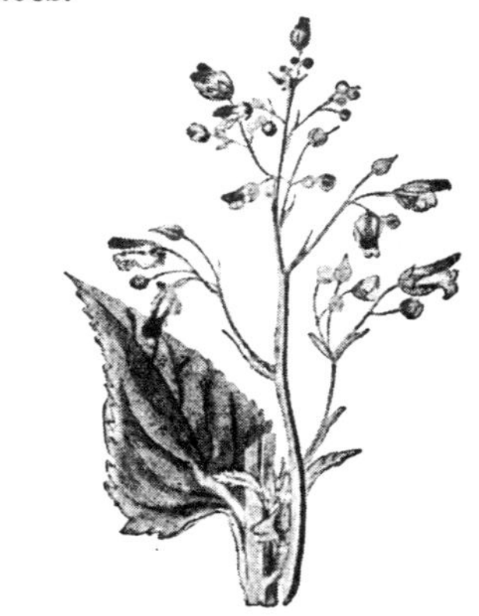

FIGWORT

Description. — Root-stock perennial, stout, fibrous and creeping. Stem erect, square, winged, branched, smooth, somewhat reddish-purple in colour. Leaves, crenate, oblong, egg-shaped, lower ones heart-shaped, smooth, veining prominent, opposite in pairs, each pair standing at right angles to the pair below, on foot stalks, rather widely separated on the stem. Flowers form a cluster of spikelets at the top of stem, with small lance-shaped bracts attached.

Corolla tinted reddish-purple, nearly globular, almost resembling small helmets. Time of blooming, July and August.

FIGWORT (WATER)

Parts Used.—The whole plant.

Medicinal Properties. — Hepatic, Anti-scorbutic, Diuretic, Remittent, Alterative, Anodyne. It is stimulating and relaxing to the glandular system, where its greatest influence is felt. It liquifies congealed blood. It soothes and allays irritation of the digestive tract. It quickly frees the blood from offending substances, such as clots, blemishes on the skin, blackheads, pimples, freckles, boils, carbuncles, abscesses, goitre and tumors, or whatsoever occurs from impurity of the blood is swiftly and surely eradicated from the blood, especially when combined with other suitable agents as given under the next heading—"Preparation."

Preparation and Uses.—Make an infusion as follows:—

Figwort (Water) Leaves. .1 oz.
Water (boiling) ....1 pint

Let it stand half-hour, strain. Dose: 1 wineglassful 4 times daily.

It has found great favour when given for blood pressure, acidity of the stomach, indigestion, dyspepsia, hepatic congestion, in the following formulæ:—

Water Figwort (Scrofularia Aquatica) 1 oz.
Nettles (Urtica Dioica)....1 "
Black Horehound (Balota Nigra)....1 "
Meadowsweet (Spirea Ulmaria)....1 "

Boil in 4 pints of water 10 minutes; strain. Dose: One wineglassful four times daily, between meals.

Use the following in cases where a tonic nervine is required:—

Wild or Wood Sage (Tehcrium Scorodonia)....1 oz.
Figwort, Water (Scrofularia Aquatica)....1 "
Scullcap (Scutelaria Lateriflora)....1 "
Lobelia (Lobelia Inflata...¼ "
Black Horehound (Balota Nigar)....1 "
Wood Betony (Stachys Betonica)....1 "

Boil in 3 quarts of water ½ hour; strain. Dose: One wineglassful four times daily, between meals.

The above will do useful service in most nervous troubles, without any serious symptoms. Would give signal results in stomach troubles of nervous origin, and in the results following bowel complaints such as chronic constipation, flatulence, and worms.

In cases of diabetus mellitus, make and use the following:—

Nettles (Urtica Dioica)..1 ounce
Mistletoe (Viscum Album)....1 "
Comfrey (Symphytum Off.)....1 "
Unicorn Rt. (True) (Aletrisfarinoso)....1 "
Night Blooming Cereus (Cereus Grandiflora)1 "
Feverfew (Pyrethrum Parthenium)....1 "
Cubebs (Piper Cubebœ)....1 "
Figwort, Water (Scrofularia Aquatica)....1 "

Boil in 4 quarts of water ½ hour; strain. Dose: One wineglassful four times daily. Add the following when strained:—

Cayenne (Capsicum Minimum) ½ teaspoonful
Ginger (Zingiber Officinalis) ½ "
Prickly Ash Berries (Xanthoxyllum Amer.) ½ "

The above is of use in diabetus mellitus; also in diabetus insipidus. It quickly stores the balance of the circulation, by its stimulating, relaxing, toning and re-invigorating the whole economy of man.

It is important to have the advice of a fully qualified Medical Herbalist to avoid quackery.

FOR PILES

Wormwood	½	ounce
Marshmallow Leaves	½	"
Horehound	½	"
Wood Sage	½	"
Yarrow	½	"
Cascara Bark	½	"

Infuse in 1 quart of boiling water.

Dose; One wineglassful three times a day an hour before meals. And also apply a little Pile Ointment to the affected part.

A THIRD EYE

A tube that claims to supply human beings with a third eye to see objects hitherto invisible and also to see in the dark was shown to the American Association for the Advancement of Science when they met at St. Louis.

While the naked eye can see 6,500 units, the tube increases the power of vision to 13,000 units.

When used with a telescope, it should revolutionise astronomy by showing us what is really on the planets, while with the microscope it should enable us to detect microbes not even suspected before, and enlarge our knowledge of biology out of all reckoning.

Meanwhile, Dr. Marston Bogert, professor of organic chemistry at Columbia University, advises Americans to increase the power of the naked eye to see in the dark by eating more carrots.

The property of visual purple which enables us to see in the dark, is supplied to the human body by carrotine, the orange colouring matter in the carrot, he says.

MOTHERWORT

Leonurus Cardiaca (Linn.). N.O. Labiate

Habitat.—Found growing under hedges, on banks, and gravelly places in many parts of Europe, where it is a native. In England it is chiefly cultivated in gardens. When found in the wilds, it is said by some authorities to be merely a garden escape. The plant will grow in any kind of soil, but particularly gravelly or calcareous; it soon spreads by allowing the seeds to scatter.

Part Used.—The whole herb.

Description. — Root perennial, long, stringy and fibrous, darkish yellow or brownish in colour. Stem, square, strong, hard, rough, 3 to 4 feet high, erect, branched, almost bushy below. Radical leaves stand on slender foot stalks, closely set, ovate, lobed, and serrate, colour dark green. They are different from all other labiate leaves, prominent leaves radiating, deeply cut into five lobes; also by the calyx teeth of its flowers, being prickly. Stem leaves, 2 to 3 inches long, with foot stalks. Upper leaves and bracts are much narrower and pointed. Flowers in whorls, pinkish-whitish outside, purplish within, stalkless, tubular upper lips of corolla almost flat, hairy above. Time of flowering, July and August.

Medicinal Properties.— Mildly stimulating and relaxing nervine. The chief influence is directed towards the uterine organs, giving tone and adding strength to the relaxed tissues. Mildly relaxing to the heart, giving to the nerves tone, and strengthening the heart exceedingly. The whole nervous system is gradually brought under the power of Leonurus. Among other uses to which this herb may be applied are inflammation of the uterus, kidneys, uterine tension, uterine irritation, thoroughly toning and strengthening the pelvic viscera. Indeed, its reinvigorating qualities properly qualify it for the office of retoring all the conditions of nervous diseases peculiarly feminine.

Preparation and Uses.—The simple infusion is made thus:—Motherwort, 1 ounce; boiling water, 1 pint. Stand covered half-hour. Dose: One wineglassful four times daily.

Make and use the following in uterine inflammation:—

Motherwort (Leonurus Cardiaca) . . 1 ounce
Scullcap (Scutellaria Off.) . . 1 "
Water Betony Scrofularia Aquatica) . . 1 ounce
Water Dock (Rumex Hydropathum) . . 1 "
Black Horehound (Ballota Nigra) . . 1 "

Boil in 5 pints of water half hour; towards the end add half teaspoonful Ginger. Strain. Dose: One wineglassful four times daily, before meals.

In cases of inflammation of the kidneys, make the following:—

Motherwart (Leonurus Cardiaca) . . 1 ounce
Gt. Water Dock (Rumex Hydropathum) . . 1 "
Valerian (Valeriana Off.) . . 1 "
Wood Betony (Stachys Betonica) . . 1 "
Plantain (Plantago Major) . . 1 "
Mugwort (Artemisia Vulgaris) . . 1 "

Boil in 6 pints of water half-hour. Towards the end add half teaspoonful powdered Ginger. Strain. Dose: One wineglassful four times daily before meals.

The above will be found to do useful service in kidney inflammation. The peculiar adaptability of the above are well suited to remove the causes of Nephritis. Having in their nature the power to purify and liquefy the blood. Make and use the following in cases of ovarian tension:—

Motherwort (Leonurus Cardiaca) . . 1 ounce
Wormwood (Artemisia Absinthium) . . ½ "
Water Dock (Rumex Hydropathum) . . 1 "

Black Horehound (Ballota Nigra..1 ounce
Sunflower (Helianthus Annuus)..1 "

Boil in 5 pints of water half-hour; sieve. Dose: One wineglassful four times daily.

This will be found to be of excellent service in acute ovaritis. The medicine is well qualified to meet such cases, being anti-inflammation, relaxing; also tones and imparts strength.

WATER MINT

Mentha Aquatica. N.O. Labiate.

Synonyms.—Marsh Mint, Hairy Mint, Whorled Mint.

Habitat. — Found throughout Russian Asia, Northern Europe, and common in this country in ditches and marshes, banks of rivers, where it grows abundantly in large masses.

Description. — Root perennial, stem square, erect, firm and strong, brownish in colour, 1 to nearly 2 feet high. Leaves stalked, roundish or oval, ovate somewhat wedge shaped at the base, acute or subacute, serrated, hairy on each side. Flowers lilac in colour, whorled, or in thick round clusters towards the top of the stem, beginning about the middle or just below. Bracts similar to leaves. The smell of the plant is agreeable, and is somewhat like those of Mint and Pennyroyal.

Chemical Contents.—The herb yields about 4 per cent essential oil, which resembles the odour of Pennyroyal.

Medicinal Properties. — Antiseptic, emetic, stimulant, carminative, astringent. Useful in all stomach and bowel disorders. Is a handy remedy for colic, pains in the bowels, and to promote menstruation. As the best of Mints, it imparts strength by its astringent quality, purifies with its antiseptic property, relieves wind, stimulates the mucous membrane of the stomach and bowels. Will cause emesis in large doses, with good results; in small doses it will relieve nausea. An infusion is the best mode of administration.

Preparation and Uses.—The simple infusion is made thus:—Water Mint, 1 oz.; boiling water, 1 pint. Steep half-hour, well covered. Sieve. Dose: One small wineglassful three times daily as required.

Make and use the following in flatulence:—

Water Mint (Mentha Aquatica)....1 oz.
Marsh Marigold (Bidens Tripartita)....1 "
Wild Sage (Teucrium Scorodonia)....1 "
Ginger (Zingiber Officinalis) ½ teaspoonful

Infuse in 4 pints boiling water, closely covered, half-hour near the fire. Strain. Dose: One small wineglassful three times daily. This will quickly remove the cause of wind in the stomach, and will gradually bring the stomach to better condition by improving the glands, blood vessels and the mucous lining of the stomach.

The following may be used for bowel troubles:—

Water Mint (Mentha Aquatica)....1 oz.
Water Agrimony (Bidens Tripartita)....1 "

Motherwort (Leonusus Cardiaca)....1 oz.
Black Horehound (Ballota Nigra)....1 "

Simmer in 4 pints water half-hour, closely covered. Strain. Add half teaspoonful powdered Ginger whilst hot. Dose: One wineglassful three times daily. This compound will give immediate and good results in complaints arising from indigestion, when the bowels are overloaded with mucous and wind.

Use the following for the stomach:—

Water Mint (Mentha Aquatica)....1 oz.
Masterwort (Imperatoria Ostruthium)....1 "
White Horehound (Marrubuim Vulgare)....1 "
Hops (Humulus Lupulus).1 "
Marsh Marigold (Bidens Tripartita)....1 "
Wood Sage (Teucrium Scorodonia)....1 "
Black Horehound (Ballota Nigra)....1 "

Simmer in 4 quarts water half-hour. Strain. Add half teaspoonful powdered Ginger whilst hot. Dose: One small wineglassful three times daily. The above will be of much service in indigestion caused by catarrh; also for wind caused by acidity.

A preparation of Water Mint and Vinegar is recommended to stop the vomiting of blood.

In influenza or cold, or any inflammatory condition where perspiration is essential, a strong tea made from this herb may be taken warm as freely as may be necessary to produce the desired results.

AVENS

Geum Urbanum. N.O. Rosaceæ.

Synonyms. — Clove Root, Colewort, Herb Bennet, Way Bennet, Goldystar, Wild Rye, City Avens, Common Avens.

Habitat.—Distributed over Europe, North Africa, Siberia, Western Asia to the Himalayas, Eastern to Western North America. Found abundantly in woods, hedges, and shady places in all parts of Great Britain.

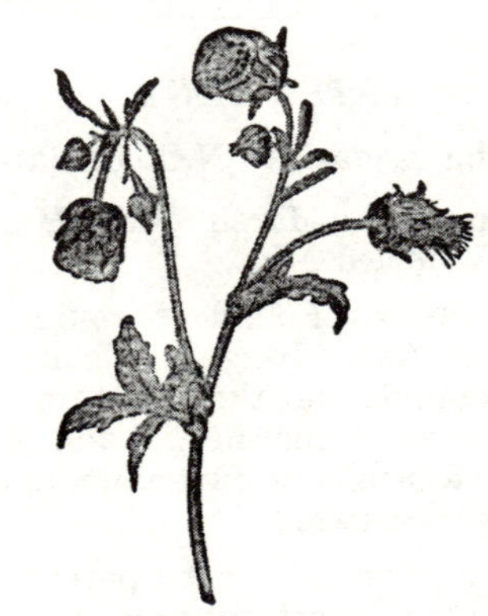

AVENS

Description. — Root perennial, woody and fibrous, odour like cloves. Stem erect, slender, firm, branched towards the top, hairy, reddish colour at the base; about 18 inches to 2 feet high. Leaves vary in form according to their position. The radical leaves stand on long channelled foot-stalks, interruptedly pinnate (a compound leaf having leaflets arranged on each side of a central rib) like the Silverweed. They are long, rough, dark green and winged. Those growing from the root have three small pairs and one large one at the end. Those on the stem are smaller with fewer parts, otherwise the same. Flowers, small, stand on separate terminal stalks. The corolla consists of 5 roundish yellow petals. The calyx cleft into 10 segments—5 large, 5 small. The plant blooms from June to December, though the green round prickly seed is more conspicuous than the flower towards the back end.

Chemical Contents.—A volatile oil, composed mainly of glucoside end eugenol, Gein Geum bitter tonic, acid, gum, resin, and muriate of lime. It yields its qualities to water and alcohol. It yields 0.04 per cent. of thick, greenish volatile oil when distilled with water.

Part Used—Herb and Root.

Medicinal Properties. — Astringent, antiseptic, aromatic, tonic, sudorific, styptic, febrifuge, and stomachic. It is employed in mild, acute and chronic cases of diarrhœa and dysentery. Its results are most positive when used in measles, scarlet fever, and stomach troubles. The herb and root form a pleasant, mild, soothing, astringent tonic. It is not drying but soothing to the mucous membranes. It will be found effective in gleet, leucorrhœa, applied locally and internally. It is quite capable of dealing with light hæmorrhages and some forms of sore mouth, used locally. Avens exercises its greatest advantage as a tonic astringent to the mucous membrane of stomach and bowels. In spring it is used as a purifier of the blood and liquefies congealed blood.

Preparation and Uses. — Make the simple infusion:—

Avens (Geum Urbanum) . . ½ oz.
Boiling Water . . . . .1 pint

Steep half-hour. Strain. Dose: One wineglassful three times daily.

Use the following in feverish conditions and stomach troubles:—

Avens (Geum Urbanum) . . 1 ounce
Brooklime (Veronica Beccabunga) . . . . .1 "
Bogbean (Menyanthes Trifoliata) . . . . .1 "
Black Horehound (Ballota Nigra) . . . . .1 "
Meadowsweet (Spirea Ulmaria) . . . . .1 "
Ragwort (Senecio Jacobea) 1 "
Mugwort (Artemisia Vulgaris) . . . . .1 "

Boil in 4 quarts water half-hour. Sieve. Dose: One wineglassful four times daily. The above will do well when given in doses as stated for measles and scarlet fever, and will prove a powerful stomachic.

The following will be found useful when employed in rupture:—

Avens (Geum Urbanum) . 1 ounce
Mandrake (Podophyllum Peltatum) . . . . .1 "
White Horsehound (Marrubium Vulgare) . . . . .1 "
White Behens (Behen Album) . . . . .1 "
Mugwort (Artemisia Vulgaris) . . . . .1 "
Wormwood (Artemisia Absinthium) . . . . .1 "
Masterwort (Imperatoria Ostruthium) . . . . 1 "

Boil in 4 quarts water half-hour. Strain. Dose: One wineglassful four times daily.

The above will be useful in all cases of rupture, spitting blood, and worms.

For diseases of women, use the following:—

Avens (Geum Urbanum) . . 1 ounce
Mandrake (Podophyllum Peltatum) . . . . 1 "
White Behen (Behen Album) . . . . 1 "
Broom (Cytisus Scoparius) 1 "
Borage (Borago Off.) . . . . 1 "

Boil in 5 pints water half-hour. Strain. Dose: One wineglassful four times daily.

This medicine is efficacious in profuse menstruation and many obstructions in women.

In most cases, seek the advice of a qualified Medical Herbalist.

PLANTAIN, COMMON

Plantago Major (Linn.). N.O. Plantaginaceae

Synonyms. — Way - broad - leaf. Englishman's foot, Way-bread, Snakeweed, White Man's foot.

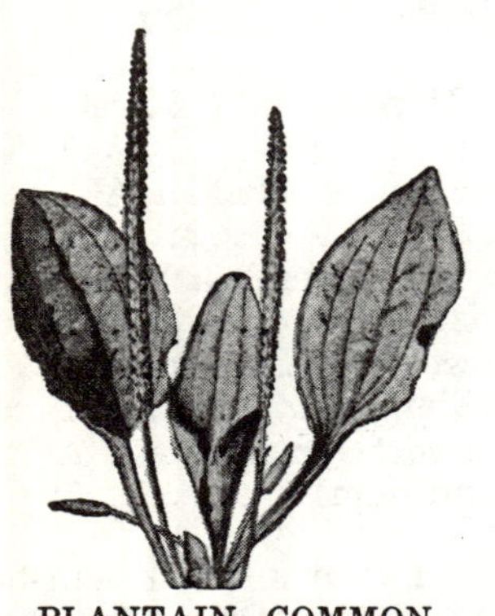

PLANTAIN, COMMON

Habitat. — Distributed throughout Europe. Common in Britain in fields, pastures, by the roadside and all waste places. Flowers May to September.

Description. — Root perennial, having many whitish, round, descending fibres, proceeding from a wood stock. The plant forms a large rosette of radical leaves, borne on channelled stalks, each leaf being broadly ovate, blunt, usually smooth, thick 5 or 11 ribbed, ribs fibrous, nearly hairless, mostly entire. Flower stem straight, leafless, simple slightly angular, slightly hairy, upwards, terminating in a slender dense flowered spike 4 to 8 or more inches long according to situation. Flowers usually purplish green, calyx four parted, small correls bell shaped and 4 lobed, stamens 4, with purple anthers. Fruit a 2-celled ovate capsule, not enclosed in the perianth, and contains 6 to 8 seeds in each cell.

Parts Used.—The whole plant, roots, leaves, and flower spikes.

Medicinal Properties. — The leaves and roots are a mild stimulating, diffusive and relaxing alterant. It exercises its chief influence over the entire urinary tract and the whole mucous membrane, together with the glandular system. It greatly increases urine, relieves its scalding, and generally relieves backache, scrofulous swellings (internal and external). Astringent, diuretic, refrigerent, deobstruent, febrifuge, vulnerary. Used in intermitants, old ulcers, ophthalmia, hysteria, inflammation of the skin and stimulates sore thereon. The leaves have proved curative in tubercular consumption, have arrested mild hæmorrhages externally. They are usually best in combination with other remedies for bleeding of the stomach and lungs. They are useful in ulcerated lungs, consumption, and dysentery. Their action is similar to Dock leaves when applied to insect stings or nettle stings. Also, they give ease to burns and scalds. The plant is considered specific against the bites of a mad dog or venomous creatures. Our broad-leaved Plantain has followed the Englishman to all our overseas settlements; indeed, some Aborigines of the Colonies name the plant "The Englishman's Foot." According to Swedish authorities, the leaves of Plantago Major are eaten by goats, sheep and swine, but cows and horses refuse them. The seeds are well known as favourite food of canaries and many other small birds.

Preparation and Uses.—

Planatain (Plantago Major)....1 ounce
Boiling Water ....1 pint

Steep half-hour; strain. Dose: One small wineglassful four times daily.

The following is useful for hæmorrhage of the stomach and lung:—

Plantain (Plantago Major)....1 ounce
Marshmallow Root (Althoea Off.)....1 "
Comfrey Root (Symphytum Off.)....1 "
Water Plantain Leaves (Alisma Plantago)....1 "
Water Agrimony Leaves (Bidens Tripartitu)..1 "

For nervous troubles make and use the following:—

Plantain (Plantago Major)....1 ounce
Water Plantain (Alisma Plantago) ...1 "
Motherwort (Leonurus Cardiaca)....1 ounce
Southernwood (Artemisia Abrotanum)....1 "
Valerian (Valerian Officinalis)....1 "

Simmer in 5 pints water half-hour. Strain. Dose: One wineglassful four times daily. The above will do good service in nervous troubles arising from whatever cause. It is calculated to give satisfaction in all cases requiring either a tonic, or a relaxing and strengthening nervine.

An ointment said to be useful for the skin is made as follows:—

Plantain (Plantago Major)....1 ounce
Southernwood (Artimisia Arbrotanun)....1 "
Black Currant Leaves (Ribes Nigrum)....1 "
Elder Buds (Sambucus Nigra)....1 "
Angelica (Angelica Archangelica)....1 "
Parsley (Carum Petroselinum)....1 "

To be chopped and simmered in enough clarified butter to cover the herbs, until the herbs are crisp. Then strain through muslin. Used for scalds, burns, and all raw surfaces.

Another excellent ointment is said to be made from:—

Plantain (Plantago Major)....1 ounce
Elder Buds (Sambucus Nigra)....1 "
Pilewort (Ranunculus Ficaria)...1 "
House Leek (Sempervivum Tectorum)....1 "

Useful for all abraded surfaces.

FIRESIDE TALKS ON HEALTH

By J. MAXWELL, N.D.

FEVERS

The thought of fever produces a scare in many minds; they are in great fear that it may be the messenger of death, and yet it is always a salutary effort of Nature to throw out of the body morbid matter that has accumulated in the system.

No matter what name may be given to the particular brand of fever that affects you, the object of Nature is one and the same, to clear the system of filth.

For instance, influenza, the flu, is a fever. It is the boiling-point of the toxins which the body has been carrying in the blood tissues for many a long day. It is Nature's grand and supreme effort to rid the system of uncleanness, to cleanse one from within, outward.

Why doesn't it affect one so much in summer?

Because in the summer people get out into the parks, they hike, go in for healthy exercise, eat more fruit, perspire freely, and thus get rid of many emcumbrances.

Of course, one may check some of the good work Nature is doing. Many frequently chill themselves with ice water, ice cream gulped down rapidly, ice cream sodas and what not. Nevertheless, on the whole, many get by with such practices; they keep the sluice gates, the eliminatory organs, fairly well open. But as the weather becomes colder they ride where they used to walk. They coddle themselves. Put storm windows and doors on their homes instead of letting more of the breath of heaven circulate through the rooms.

They wear heavy underwear and outer clothing, to conserve the heat of the body, instead of generating heat by exercise. They stew in their own juice. The carbonic acid wastes are piling up inside instead of being expelled vigorously and regularly.

The winter is the time of banquets, dinners, sociables. The 57 varieties on the menu at big banquets are enough to floor a Samson. Those who run the whole gamut, who taste every dish, have sometimes a seething putrefying mass in their intestines. During the night it may be fermenting in the body, and then comes the attack of 'flu; the heat of the body creeps up to 100 or higher.

It was bad enough to be so gluttonous, but even then one might have obtained some relief before going to bed, by a simple expedient; have tickled the throat and produced a vomit just after leaving the dinner room, as the ancient Romans did when they visited the vomitorium, and thus avoided the splitting headache which might come the morning after.

Of course, everybody cannot afford to attend big banquets. We have the poor always with us, and among them many are stricken with 'flu. But every church has its socials, and there are many family parties. They have their suppers and entertainments even if it is nothing more than a hot dog sandwich, cakes made from white flour, coffee, candy for the girls, ice cream and what not. Then the bridge parties are often followed by eats.

Mrs. Robinson tries to outvie by a sumptuous repast, and many extra dishes, the party which Mrs. Jones gave the week before. Many, in the cold weather, fancy they need lots of hot, nourishing food, stuff more heavily to keep out the cold. Many eat freely of denatured starches, drink lots of coffee sweetened with refined sugar. Then their food ferments and whisky is manufactured in their stomachs. Their bodies become enervated by such practices.

Along comes a strong, cold North wind, which pierces the body like a dart. They are vulnerable, their vitality has been lowered, then down they come with a severe cold; the toxic body has little resistance, and presently fever develops; they are told they have the 'flu.

Nature is anxious to cleanse them, for the toxins have almost reached the saturation point in their bodies. Appetite departs, they no longer have any desire for food. The fever is busy, and should not be suppressed.

We talk of typhus fever, typhoid fever, acute fevers, scarlet fever, hay fever and febrile conditions in general.

Hippocrates declared that if his patient came into a feverish condition, it was easy to effect a cure. The danger is not in a fever, but in a suppression of that fever by drugs or other means. Fever is a cleanser; it is a supreme effort of Nature to rid the system of accumulated impurities.

The temperature rises, heat is generated, there is a hot condition of the skin, whilst the body seems to be making keen efforts to produce a violent perspiration, whereby to throw out of the system toxins that have endangered one's life.

Unfortunately, many practitioners, dealing only with symptoms, are mainly concerned about decreasing the temperature by some depressent drugs, failing to see what Nature's efforts are leading to; thus they simply thwart Nature's processes, and whilst the temperature is lowered, the heart is depressed, and the poisonous wastes are driven deeper into the tissues, instead of being eliminated.

If we can assist Nature in her work, well and good. Otherwise most people would fare better under such conditions if left entirely without interference. All appetite for food would probably vanish. There would be a great craving for water, which they would satisfy if possible, and Nature, taking its course, would bring about good elimination of the accumulated waste material.

In some fevers there may be acute stomach and bowel disturbance, in others much lung distress, in others skin eruptions; again the nasal passages, sinus and bronchial tubes may be in trouble. But in each and every case Nature is making great efforts to clear the body of poisons which threaten life.

How can we assist Nature? How can we further her efforts at house cleaning?

A dog when sick or feverish will crawl away under some bush or anywhere that it can be left alone and rest. It will not eat at such times. It will take nothing but water, until it feels a natural urge for activity. Then it becomes an absolute vegetarian for a while. It eats grass, which seems to act as an emetic, and it vomits foul material.

Wounded soldiers, overlooked on the battlefield, not picked up by the medical corps, frequently fare better and recover more quickly where Nature's healing forces carry on their work unhampered, than in many cases where others have had the latest so-called scientific care in hospital.

How can we assist Nature to bring the acute distressing stage to a climax and thus get the temperature down to normal, after the copious discharge of poisons through the skin and bowels, by profuse perspiration and bowel action?

First, absolutely stop the intake through the mouth of anything but water.

Put the patient to bed, see that the body is kept warm and there is plenty of fresh air without a draught. Arrange for absolute quiet and no outside disturbance. Well-meaning friends, by meddlesome tactics, frequently do much harm to the nervous system of the patient.

Wash out the bowels by an enema. Use two quarts of tepid water to which the juice of a lemon has been added. Then give a warm bath. If the patient is strong enough, a vapour bath would be better if a vapour bath cabinet is available. Then put patient to bed and cover up warm.

Give all the water to drink that thirst calls for. Hot lemonade sweetened with honey may be taken as soon as patient is put to bed. If the fever persists after the enema and bath and patient has gone to bed, put a cool wet pack over abdomen. Apply a fresh one every five minutes, or as soon as they become warm from the heat of the body. At the same time put the feet in warm water when convenient, or put a hot water bottle to the feet. Repeat this treatment each following day until all feverish symptoms have subsided.

Take the temperature occasionally to note conditions. Normal mouth temperature is 98.6. Rectal temperature is 99.5.

It is imperative that no food—save weak hot lemonade referred to—should be taken during the acute symptoms, or until the temperature has finally settled down to normal; even for 24 hours after that.

Do not be tempted to give any food under the impression that it is necessary to keep up the patient's strength. It is positively dangerous to feed during a fevered condition, and in many cases might have a fatal result. The body has all it can do in tackling the cleaning processes, in the elimination of accumulated poisons, without being called upon to digest food, or attempt to digest food, which, under the circumstances, it has no use for.

"THE GARDEN OF THE LORD"

Our chief aim in this "Garden" is the "Prevention" of illness, believing that Prevention is better, and also easier, than Cure. So our endeavour shall be to erect a Battlement at the top of the cliff, and not to arrange an expensive "Red Cross Ambulance" at the bottom!

We trust that it will be no offense to broadcast the published sentiments of two of our eminent medical men. Sir W. Arbuthnot Lane, referring to the astounding cost of ill-health, says: "Avoidable ill-health costs the country the astounding sum of £1,000,000,000 a year! Nearly 90 per cent of the health troubles and diseases of civilisation could be avoided. I have no hesitation in stating that the financial burdens of avoidable ill-health, and disease, is very much heavier than that imposed by our War Debt. Our heaviest tax of all is our tax on health!

I have come to the conclusion that of the health troubles and diseases of civilisation, approximately 90 per cent are quite unnecessary, and are comparatively easily avoidable."

Sir William blames injudicious feeding, and faulty methods of living, for the ill-health of the civilised world. His cry is—**Back to Nature.** He asserts that we throw away the most valuable part of our food, and over-boil our vegetables.

The other great man we wish to quote, from the "Daily Express," is Dr. Harold Dearden:—"My greatest hindrance in what I considered a full and adequate life was the inheritance of an income which rendered me independent; but the Great War having lifted that burden from my shoulders, I have never known a dull day since. It is undeniably a fact that life is difficult, but if you have to get up at 6 o clock in the morning you are very apt not to notice it. To be continually constructive mentally and physically, and to leave to-morrow till to-morrow, is to do all that is possible to assure health and happiness. It is a programme which, if universally adopted, would, in my sober judgment, plunge into the deepest gloom half Harley Street and its neighbourhood! The greatest success is to understand and love mankind; and only by sharing their troubles can love come into its own! I believe that to be the purpose of life, and not money, nor power, nor honours. In that belief is the whole of my religion; and that life is an adventure is the whole of my philosophy!"

Let us further quote Sir William Arbuthnot Lane:—"We boast of this age as being the 'Health Age'! Yet there was never a time when disease, in the true meaning of the word, was more prevalent than it is now. Of ten people one meets, nine complain of more or less impaired health. At no time in the world's history was the taking of medicaments as much in evidence as it is to-day. To millions of people medicaments have become as necessary as their daily bread! Among primitive races, leading primitive lives, Indigestion is almost unknown, and so are Appendicitis, Colitis, Gastric and Duodenal Ulcers, Gall-Stone, etc. Cancer, the various diseases of the Digestive tract, Arteriosclerosis, Heart Disease, Insanity, and others increasing in a very alarming manner!

"The most nerve-worn among the people are not the rushing City men, who gamble with fortunes every day, but are seamstresses and other people who lead a quiet life, and who subsist on white bread, margarine, jam, and strong tea, with plenty of white sugar."

Sir William suggests:—"Scrap the Hospitals; and let our efforts be to make the present generation well. And confine the efforts to the education of the children in the right way of living."

And yet that is easier said than done.

Even enlightened people will insist upon gratifying their lust, and feed the beast!

Are not medical men well aware that strong drink destroys health and life? And yet, how many of them fall a prey to their craving for it? The masses will not come to the light. They hate the light! And love darkness!

"A man convinced against
his will
Is of the same opinion stiil."

The most common ailments of the human body are those of the Liver, Kidneys, Bladder, Ovaries, and the Womb. Liver and Kidneys are near relatives, and are therefore in deep sympathy with each other. As long as these organs are in a good form, as a rule, it is well with the whole system. But when they fail, all the other organs become erratic. Liver trouble is caused by errors in eating and drinking. Eating too much of even the proper food would give too much poison in the body for the Liver to dispose of. And worse still are improper food and drink. Wrong living is the cause of all our ailments. As long as we persist in our wrong habits, in vain we treat the symptoms!

A doctor in a Mental Institute had a very ingenious way of testing whether an inmate was sane enough to leave or not. He would turn the water tap on in a certain room which he had for that purpose, and handed a broom to the person that maintained he was fit to leave, and told him to sweep the water out of that room and then he would be allowed to go. One would sweep and sweep, and the room is still as full as ever. That one was retained as unfit. He would give the broom, with the same promise, to another. This one takes the broom, and ere he begins to sweep he looks around; he sees the open tap, he turns it off, and in a short time the room is dry! And he's allowed to go! The human system cannot be cleared of the poison until the tap of wrong habits is turned off!

We want to state here the Principle on which the Herbal Remedies are administered. There are two theories of Life Process, namely:—

1. The **Materialistic**—that Life results from the activities of Matter.

2. The **Vitalistic** — that the Living Organism (the body) is essentially a Vital realm of an immaterial directive entity, which is

called **Vital Force.** It is the Vital Force which appropriates to itself anything of utility in the Life process, or rejects it as unsuitable and injurious.

Herbalism is the only School of Medicine that is based on the Vital theory of Life. Its aim is:—

1. To relax contracted tissues.
2. To contract relaxed ones.
3. Stimulate the sluggish.
4. Tone up the debilitated; and
5. Soothe the irritated conditions.

So Herbalism goes for all its Medicaments, not to the "Mines of Man," but to the

GARDEN OF THE LORD

In a Garden man was placed by God,
To live on produce of the sod;
And there God meant for him to stop,
Not in a Club, nor Butcher Shop;
God made a Temple for man and spouse,
But Satan built them Public House!

The Allopaths, with flaming sword,
Now guard the "Garden of the Lord,"
So that the sick shall not have free,
Straight entrance to the healing Tree;
And to the Flowers of the land,
Which God has planted with His hand!
In such variety and wealth,
To keep mankind in perfect health!
That they might gamble with health and life
Of fellow men, by drug and knife!
Yes, we are treated now, by knaves,
In our free country, just like slaves!
We want the men in bondage, know—
Who would be free must strike the blow!
The problem—friends of freedom, face,
Once more the Altars set ablaze!

The Garden of Nuts and The Green Plants of the Valley

("The Song of Songs," vi. 11)

1. Fifty per cent of our young people commence the struggle for life with Heart Disease, and accounted for chiefly by sweets and cigarettes.

2. Prunes and Currant juice will cure Constipation.

3. Drugging increases Constipation, interferes with digestion, sets up irritation, and may lead to fatal consequences.

4. No fruit is **acid** except **unripe** fruit. (Comyns Berkely.)

5. Don't skin the nuts.

6. Wash fruit and nuts, always in cold water.

7. Grapes, Muscatels, Sultanas, and Raisins; Apples, Lemons, Oranges, and Nuts can be relied upon to bring about improvement in health.

8. For Ulceration and Dilatation of the Stomach: Dry feeding, and a course of fruit-liquor. Grapes, grated Apples, Orange and Lemon juice, Sultanas, Muscatels, Raisins, Dates, mashed Bananas, grated Almonds, should form the sole diet till the stomach is healed. Fruit is the cure. (Reddie Mallett.)

9. Piles are cured by injections of undiluted Lemon juice. Use a small syringe to hold a tablespoonful.

10. For Blood Pressure, etc., Dry feeding, and the fruit-liquor.

11. For Earache, put a few drops of undiluted Lemon juice, warmed, in the ear.

12. The best way to cook an egg: Put it in a pint of boiling water, take off the fire, let it stand 6

or 7 minutes; then it will be congealed—**but not killed.**

13. It is wrong to eat and drink at meals. Only man and duck do it. It is right for the duck, but wrong for man.

14. Ringworm: Paint it with equal parts of Fluid Ext. Blood Root and Eucalyptus, or try strong Acetic Acid.

15. "The wise for cure on exercise depend."

16. The Botanic and Eclectic Practice of Medicine embraces everything rational and useful.

17. Vaccination is a cruel humbug! There is no test in existence to distinguish a harmful from a harmless Lymph. During the last 21 years, 207 children under 5 years of age died from Vaccination, against 60 from Small-pox! (Miss Loat, of the Anti-Vaccination League, London.)

18. Each mouthful of food should be masticated 32 times—once for each tooth.

19. Sleep: The physiology of sleep is not fully understood, but it seems evident that it is brought about by cutting off the blood supply from the brain. It is during sleep, and then only, that the nutritive material gathered into the blood is delivered to the expectant tissues. (Dr. Leonard Williams.)

20. Water is to the human system what oil is to a machine; an insufficiency gradually but surely ruins the bearings. A glass on waking, another before luncheon, another before dinner, and one at bedtime is a fair allowance. (Dr. L. Williams.)

21. The warm and stagnant air, not the cold and circulating, holds the germs of deadly disease. (Dr. L. Williams.)

22. The two curses of modern dietaries are cookery and concentration. Cookery destroys the Vitamins in the food. The crime of concentration is well exemplified by a consideration of sugar. It requires 20 sticks of sugar-cane to make one pound of loaf-sugar. This means that an ordinary lump of sugar is equal to about 2 feet of sugar-cane. Children in these islands eat the equivalent of 4 yards of sugar-cane in a few minutes, and the amount of sugar dissolved in an ordinary cup of tea or coffee represents about 6 feet of the article supplied by Nature. An indication that Nature never intended us to use sugar in this form is afforded by the fact that the variety of sugar called Fructose, which provides the sweet element in all fruits except Grapes, is so combined with the other substances that it cannot be extracted, crystallised and refined. (Dr. L. Williams.)

23. Alcoholic drinks, when the worst has been said against them, the harm which they impose upon the health of the community is as nothing compared to the disaster attendant upon meat eating and sugar sucking. These devastating poisons begin their sinister strength-sapping work in the earliest sapling stage. (From Dr. Leonard Williams' noted book.)

24. Syrup of Lobelia, to make: One pound best Molasses, 2 ounces Tincture of Lobelia, 2 ounces Aniseed Water. Shake all up together. Dose: A teaspoonful. Good for all chest troubles.

25. Rheumatic Liniment: Spirit of Turpentine, Spirits of Camphor, Spirits of Hartshorn, 1 ounce of

each, in 4 ounces of Olive Oil. Shake all well up together.

26. A London M. D., denouncing patent medicine, asks: "Would any mother give Teething Powder, so advertised, to her children, if she really knew they were composed chiefly of Mercury and Opium—two deadly poisons, which should be prescribed only with care and caution by a physician?" And we ask: "Why should any physician prescribe such deadly poison to anyone?"

27. The only food that's good is food that's perishable.

28. Marshmallow.—Pliny says: "Whosoever shall take a spoonful of its juice shall that day be free from all diseases."

29. No agent has the faculty of elaborating red blood so rapidly as Cinchona (Peruvian Bark), good diet and fresh air. ℞ Comp. Tinct. Cinchona, 1 ounce; Simple Syr., 3 ounces; Water, add 2 ounces. Mix. A teaspoonful every 3 hours.

30. Marshallow leaves: A decoction has a splendid action in all obstinate cases of Constipation, whenever the stools are lumpy and hard. Combined with Agrimony, it has a splendid action on the whole of the intestinal tract. Where there is a tendency to Appendicitis, use them, and they will save many an operation if taken in time.

31. Cubebs: In Bronchitis use the Fluid Extract, 5 to 10 drops on sugar. Use it in Prostatic troubles. It gives good results in Catarrh of the Bladder, and Spermatorrhœa. Employ it when there is a constant desire to pass urine, attended with pain.

32. Blue Flag has a special action on Prostate Glands and Testes.

33. Golden Seal Root, Calendula, Collinsonia, Pulsatilla, and Cactus are all good heart tonics.

34. Yellow Dock Root and Burdock Root to purify the blood.

35. Dr. Richard Ackerley, in an address to a section of the Royal Society of Medicine, quoted the following:—

"Tickle the public and make them grin,
The more you tickle, the more you win,
Teach the public, you never grow rich,
You'll live like beggar and die in the ditch."

Is it the chief aim of the Doctor to get rich?

36. Elder Flowers, Peppermint, and Boneset will cure the 'Flu. And no danger of an overdose or harmful action on the heat.

37. "Death from Disease. There is no need for people to die from diseases. It is possible to bring about in a community such a high state of health that disease can be kept away." (Quotation of Sir W. A. Lane.) Cayenne, Lobelia, and Bayberry keep the system clean and active. Cayenne stimulates the whole body. Lobelia relaxes the whole body. Bayberry astringes the whole body.

38. The most natural foods are uncooked salads, fruits, nuts, lean mutton, fish and wholemeal bread.

39. Ergot. What is used by the Physio-Medicals instead of the Ergot drug is Golden Seal and Shepherd's Purse; these do all that is claimed for the drug Ergot, but without any of the injurious effects.

40. Cause of Disease.—Disease arises from Obstruction. Until the obstruction is removed and the injury is repaired, there is always a disturbance of the equilibrium of

the blood circulation and of the Nerve Force. Black Horehound is very good for it.

FLESH FOODS

They increase the normal wear and tear of the body-cells considerably. They place an extra strain upon the kidneys, which are called upon to eliminate the uric acid, and waste effete poisons in the flesh of slaughtered animals. Flesh foods tend to putrefy in the large bowel, hence the liability of meat eaters to appendicitis, colitis, dysentery, and chronic constipation. Flesh foods are also largely responsible for such serious diseases as apoplexy, arterial degeneration, high blood pressure, epilepsy, rheumatism, arthritis, and congestion of the liver.

And the terrible increase in the dread disease—cancer—is due in no small measure to the great increase in the consumption of animal foods throughout the civilised world.

PROTEIN FOODS

Is that which builds muscle, repairs tissue-work, helps digestion, and is probably the least dispensable element in our food. "Without protein we die." A deficiency of this in our diet leads to weakness, loss of energy, and loss of weight.

And excess of protein causes kidney trouble, plethora, leading to arterial degeneration, apoplexy, etc., over acid condition of the blood.

Protein is found mainly in eggs, cheese, nuts, milk, and the pulse foods; peas, beans, and lentils. In much less pure form it is found plentifully in flesh foods.

CARBOHYDRATES — Starch and Sugar

They are muscle foods, and are also thought to be capable of producing heat and energy.

The cereals and root vegetables have a large proportion of Carbohydrates, also the pulse-foods. Lack of force, thinness and physical exhaustion is caused by a deficiency of that class of food. Yet, too much of it, which is the more common mistake, causes skin troubles, clogged glands, indigestion, flatulence, dilatation of the stomach, rheumatism and gout. They are especially mischievious when taken in a mushy form, like porridge, bread soaked in milk, or when combined with stewed sugary acid fruit, such as bread with stewed apples, and in white flour, corn-flour, polished rice, etc.

HYDROCARBONS—Fats

These foods are used in the nutrition of nerve tissue, for the oil-glands of the skin, partly as lubricants of the digestive organs, and for making the red marrow in the centre of the larger bones, are similar to the starchy and sugars as "fuel foods."

One part of **fat** is equivalent to three or four parts of **starch,** the making of red marrow. Nuts, not butter, and nut oil, cream, and fresh dairy butter, are the purest and best sources of fat. A deficiency of **fat** in diet results in nerve weakness, neuralgia, and mental exhaustion. An excess produces billiousness and sluggishness.

SALTS

Salts are the various kinds of organic elements and food minerals, such as iron, lime, potash, soda, etc. They are of great importance in keeping the blood from becoming over-acid, or sticky. Organic iron is needed by the **red cells** of the blood as oxygen carrier to the tissues.

Potassium is essential to the building up of all forms of living tissues; it is an indispensable solid tissue-base.

Soda neutralises harmful acids in the blood and tissues.

Lime is essential for bone building and replenishment; and for maintaining the proper consistency and power of coagulation of the blood. A deficiency of this element is the cause of that peculiar condition known as a "Bleeder"; that is, a person who bleeds profusely from the slightest cut. Deficiency of lime accounts for that terrible affliction, Rheumatoid Arthritis.

Magnesium is needed for bone and cartilage formation.

Sulphur is used in the construction of hair and nails and skin.

All these organic "Salts" are particularly abundant in greenstuffs, salad, and conservatively cooked vegetables. In a lesser degree in fresh raw, ripe fruit, and in the outer layers of grains such as Barley, Wholemeal Flour, unpolished Rice, and peel of Fruits. There is no need of table salt, and the harmful chemical mixtures of these salts in the form of crude doses of medicine.

The problem of balanced meals, then, is to combine foods in such a way that the daily meals shall furnish, in right proportions, the above-named constituents of proteins, carbohydrates, fats, organic salts, and vitamins, with the addition of water. The orthodox meal will usually approach more nearly to a well-balanced meal if the starchy and sugary items such as white flour, soft mush, sweet puddings, porridge, etc., are ruled out, and replaced with plenty of greenstuff, pure oil and lemon juice, and twice-baked bread.

Does Meatless Diet Suffice for the Need of One Following a Laborious Occupation?

All the hardest worked beasts of burden—the horse, the ox, the camel, and the elephant—are vegetarian feeders.

And in the matter of endurance and stamina the vegetarian feeding animals far outmatch the carnivora.

As regards human strength and endurance on a meatless diet, the record of vegetarian athletes puts the issue beyond any doubt.

Bad Combinations in the Same Meal

Stewed fruit and vegetables; milk and meat; milk and sugar in combination with a soft mushy cereal like porridge or cooked rice, etc.; or starchy food like bread (which demands an alkaline digestion) eaten with acid fruit cooked with a lot of sugar (which gives an acid result in the stomach). Such mixtures can scarcely fail to produce either flatulence or fermentation, or intestinal putrefaction in the food tract.

Vegetables containing Lime — The Onion (says Broadbent) has 22 per cent.; Cabbage, Lettuce and Radishes, 14; Celery, 13; Turnips and Carrots, 11; and Eggs, 10.

Root Vegetables should be avoided for those who suffer from Rheumatism, Gout, or Stone; green used instead.

FOR THE CHILDREN

By "AUNT BEC."

Dear Boys and Girls,—How are you? All well, happy and jolly, I hope. I would so much like to see all of you together. It would be great fun, and especially if we had a huge party.

Now, I guess you are looking forward to Christmas. I am! although I am now too old to hang up my stocking for Santa Claus.

Christmas is a lovely time. I love it; don't you? Just think of oranges, nuts, crackers, toys (lots of them), sweets, cake, pudding, Oh-h! and then all the decorations of paper streamers, Holly and Mistletoe.

I am Aunty to lots of boys and girls up here in Durham, and we all endeavour to keep up old customs. When Christmas comes along and I go visiting, sure as sure someone catches me under the Mistletoe, and then I have to hunt up my purse and pay my footing. It is great fun. I love to pay up to these jolly children.

Let me tell you something about Mistletoe. I am sure you will know it well. Uncle Jack is adding a picture, so you see what it is really like.

Viscum Album is the Latin name for Mistletoe. It is a parasite; this means, it lives on others. Having no root, it grows not in the soil but on other trees, such as the apple-tree, and rarely on the oak.

Long, long ago, the Druids thought the Mistletoe possessed magical powers. At a certain time of the year, the priest, dressed in a long robe of white, and followed by a procession of people, cut the Mistletoe with a golden knife. The Mistletoe was then shared out among the people, who then kept it as a charm against disease.

Then you remember the myth of how Baldur the White Sun God was slain with a twig of Mistletoe. So you see the Mistletoe was well known in the days of long ago.

Like the Druids of old, we Herbalists think the Mistletoe a wonderful plant. Not for its power of magic, but for its medicinal value, for it is a valuable nervine.

No doubt you know someone suffering from fits. Just let them know Mistletoe can help them. Of course, it must be specially prepared first and made into medicine.

Sometimes Daddy is worried about his work and feels tired out, and cannot remember things; just whisper that Mistletoe would help him such a lot.

And Mam, what about her; does she suffer with headache, or maybe she cries because everything seems to go wrong, and feels awful because others don't seem to understand? Just put your arms around her and say: "Mam, I love you; will you try Aunty Bec's remedy of Mistletoe and get well?"

Oh! the good you boys and girls can do. Learn your Botany well; then learn what all the various plants are used for, and, as you grow up, try to help all who suffer from disease. Be kind and gentle, be an example to all, and then when you eventually grow up you will do wondrous things and be a credit to your teachers.

MEANING OF MEDICAL TERMS

Acrid.—Biting, caustic, for dissolving warts, corns, and other hard substances: Celandine and Wake Robin.

Alteratives, which gradually alter and correct a bad condition of the blood: Burdock, Yellow Dock, Sarsaparilla, Poke Root, Celery, Chickweed.

Anodynes, which alleviate pain: Figwort, Gelsemium, Bittersweet.

Antacid.—Alkaline agents, which correct acidity of the secretions in a chemical manner, such as the Burnets, Kidney Wort, Wood Betony, Agrimony, Wood Avens.

Antalkaline.—Those which neutralise excess of alkaline matter in the alimentary canal and urinary passages. This is most frequently due to relaxed and sluggish conditions of the tissues.

Anaphrodisiacs, which diminish excessive or unnatural sexual desire: Damiana, Groundsel.

Anthelmintics, which destroy and expel worms: Santonica, Tansy, Rue, Senna, Male Fern.

Deodorants, which correct unhealthy smell: Eucalyptus, Peppermint, Wintergreen.

Disinfectants, which act chemically upon the special poisons of communicable diseases, preventing their spread: Camphor, Eucalyptus, Terebene, Thyme.

Antibilious, which increase the flow of bile: Tansy, Pomegranate Bark, Hyssop, White Poplar Bark, Balmony, Barberry Bark, Bitter Root, Centaury, Golden Seal, Mandrake, Fringetree Bark, Dandelion, and Cayenne Pepper.

Anti-scorbutic.—For scurvy and blood disorder: Bogbean, Burdock Root, Chickweed, Clivers, Cubebs, Yellow Dock, Sarsaparilla, Blue Flag Root.

Aperient.—Bitter Root, Black Root, Centaury, Clivers, Curcuma, Dandelion Root, Cascara Sagrada, Mountain Flax.

Aromatic. — Agreeable, spicy, such as Aniseed, Cinnamon, Cloves, Cubebs, Orange Peel, Nutmeg, Pimento, Pennyroyal, and the Mints.

Cephalic.—Snuff for pains in the head: Bayberry Bark, Wood Betony, Blood Root.

Antispasmodic, which prevent the recurrence of spasms and excessive contractions when the nerves fail to respond to the vital force, such as Cayenne, Lobelia, Cramp Bark, Skunk Cabbage.

Anthrodisiac, which excite sexual desire.

Astringents, which induce greater density and firmness of the tissues, such as Agrimony, Angelica, Great Burnet, Bistort Root, Blackberry Root, Bayberry Bark, Cranesbill, Lady's Mantle, Raspberry Leaves, Shepherd's Purse, Yarrow, Tormentil Root, Wild Mint, White Pond Lily, Oak Bark, Burr Marigold, Purple Loosestrife.

Carminatives, which remove wind from the stomach and intestines. The Aromatics and Carminatives are the Mints, Cloves, Ginger, Angelica, Calamus.

Cathartics. — To evacuate the bowels: Mandrake, Aloes, Mountain Flax, Senna Leaves; combine them with a small proportion of the Carminatives.

Chologogues, which cause the excretion of the bile into the intestines: Bayberry Bark, Cascara Sagrada, Juglans—Walnut.

Demulcents, which soften and allay irritation of mucous membranes. Applied outwardly as poultices. Inwardly, they lubricate the mucous surfaces, and soothe inflamed conditions of the stomach, bowels, uterus, vagina, etc. They pass through the kidneys; so they are always of much service in acute irritation of the kidneys and urinary passages. They are: Chickweed, Comfrey Root, Irish Moss, Gum Arabic, Coltsfoot, Liquorice Root, Marshmallow (root and leaves), Common Mallow Root and Leaves, Slippery Elm, Gum Tragacanth.

Discutient.—Dissolving tumours, etc.: Camomile Flowers, Chickweed, Comfrey, Elderflowers, Marshmallow, Common Mallow, Ragwort, Sanicle, Wormwood.

Diaphoretic. — To increase perspiration that is not great or visible. Those which induce a very abundant perspiration are called Sudorifics.

Where the use of a relaxing Diaphoretic is followed by a cold perspiration, its continued use would be very inadvisable.

Given in warm infusion.

Warm gruels also help very much.

The Sudorifics are: Angelica, Cayenne, Ginger, Red Sage, Virginia Snakeroot, Crawly Root, Boneset.

The Diaphoretics are: Balm, Germander, Guaiacum, Lobelia, Wood Sage, Yarrow, Hyssop, Aniseed, Dill Seed, Cinnamon, the Mints, Ginger, Cayenne, Cloves, Fennel Seed, Pennyroyal.

Diuretics, which promote the secretion of urine: Parsley Piert, Pellitory, Uva Ursi, Buchu, Juniper Berries, Clivers, Shepherd's Purse, Meadowsweet. There is danger of overdoing them!

Emetics, which promote the expulsion of the contents of the stomach by vomiting. Emetics may be given to babes a few hours old, and to people 90 or more years old, but should not be given to any age when there is organic disease of the heart: Lobelia, Boneset, Ragwort, Groundsel.

Emmenagogues, which promote the menstrual flow, such as Blue Cohosh, Camomile, Feverfew, Black Horehound, Stinking Arrack, Black Cohosh, German Camomile, Motherwort, Pennyroyal, Tansy, Southernwood, Water Mint, Red Sage.

Emollients — Softening, causing warmth: Chickweed, Marshmallow, Slippery Elm.

Expectorant, which cause the increased secretion of bronchial mucous and tone the relaxed part: Angelica, Chickweed, Coltsfoot, Horehound, Lungwort, Lobelia, Mouse-ear.

Hepatic.—For the liver.

Nervines.—For the nerves: Mistletoe, Sea Holly, Scullcap, Valerian, Passion Flower, Wood Betony.

Stimulants.—To help the circulation of blood and functional action: Blood Root, Cayenne, Cinnamon, Cloves, Ginger, Peppermint, Sage, Wood Betony.

Stomachics, which improve appetite and digestion: Agrimony, Gentian, Columba Root, Centaury, Meadowsweet.

Tonics, which impart fuller vigour to the system. It should not be overdone: Barberry, Bitter Root, Centaury, Bogbean, Agrimony, Peruvian Bark, Gentian, White Poplar, Great Waterdock.

Vulnararies, which are healing to wounds: Chickweed, Comfrey, Purple Loosestrife, Slippery Elm, Clown's Woundwort, Plantain Leaves, Marshmallow, Burr Marigold, Ragwort.

Sea Holly

Eryngium Maritium. Class 5. Order 2

JOHN BIRCH, M.N.A.M.H.

This plant is also called "Sea Eringo."

The therapeutic principles of Sea Holly are a resin and two alkaloids.

Medical Properties.—Stimulant, aromatic, expectorant, diaphoretic, diuretic, nervine, hepatic, mild astringent, antacid.

It rises one to two feet in height; the leaves are roundish, plaited,

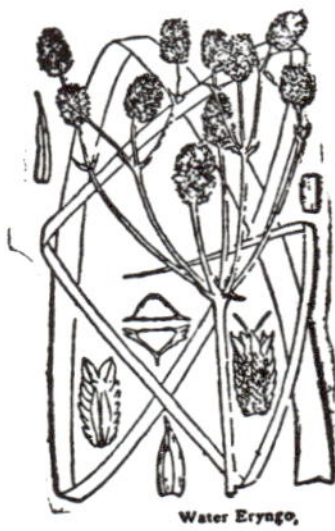

SEA HOLLY

firm; spiney like those of holly, marked with white reticulated veins, of a pale bluish green colour; the flowers are of a blue colour and terminate the branches in round heads. The calyx consists of five erect sharp pointed leaves; the corolla is composed of five petals which turn inward; the germen is beset with short hairs.

It grows abundantly on the sea coast, from July till October.

The root is mild and mucilaginous, and aromatic in a small degree. It is a mild balsamic pectoral, and enters as an ingredient into what is commonly called mild artificial asses' milk, and is made thus:—

Mock Asses' Milk.—Take an ounce of Hartshorn shavings, put into a quart of boiling barley water, boil down to one pint, add two ounces of candied Eryngo Root and a pint of new milk; boil for a quarter of an hour and strain it for use.

Another method.—Boil in three pints of water till half evaporated one ounce each of Eryngo Root, Pearl Barley, Sago and Rice. Strain it off. Put a tablespoonful of the mixture into a coffee cup of boiling milk so as to render it of the consistency of cream, and sweeten with loaf sugar to taste. This is a good food for consumptives, and is valuable for weak people.

Sea Holly is good and valuable in obstruction of the Liver and Spleen; also dropsy, pain in loins, gravel, and bladder trouble.

It is good for coughs and in the debility accompanying advanced stage of rheumatism. To use singly the decoction is made by boiling one ounce of the herb or root in one pint of water for 15 minutes; when cold, strain and bottle for use. Dose: One wineglassful an hour before each meal. A Compound of Sea Holly is as follows: Take one ounce each of Sea Holly, Wild Carrot, Barberry Bark, Meadow Sweet, Yarrow, Bruised Ginger Root. Add 6 quarts of water and boil down to 3 quarts; strain and sweeten with honey, and when cold, bottle.

Dose: One wineglassful an hour before each meal.

THE SOYA BEAN

During the course of many years the Soya Bean, botanically known as Glycine Max, has sprung from the straggling, uncultivated species to an upright, sturdy Leguminous annual. Originally a native of Manchuria, where it has been known for many hundred years, it is now cultivated in many parts of the world; but as yet for commercial success has to be proved in this country.

Its value is far in excess to any other legume or cereal, and new uses are being discovered all the time.

Two of the best types for growing in this country are Glycine Max, and Glycine Max var ochroleuca, although in some countries as many as 60 varieties are cultivated. It has been proved that it grows best in Southern England, as the Soya Bean flourishes best in warm conditions, with good, well drained soil.

Among the many by-products of the Soya Bean, the oil is most important.

Soya oil is widely used in industry, especially in the United States. About 380 pounds of oil is yielded by a ton of beans, having an average oil content of 17 per cent.

Soap-making and margarine industries are the largest consumers of Soya oil.

For thousands of years this bean has been an article of food in the life of the Orient. It supplies substitutes for milk, butter, cheese, coffee, and flour; also forms the basis of most sauces.

In the United States, Soya milk has now been employed in infant feeding tests for several years, with excellent results.

For vegetarians, the Soya Bean is an important article of food, containing essential elements of human nutrition as iron, magnesium, calcium, and mineral salts.

The oil is also used commercially in the making of paints, enamels, varnishes, printing ink, celluloid, rubber substitutes, and glycerine for high explosives.

The cake left after the oil is extracted from the bean has a high feeding value for cattle.

The Soya Bean is unquestionably the crop of the future, being only in its infancy. JOHN PASKE.

Nerve Troubles

Scullcap	½ ounce
Motherwort	½ "
Wood Betony	½ "
Black Horehound	½ "
Hops	¼ "
Mistletoe	¼ "
Valerian Root	¼ "
Ginger Root	¼ "
Senna Leaves	as required
Spanish Licorice	½ ounce

Snuff for Watery Catarrh

℞ Witch Hazel, in fine powder—1 ounce
White Oak Bark powder . . ½ "
Wild Cherry Bark powder . . ½ "

Mix thoroughly and sift.

INFUSIONS

By HUBERT B. FIGG,
F.F.Sc., M.I.C.A., M.P.S.

Few forms of preparation are more convenient from the vegetable world than that of Infusions. The greater number of vegetable drugs are easily exhausted of their active ingredients in this way, the process is exceedingly simple and speedy, more especially as it is seldom necessary that the solid materials be in a state of fine division, and the form in which the active constituents are presented is one of the best for administration.

Degree of Comminution

The degree of comminution depends upon the nature of the drug and the constituents to be extracted; it is usual to coarsely comminute, slice or bruise. Very fine powders must be avoided, because it is difficult to separate the fine particles from the infusion, and if percolation is resorted to, so much time is consumed in the operation, owing to the swelling of the powder, that decomposition may set in before the preparation is finished.

Hot or Cold Water

Infusions are dilute solutions containing the water soluble extractive of vegetable drugs. In very early days, boiling water (note, the drug is not subjected to the boiling process) was entirely used, but as advance and research has come along, the choice between hot and cold water now depends on the nature of the drug and the constituents to be extracted. While the use of hot water has the advantage of saving time, it has the frequent disadvantage of dissolving along with the active ingredients, starch and other inert principles whose presence renders the infusion more apt to become acid or mouldy, and also, as the infusion cools, a precipitate occurs in such a finely divided condition that there is great difficulty in removing same by filtration.

Cold water should be selected as the menstrum when the drug contains a volatile (valuable) principle, when the active principle is easily soluble in water at ordinary temperature, when the active principle is inured by heat or where the drug contains an appreciable quantity of starch.

How Are They Prepared?

Infusions are usually made by one of the following methods:—(1) By Maceration. (2) By Digestion. (3) By Percolation.

(1) **Maceration.**—This is the process most frequently used, and when the strength is not otherwise directed, they may be prepared by infusing for fifteen minutes one ounce of the drug in one pint of distilled water and straining.

Infusions should always be prepared in earthenware vessels; tinned or metallic vessels are unsuitable for infusions; they are particularly objectionable when the drug used for making the preparation contains tannin, gallic acid, or an astringent substance.

The drug should be introduced

into a suitable vessel provided with a cover, and the boiling water poured in and the vessel covered tightly; allow to stand for the requisite time, then strain, slight pressure should be given to the marc.

It is preferable that the drug should be suspended by some suitable contrivance, or enclosed in a muslin bag, so as to be immediately below the surface of the water; if, however, the drug is allowed to sink to the bottom of the vessel, the mixture should be stirred occasionally.

(2) **Digestion.**—The process of digestion consists in subjecting the substance to the continued action of moderate heat, below the boiling point. In making infusions, digestion is often very useful, although it may not be directed in the formula. It generally suffices to place the infusion vessel upon a moderately hot portion of a stove or near some other source of heat.

(3) **Percolation.**—This method of making infusions is by far the most satisfactory, and should be used whenever possible; it is observed that cold water infusions generally have less tendency to decay than those made with boiling water. Details of the process are adequately described in the various text books; suffice to say that the process of Percolation is nothing else than the gradual transmission of the menstruum through the solid materials in a state of moderately fine division; it also presents the advantage of furnishing a finished product, straining being unnecessary.

Infusions must always be allowed to cool before being used, and fresh infusions should be dispensed within twelve hours of their preparation.

"The British Pharmaceutical Codex, 1936," states:—"When an infusion is ordered, the fresh infusion not being specified, either the fresh infusion or the concentrated infusions suitably diluted may be dispensed." "Concentrated infusions, when diluted with seven times their volume of distilled water, yield a preparation which is approximately equivalent in strength, **but not in flavour,** to the corresponding fresh infusions; they differ also in containing a small proportion of alcohol." "Concentrated infusions of drugs such as Digitalis and Ergot are unstable, and only the fresh infusions should be used."

There is no doubt in my mind that all infusions, in order to obtain the full natural therapeutic value, should be freshly prepared, and the substitution of a fluid extract made infusion when a fresh one can so easily be prepared is inexcusable.

ADDER'S TONGUE, ENGLISH

Ophioglossum vulgatum, Linn.
(N.O. Filices)

Action.—Antiseptic, detergent.

Distinctive character.—Leaf solitary, lanceolate, with forked veins, bearing a stalked linear spike of spore-cases in a double row. Root fibrous.

"The Garden of the Lord"—Cont.

By REV. T. GWERNOGLE EVANS, M.N.A.M.H.,
and
MR. ALFRED HALL, M.P.S., F.N.A.M.H.

NAMES OF HERBS—SOME OF THEIR VIRTUES

(The words in parenthesis are Welsh equivalents).

Adrue.—Dyspeptic disorders. Very good in vomiting of pregnancy.

Agar-Agar.—Japanese Isinglass. The powder, 1 dram, with stewed fruits for constipation.

Agrimony (Crimp y Dryw).—Tonic and diuretic. For the kidneys and liver.

Allspice.—Jamaica Pepper. Carminative.

Aloes.—Purgative.

Ammoniacum.—Good for asthma and catarrh.

Angelica (Llysiau'r Angel).—Carminative and diuretic. For stomach disorders.

Arbutus, Trailing.—Superior to Uva Ursi and Buchu in diseases of the urinary organs.

Arrach.—Menstrual obstructions.

Arrowroot.—Food for infants and invalids.

Asparagus.—For heart and dropsy.

Avens, Herb Bennet, Colewort (Llygad y Sgwarnog).—Useful in children's diarrhœa.

Bael.—A specific for diarrhœa.

Balm.—Makes a pleasant and cooling tea. For headache and the nerves.

Balm of Gilead.—For chest and kidneys.

Balmony.—Constipation and jaundice.

Barberry (Y Pren Melyn).—One of the best for jaundice.

Bayberry.—One of the best, if not the best, in herbal practice for the cure of jaundice, indigestion, and diarrhœa.

Belladonna.—Deadly Nightshade.—Poison.

Beth Root.—Good for female disorders; medicine and enemata.

Bilberries (Llyse Duon Bach).—For dropsy and gravel.

Bittersweet—Woody Nightshade.—Kidneys and rheumatism.

Blackberry (Mwyar Duon).—Root and leaves are used.

Black Currant.—Diuretic and detergent.

Black Horehound.—One of the most efficacious remedies for biliousness, bilious colic and sour belchings. In coughs, bronchitis and asthma it is exceedingly useful; alone or combined with Lobelia, Hyssop, Marshmallow, etc.

Black Root.—Cathartic, without griping.

Bladderwrack.—Anti-fat.

Blood Root.—Of great value in chest and lungs and polypus.

Blue Flag.—For blood and urine.

Blue Mallow (Malws).—Demulcent and cough.

Boneset.—Diaphoretic. Best for all fevers and in liver disorders.

Borage.—Diuretic and chest.

Brooklime (Llysiau Taliesyn.—Diuretic and blood.

Broom (Banadl).—Dropsy.

Bryon, Black—Blackeye Root (Bloneg y Ddaear).—Bruises.

Bryony, White—English Mandrake.—Cardiac, rheumatism.

Buchu.—Very good for urinary organs.

Buck Bean (Ffa'r Gors).—Good tonic and rheumatism.

Burdock (Cyngaw).—One of the finest blood purifiers.

Burnet, Greater (Y Gwlydd Lwyn).—Tonic and astringent.

Burr Saxifrage. — Good for gravel.

Burr Marigold.—Dropsy and gout.

Butterbur.—Cardiac, tonic and asthma, and gravel.

Cajuput.—For all pains, internal and external.

Calamint—Mountain Mint.—Diaphoretic.

Calmus.—Carminative and stomachic.

Calumba.—In all cases of dyspepsia.

Cardamoms.—Carminatice and stomachic.

Cascara Sagrada. — Laxative, tonic.

Catnip, Catmint.—Carminative, diaphoretic and tonic.

Cayenne.—The purest and most certain stimulant.

Celandine (Llysiau'r Wennol).—Diuretic and jaundice.

Centaury.—Stomach and liver Give with Barberry Bark in jaundice.

Chamomile (Gawmil). — Stomachic and tonic.

Chekan.—Excellent in winter coughs of elderly people.

Chickweed (Gwlydd).—Excellent for poultice and ointment.

Chiretta.—Bitter, tonic.

Cineraria Maritima.—For cataract of the eye.

Cinnamon.—Weakness of stomach and diarrhœa.

Clivers (Llaw'r Ffeirad).—For blood and urine.

Clownswort.—For wounds, even on the lungs.

Cohosh, Black.—Astringent, diuretic.

Cohosh, Blue.—Rheumatic and female troubles.

Coltsfoot (Troed yr Ebol).—Popular for cough and asthma.

Columbo Root. — Tonic, stimulant.

Comfrey (Cwmffri — Llysiau'r Lloi).—Lungs.

Coolwort.—Diuretic and tonic.

Corn Silk.—For bladder.

Cotton Root.—To contract the uterus; safer than Ergot. Especially useful in sexual lassitude.

Couchgrass—Dog-grass. — Urinary and bladder.

Cramp Bark.—Nervine and for cramp.

Cranesbill Root, American.—Injection for whites.

Cubebs.—Part used, unripe fruit. In gonorrhœa, etc.

Cudweed.—Astringent; good.

Damiana.—Aphrodisiac, diuretic and tonic.

Dandelion (Dant y Llew).—Kidney and liver.

Deer's Tongue (Tafod yr Hydd).—Diuretic, tonic.

Devil's Bit.—Diaphoretic, demulcent, febrifuge.

Dwarf Elder (Ysgawen Bach).—Diuretic etc.

Echinacea.—For al' impurities of the blood.

Elder (Ysgawen).—Alterative, diuretic.

Elecampane, Root (Y Llwyg Las).—Blood, tonic.

Eryngo—Sea Holly (Celyn y Môr).—Diaphoretic, bladder.

Euphorbia.—Asthma.

Evening Primrose.—Astringent, sedative.

Eyebright (Y Llygad Eglur).—For the eyes.

Feverfew (Wermwoodwen).—Aperient; promote the menses.

Figwort (Gwenith y Gô).—It is called the Scrofula plant. Wounds, etc.

Fireweed.—Astringent. Remedy in relaxed throat and mouth.

Fleabane (Chweinllys).—Astringent, gravel.

Fluellin — Speedwell (Llysiau Llewelyn).—Profuse menstruation.

Foxglove (Bysedd y Cwn).—Poison, cardiac, sedative, diuretic.

Fringetree—Old Man's Beard.—Liver, and female troubles.

Fumitory (Mwg y Ddear).—Tonic, diuretic, liver, skin.

Garlic.—Made into syrup with honey for coughs and asthma.

Gentian (Y Goesgoch).—Most popular tonic.

March Gentian, or English Gentian.—It ought to be far better known. In many derangements of the urinary apparatus, English Gentian is admirable, combined with common Plantain leaves. In chronic inflammation of the bladder it is one of the most reliable agents. It should be given in full, and repeated doses of half-a-teacupful every three hours. In congestion of the ureters, chronic suppression of the urine, and gravelly affections, it should be combined with Marshmallows, Comfrey, Yarrow, or Buchu leaves. Also in incontinence of the urine and diabetes.

Gold Thread. — Bitter tonic. Ought to be better known.

Golden Rod (Y Wialen Aur).—Carminative, kidneys.

Golden Seal.—Biliousness and debility of the system.

Goutwort.—Diuretic, aches in the joints, gout and sciatica.

Gravel Root.—Is the best to relax the kidneys.

Grindella.—Asthma. Guy's Hospital uses. Fluid Extract Grindella, ½ dram; Fl. Ext. Liquorice, 1 dram; Mucilage, to 1 ounce.

Ground Ivy (Llysiau'r Gerwyn).—Kidney and indigestion.

Groundsel.—Diuretic, emetic and purgative in strong doses.

Guaiacum.—For gout and rheumatism.

Hart's Tongue (Tafod yr Hydd).—Gravel, spleen.

Hawthorn (Drain Gwynion).—Cardiac, tonic.

Heartsease (Dauwynebog).—Diaphoretic, diuretic, asthma.

Hedge Hyssop (Gras Duw).—With yellow blossom shape of Foxglove.

Hemlock (Cegid).—Poison, sedative, good for cancer.

Hemp Agrimony (Byddon Chwerw).—Cathartic, blood.

Henbane (Llewyg yr Iâr).—Poison.

Hollyhock (Hocs Bendigaid).—Emollient, chest.

Holy Thistle (Ysgallen Fendigaid).—Diaphoretic, emmenagogue. Blood purifier and useful in headaches.

Honeysuckle—Woodbine (Gwinwydd y Perthi).—Asthma.

Hops.—Tonic, anodyne, diuretic.

Horehound (Llwyd y Cwn).—Most popular pectoral, chest.

Horehound, Black.—Stimulant, antispasmodic, vermifuge.

Horsemint, American.—Carminative, diuretic.

Horseradish.—Stimulant, diuretic, diaphoretic.

Horsetail (Rhonell y March).—Astringent, kidney.

Houndstongue (Pigl).—Demulcent, astringent.

House Leek (Y Fyddarllys).—Refrigerant, ears, warts, corns.

Hydrangia.—To prevent gravelly deposits. Excellent for the removal of stone deposits in the bladder.

Hyssop (Isop).—Chest, lungs.

Irish Moss. — Pectoral, nutritious; bladder, kidneys.

Ivy (Iorwg).—Good as poultice, and fomentation in glandular enlargements.

Jaborandi.—Very good in asthma and diabetes.

Jacob's Ladder—Abcess Root.—For pleurisy and coughs.

Jambul.—Diabetes.

John's Bread.—Nutritive; good for the voice.

Juniper Berries. — Kidney complaints.

Knapweed (Pengelyd). — Diuretic, diaphoretic, tonic.

Kola.—Nerve stimulant, diuretic, cardiac, tonic.

Ladies' Bedstraw (Brigau'r Twynau).—Popular in gravel.

Ladies' Mantle (Mantell Fair).—Excessive flooding.

Ladies' Slipper (Esgid Fair).—Nervine; sleeplessness, headache.

Lavender.—Seldom used as medicine.

Lavender Cotton. — Emmenagogue and worms in children.

Lemon.—One of the best of fruits for everything.

Lily of the Valley.—Cardiac, tonic, diuretic. Better than Foxglove.

Life Root.—Suppress menstruation.

Lime Flowers (Blodau'r Bisgwydden).—Headaches, indigestion.

Linseed (Hâd Llin).—For cough medicine.

Liquorice Root.—One of the best for chest complaints.

Liverwort, American (Llysiau'r Afu—Clust yr Asen).—For liver.

Liverwort, English—Ground Liverwort.—For liver complaints.

Lobelia.—One of the most valuable of herbs; emetic, asthma. Given in all cases when system is in a relaxed state.

Loosestrife.—Astringent; useful in bleeding, flooding.

Lungwort (Llysiau'r Ysgyfaint).—Coughs, and asthma.

Maiden Hair (Gwallt y Forwyn).—Coughs and kidney.

Male-Fern.—For tapeworm.

Mandrake, American.—Dropsy and liver.

Manna.—Nutritive, laxative; infants and pregnancy.

Marigold.—Stimulant and diaphoretic.

Marshmallow.—For coughs, and urinary organs.

Masterwort.—Asthma and menstrual complaints.

Mayweed.—Sick headache.

Meadow Lily.—Prolapse of the womb; female troubles.

Meadowsweet (Brenhines y Waen).—Children, diarrhœa, stomachic.

Mezereon (Briwlys). — Alterative, diuretic, rheumatic.

Mistletoe (Ucelwydd).—For nervous diseases.

Motherwort (Llysiau y Fam.).—Nervine, heart tonic.

Mountain Ash (Cerdinen).—Astringent; vaginal injections.

Mountain Grape.—For chronic constipation with Cascara.

Mousear—Hawkweed (Clust Llygoden).—Whooping cough.

Mugwort (Bydiawg Llwyd).—Obstruction of menses.

Muira-puama (from Brazil).—Strongest aphrodisiac.

Mulberry (Morwydd). — Nutritive, laxative.

Mullein (Dail y Melfed—Clust y Fuwch).—Astringent; warts.

Myrrh.—Stimulant, tonic; ulcers, bad legs.

Nettle (Danadl Poeth).—Diuretic, astringent, tonic.

Night-Blooming Cereus (Y Glydlyd Nosflodeuol).—Cardiac, prostatic.

Nutmeg.—Powder is good for piles (bleeding), skin eruptions, and hæmorrhage.

Nux Vomica. — Tonic, bitter; poison, strychnine.

Oats (Ceirch).—Good for muscles of the heart.

Olive. — Emollient, nutritive, aperient.

Onion.—Diuretic, nervine.

Ox-eye Daisy (Llygad yr Ych).—Diuretic, asthma.

Pareira.—Chronic inflammation of bladder.

Parsley.—Gravel, stone.

Parsley Piert.—For all bladder troubles.

Peach.—Almost a specific in gastric surfaces.

Pellitory, Spanish.—Good for toothache.

Pellitory of the Wall (Pelywr y Mur).—Stone, with Wild Carrot and Parsley Piert.

Pennyroyal. — **(Organs);** obstructed menstruation.

Peppermint.—Stimulant, carminative.

Peruvian Balsam.—Catarrh, dysentery.

Peruvian Bark. — Astringent; overdose gives giddiness.

Pilewort (Llygad Ebrill).—For piles.

Pimpernel, Scarlet (Gwlydd Mair).—Diuretic, diaphoretic.

Pine (Pinwydd).—Kidney and-der.

Pine, White. — Urinary apparatus.

Pinus Bark.—For the womb.

Pipsissiwa.—Rheumatic and kidney.

Pitcher Plant—Fly Trap.—Kidney, laxative.

Plantain.—Pounded and applied direct to wounds and stings.

Pleurisy Root.—For pleurisy and lungs.

Poke Root.—Rheumatism,

Poplar, White.—Universal tonic.

Poppy.—Not much opium in the European.

Prickly Ash, Berries.—Rheumatism and skin.

Primrose (Briallu).—Insomnia, muscular, rheumatic.

Pulsatilla.—Nerve exhaustion in women due to menstruation trouble.

Pumpkin.—Diuretic and worms.

Quassia.—Digestive apparatus, and worms.

Quebracho.—Tonic, anti-asthmatic.

Queen's Delight.—Alterative, laxative, blood.

Quince.—Gonorrhœa, dysentery, diarrhœa.

Ragwort (Llysiau'r Gingroen).—Coughs, for bathing.

Raspberry (Afanscoch). — Astringent; easy childbirth assured by its use; also for colds, ulceration.

Red Clover.—For blood and cancer.

Red Root.—Asthma; sores in the mouth.

Red Sage (Sage yr Ardd).—Aromatic, astringent.

Rhubarb, Turkey.—In small doses cures diarrhœa; large, purgative.

Rose, Red (Rhosyn Coch).—In lotion for ophthalmia.

Rosemary.—Nervine; hair wash with Borax.

Rue.—For the menses; should not be taken in large doses.

Rupturewort (Llysiau'r Llengig).—For catarrhal bladder.

Saffron.—It arrests chronic discharges of blood from the uterus.

Sandalwood.—Antiseptic; inflammation bladder.

Sanicle (Clust yr Arth).—With other herbs for the blood.

Sarsaparilla, Jamaica.—With Sassafras and Burdock for the blood.

Sassafras.—For skin; wash for the eyes; gout and rheumatic.

Saw Palmetto.—In wasting diseases increasing flesh.

Scullcap.—About the best nervine; headache.

Scurvygrass.—Strong anti-scorbutic.

Self-Heal—Heal-All (Dail Du).—Astringent.

Senega.—Catarrh, asthma.

Senna.—Laxative.

Sheep-Sorrel (Dail Surion). — Diuretic.

Shepherd's Purse (Pwsy Bugail).—Kidney and dropsy.

Silverweed—Wild Tansy.—Useful as outward application in painful rheumatic joints; astringent.

Skunk-Cabbage.—½ ounce powder in 4 ounces of honey makes good remedy for asthma.

Slippery Elm, Powder.—Bleeding of the lung; best food.

Smartweed.—Obstruction of the menses.

Snake Root.—In fevers.

Soap Tree.—Pulmonary complaints.

Solomon's Seal (Deilen Solomon).—Fluor albus.

Southernwood (Yr Hen Wr—Shilicapwd).—Emmenagogue.

Spearmint.—Stimulant, carminative.

Speedwell.—Good for urine and blood; best fresh.

Squaw-Vine.—Parturient, diuretic.

Squill.—Diuretic, emetic.

Stonecrop, Virginia.—Astringent; gastric disorder.

Stone Root.—One of the best for bladder and stone.

Stramonium.—Good to smoke in asthma.

Strawberry.—Children's diarrhœa; diuretic.

Strophanthus.—Cardiac, tonic.

Sumach, Sweet.—Diabetes, kidney and bladder.

Sundew.—Respiratory organs.

Sunflower.—Bronchial.

Tag Elder.—Astringent, emetic.

Tamarac.—Jaundice.

Tansy (Ystrewlys).—Worms, kidney, heart.

Thyme.—Tonic, astringent.

Thyme, Wild.—Whooping Cough.

Toad Flax.—Jaundice.

Tolu Balsam.—Used in chronic catarrhs.

Tonka Beans.—Cardiac, tonic.

Tormentilla.—Astringent; used in diarrhœa, piles and ulcers.

Tragacanth.—Demulcent.

Tree of Heaven.—Poison; heart and asthma.

Turkey Corn.—Alterative.

Turpeth.—Like Jalap.

Unicorn Root, False.—Weakness of reproductive organs.

Uva-Ursi.—Specific for the urinary organs.

Valerian (Llysiau Cadwgan).—Nervine.

Vervain (Cas gan Gythraul).—Nervine, emetic.

Violet (Y Feddyges).—Good for cancer.

Wafer Ash.—Tonic.

Wahoo.—Liver, laxative.

Wake Robin, American.—Chest, asthma.

Water Betony.—For sores.

Water Dock, Red (Tafol y Dwfr).—Alterative.

Water Fennel.—Diuretic; asthma.

Water Germander.—Inflammation.

Water Plantain.—Good for gravel.

White Pond Lily, American.—Bowel complaints.

White Poplar Bark.—It is diuretic. It is the best universal tonic. It takes the place of Peruvian Bark and Quinine, with none of the drawbacks of the last-named drug. For all cases of debility, indigestion, etc., use the powdered bark with other remedies.

Wild Carrot.—Retention of urine.

Wild Indigo.—Laxative, emmenagogue.

Wild Mint—Marshmint.—Painful menstruation.

Wild Yam.—In all forms of colic.

Willow, Black, American.—Ovarian pains.

Willow, White (Helyg).—Tonic, rheumatism.

Winter's Bark.—Flatulence.

Wintergreen (Y Goedwyrdd).—Rheumatism, urine.

Witch Hazel.—Hæmorrhages.

Wood Betony (Cribau St. Ffraid).—Best for the head and nerve pains; also for diseases of the brain.

Woodruf (Llysiau'r Eryr).—Liver, kidney.

Wood Sage (Sats Gwyllt).—Tonic; promote flow of urine.

Fresh plants applied to tumours as poultice.

Wood Sorrel (Bwyd y Gog).—Catarrhs, refrigerant.

Wormwood.—Stomachic, worms.

Woundwort Marsh (Dail Du).—Gout, cramp, joints.

Yarrow (Milddail). — Diaphoretic; good for colds.

Yellow Dock (Tafol y Dwfr).—Laxative, blood.

Yellow Flag.—Astringent, lotion.

Yellow Parilla.—Better than Sarsaparilla for the blood.

Yerba Santa. — Asthma, expectorant.

Zedoary.—Aromatic, stimulant; milder than Ginger.

HERBS—WHEN TO GATHER

Collect after they are fully developed and begin to fall back—**not** at the time of full-bloom. Dry them in small bunches hung down over a wire line in a current of air. Gather roots when the plants have died down.

DISEASES AND THEIR TREATMENT

Abscess (Common or Bealing).—This is a collection of pus or matter in the cellular membrane, the viscera, or the bones, preceded by inflammation, which terminates in the suppuration. The symptoms are a throbbing pain, as well as heat, redness of the part, and if the matter be near the surface, a cream-like whiteness is seen, with a prominence about the middle. Abscesses should be brought to maturity quickly, since, if they are in the neck or immediately above a joint, the matter is apt to descend into the cellular tissue or membrane and occasion a serious extension of the disease. If the abscess is large, and the patient labouring under debility, give a decoction of Peruvian Bark. It is improper to give purgatives during the formation of matter, or till ripe, unless the inflammation is very violent.

Treatment.—Mix together one ounce each Slippery Elm powder, Resin Ointment and Olive Oil, previously melting the ointment in the oil, and apply to the part on lint. For internal use, take Blood Mixture three times daily.

Abscess of Breast.—The breast is liable to many diseases from irritation during nursing and inflammation of the breast is due chiefly to bruises, undue pressure from tight clothes, or from superabundant secretion of milk. The symptoms are pain heat and followed with hardness, the skin becomes red and glistens with pain intense. If active measures are not taken, it terminates in suppuration (milk abscess), when the patient develops general fever. The treatment consists in drawing off the milk by means of a breast pump, and apply the following oils:—

Olive Oil	4 ounces
Raw Linseed Oil.....	4 "
Camphor	1 "

Cover the part with a piece of flannel saturated in the oils, and over this place a piece of rubber sheeting or oiled silk. Even should the breast gather, this oil is an excellent outward application. It is advisable that the patient take a laxative also, such as Compound

Licorice powder or liquid Cascara. We know of severe cases treated successfully.

Ague (Intermittent, or Marsh Fever.)—This form of fever is generally the result of inhaling the product arising from marsh lands, stagnant water, or decayed vegetable substances; it occurs also in debilitated people, from poor diet and from cold united with moisture. It is obvious from these few remarks how our brave soldiers contracted the disease. The symptoms are languor, debility, yawning, the extremeties become cold, the tips of the fingers are of a bluish tingue, the features are shrunk and livid, the patient has a sensation as of cold water being poured down the back, the teeth chatter, and there is an uncontrollable tremor of the whole body, with headache and oppressed breathing; after a time the feeling of cold diminishes, the features become flushed, the pulse rises, violent headache, hot and dry skin, and there is a violent headache; soon a sweat breaks out on the head and face, extending over the rest of the body from above downwards, when the patient becomes relieved.

Treatment.—During the cold period, apply heat to the stomach and spine; a hot-water bottle is most useful, and give a warm drink of Composition Essence. It is advisable to give an injection of warm water to empty the bowels; by this treatment the severity of the hot stage will be diminished. In the subsequent stages, one must tend to prevent organic affections which so frequently follow this disease, and if the patient be weak, administer a little brandy. The following mixture will soon stimulate the system, and if taken occasionally after the attack, often wards off other attacks or paroxysm:—

Peruvian Bark ......2 ounces
Scullcap ....1 ounce
Barberry Bark ......1 "
Cayenne Pods......½ drachm

Boil slowly in a point of water for 20 minutes, press and strain, and give one tablespoonful after each meal.

Anus, in Anatomy, is the external orfice of the lower intestines, the extremity of whose office is to form an outlet for the fœces. The Anus and Rectum are subject to a variety of diseases, the most common of which are abcesses, piles, ulcerations (see notes on), and prolapsus, or falling down.

The Prolapsus of the Anus consists in an eversion of the Rectum, occasioned by relaxation or irritation, and frequently occurs in children who are affected with worms, which lodge and irritate the lower part of the bowels, or straining at stool. In adults it sometimes occurs in pregnant females, and in other instances induced by piles, diarrhœa, constipation, and the use of drastic purges.

The treatment for replacement of the protrusion consists in placing the person on the face over a table, or in case of a child over the thigh of its attendant, and the gut gently anointed with Olive Oil. The hips are then to be separated as far from each other as possible and quickly shut, pressing on the hips on each side; during this later part of the operation, the intestines will frequently return.

If this method fails, smear the finger with oil or vaseline and introduce into the gut, gently press against the upper part of the protrusion, so as to retain it, when the remainder will quickly follow. In cases where inflammation as well as swelling and pain occur, the application of fomentations will be necessary, then on replacement constantly apply wetted pledgets to the part, using decoction of Oak Bark.

In all cases, once replacement has been brought about, saturate a piece of flannel in the following lotion and renew often, keeping the flannel in position with a bandage; by so doing, the muscles will be strengthened and the intestine then will be retained.

Use Witch Hazel, Oak Bark and Yarrow, 1 ounce of each. Boil in a quart of water, and when strained apply to the part, cold, as mentioned above. If the trouble is brought about by diarrhœa or worms, remove the cause and treat as above, and give the following tonic:—

Fluid Ext. of Peruvian
Liquid Ext. of Malt. .8 ounces

A dessertspoonful three times daily according to age.

Apoplexy. — Cerebral Apoplexy may be defined the cessation of voluntary motion, the loss of feeling, consciousness of existence, and perhaps a real suspension of the functions of the brain, the respiration and circulation furnishing the only evidence that the sufferer is alive. When a person is attacked, often no warning is given; he suddenly falls, though often a previous warning, such as giddiness, confused vision, imperfect memory and sleepy inclination, are tokens of a deranged state of the brain.

The disease most commonly occurs between the ages of 35 and 60, though a premature and immoderate indulgence in spirituous liquors brings it about at a much earlier period.

The most fruitful sources of the disease are luxurious living, and a habitual intemperate indulgence of temper, passions, and appetites, excessive sexual intercourses, severe bereavements, over and long-continued exertion, and the over-indulgence of tobacco. All these things compress the medullary portion of the brain.

Treatment.—The first object is to slacken all tight articles about the neck and stomach, and the patient placed in a sitting posture, with the head considerably elevated. Place the feet in hot mustard and water and massage the legs, and give as soon as possible Composition Essence or Cayenne Tea, for this will bring about circulation and stimulate the heart's action. Repeat the dose of the tea, say, a tablespoonful, every ten minutes, and give an injection of Asafoetida, Myrrh, and Cayenne, about a teaspoonful of each in a pint of warm water, straining before use. This will evacuate the bowels and cause perspiration, when the patient will recover. Now give the following mixture:—

Fluid Ext. of Skullcap 2 drachms
Bark. . . . . .2 "
Fluid Extract of Oats. 2 "
Fluid Extract of
Valerian. . . 4 "
Milk of Asafoetida. . . . 4 ounces
Syrup of Rhubarb. . . . 4 "

Two teaspoonsful three times daily in water if necessary.

Asthma.—Popularly, shortness of breath or difficulty of breathing is called Asthma. There are three kinds of Asthma—the Nervous, the Spasmodic or Dry, and the Catarrhal or Spitting Asthma.

The first, or Nervous, occurs in persons affected with chronic mucous catarrh, and is accompanied with slight cough and free expectoration.

The second: The respiration is imperfect, cough is dry, with scanty expectoration.

In the third, the cough is severe and suffocating, with early expectoration, at first scanty, but later copious, and affording relief; such depends upon the congestion of the mucous respiratory surface.

The symptoms are drowsiness, headache, a sense of fullness, tightness, and flatulance in the region of the stomach, with depression of the spirits, and a sluggish state of the bowels. The patient is unable to lie down and struggles and gasps for air, presenting a pathetic picture of distress. The duration of these attacks varies, often seizing the patient after the first sleep and abating towards the morning. These returns are most frequent on any sudden change of the weather; indeed, the asthmatic feels severely every atmospherical vicissitude.

Treatment.—Take the following ingredients:—

Euphorbia Herb .....1 ounce
Skunk Cabbage ......1 "
Hyssop ....1 "
Elecampane Root ....1 "
Coltsfoot ....1 "

Boil in two pints of water down to one, strain, and dissolve 8 ounces of honey in the liquid. When cool, add half-an-ounce of Tincture of Cayenne and one ounce of Tincture of Lobelia. Take a teaspoonful every four hours. It is advisable to keep the temperature of the room constant, the diet light and nourishing, and during the attack, the sitting posture is preferred, and during sleep the pillows should be more elevated than usual. Give two Compound Asafoetida pills night and morning for the bowels, if necessary.

"SCIENTISTS GET LOP-SIDED

" 'Money and Brains for War'

" 'While vast sums of money and some of the best scientific brains in the country are employed in the interests of war and destruction, almost nothing is being done in the direction of sociological and psychological research.'

"That was a phrase of Professor Julian Huxley, the biologist, when he spoke of 'lop-sided scientists' at the luncheon of the National Institute of Industrial Psychology in London yesterday.

" 'Inertia in official quarters and the pressure of vested interests,' he said, 'are making us a nation of lop-sided scientists.

" 'We pride ourselves on living in our scientific age, yet we are miserably content to exist most unscientifically, enduring a farcical situation of economic waste and artificial shortage in the midst of plentiful production.

" 'One hears a great deal about the progress of the scientific breeding of agricultural crops, plants and livestock. But to make commercial ends meet valuable foodstuffs have to be thrown away or destroyed, and this with a large section of the population toeing the hunger line.' "

—(Press cutting).

MENTAL AND PHYSICAL REGENERATION

By J. MAXWELL, N.D.

GENERAL REMARKS CONCERNING DIET

Food, to be healthy, must come from fertile, clean, well-drained, well-situated soil. It must have been bathed with sufficient sunshine and shower. If of superb quality, it will not have been "fertilized" with animal manure or any other animal slop, no rits growth forced by commercial nitrates. See my article on "Clean Culture."

We are what we eat. In God we live and move and have our being. Our very life depends upon the fact that we are a very integral part of the natural world around us. We cannot live unto ourselves and separate ourselves from other parts of creation.

Air is our most important food; therefore, let us have it as fresh and uncontaminated as possible; less and less of the steam heated variety; not the stale kind found in ill-ventilated rooms and crowded assemblies, or that which is mingled with noxious fumes such as tobacco smoke.

Human food, to be healthy, should not be associated with death and corruption; hence, I told that meat, fish and poultry should form no part of our dietary. For further reasons, see my article, "Why I am a Vegetarian."

ALKALINE FOODS NECESSARY

Our food should always preserve the alkaline balance of the body. Normally we are eighty per cent alkaline, twenty per cent acid.

The acid elements, phosphorus, sulphur, chlorine, silicon, iodine, etc., so long as they are in the organic form, in plant life, should have a place in our diet. They have specific, important, vital parts to perform in our economy, and are intimately associated with the work of other organic minerals, but care must be taken that our foods are such as give predominance to the alkaline minerals, potassium, sodium, calcium, magnesium and iron —that the alkaline balance of the body be preserved.

NEVER EAT WHEN TIRED

We should eat only when we are hungry; never when we are much enervated, very tired, feverish, or when we are emotionally disturbed by fear, worry, anger, jealousy, hatred or what not. Composure and a happy, cheerful state of mind are necessary to good digestion.

We eat to promote growth and repair, to produce energy, to assist in producing heat and the necessary warmth of the body.

We drink to supply the fluids necessary for the blood and normal body functioning, for all the internal activities of the body are carried on in a liquid medium. Seventy per cent of our make-up is water. Therefore, let that water be clean, not mixed with alcohol or meat extractives—as in beef tea—nor with synthetic essences as are many soda fountain drinks, nor saturated with alkaloids, or nerve disturbers, as in coffee and tea.

Don't flood the body with water. Drink whenever thirsty.

AVOID DENATURED FOODS

Our foods should be whole foods, not emasculated, not robbed by any commercial processing. They should be natural foods, unsophisticated foods, served up in all their pristine purity. Therefore, we should discard and refuse to eat such emasculated provender as white flour in any of the forms in which it is served, as in bread, pastry, cakes; white refined sugar, no matter how served, in drinks, ice cream, candies, cakes, or what not. Use honey instead of white sugar.

Polished rice, flaked oats from which the germ has been removed, pearled barley, tapioca, salted foods, should be taboo.

BE TEMPERATE

Gluttony should be avoided. Weak people often stuff themselves, thinking to gain strength. But it is a mistake. Temperate eaters, who choose whole foods, are the stronger. It is not how much we eat, but how much we assimilate that counts. If we eat more than the digestive organs can handle at one time, the surplus is a drag upon the whole system, and the body usually ferments the useless mass, which disorganises the works for a time and gives rise to gas pains and auto-intoxication. One becomes more or less inebriated, and it takes two hours' extra sleep to sleep off that drunk. Further, gluttony produces over-stimulation, which may lead to high blood pressure or other maladies.

VALUE IN FASTING

Nearly every religion has ordered fast days. One can be very religious, and do well by instituting a fast day or days occasionally. It is a good habit. Always fast if there is a fever. Never eat whilst the temperature is at any time even one degree above normal. Make that a fixed rule.

Never resort to pills, inorganic mineral drugs or any poisonous medicine, serum or vaccine, to correct errors at the table or any other errors.

FACTS ABOUT NUTRITION

Away back in 1928 a friend of mine, Mr. W. C. Morse, presented me with a copy of his book, "The Wonders of Nutrition," from which I take the liberty of extracting the following pregnant passage:—

"All natural law, phenomena, is related and underlies nutrition even in plant as well as in animal life. Food, including water, sunlight, air, limited to actual requirements, compose the essentials for normal growth, and provide immunity from disease in all of its aspects, because the normal digestive secretions, charged as they are with the vitamins, dispose of and digest the reproductive products of all parasites. This automatic immunizing, cleansing process, is, pursuant to Nature's utilitarian, compensatory scheme, the appointed work or function of these secretions. They are the body's defenders, its citadels. Nature manufactures her own 'serums' out of the products of her own laboratory. The vitamins or enzymes, which are synthesized in plant and animal growth, are a part of the product of her laboratory and their genesis; their elaboration is as far above and beyond man's understanding as is the spark or flash of consciousness, called life. Man-made drugs are too coarse for Nature's use. They are, in truth, metamorphically, the 'bulls in the china shop.'"

The Marshmallow

H. R. BLUNT (Late Hon. Treasurer, N.A.M.H.)

The Marshmallow (Althœa Officinalis) is a tall wild plant frequently found growing with us about salt marshes and the sides of

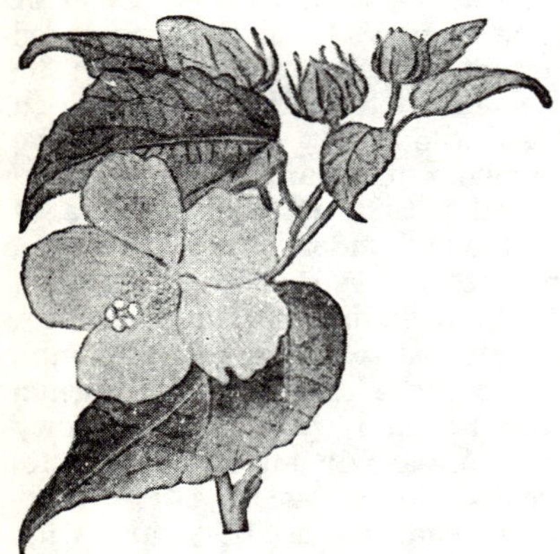

MARSHMALLOW

rivers up which the tide comes. It grows to about four feet in height, the stalk is round, upright and somewhat hairy, the leaves are large, broad at the base, small at the point, of a figure approaching the triangle, and indented round the edges; they are of a whitish green colour, and are soft to the touch like velvet; the flowers are large and white with sometimes a faint shade of reddish.

The Mallow family seems to have been known to the ancients, and has continued in very general use in every country where the science of medicine has been cultivated.

The dry roots of the plant boiled in water, give out about half their weight of a gummy matter which, on evaporating the aqueous fluid, form a flavourless yellow mucilage. The leaves afford scarcely one-fourth their weight, and the flowers and seeds still less. This glutinous or mucilaginous matter with which the Mallows abound is the medicinal part of the plant, and is commonly employed for its emollient and demulcent properties. Its use is recommended when the natural mucus of the membranes become acrid; in tickling coughs, erosion of the stomach and intestines, strangury, and for lubricating and relaxing the passages, it is most valuable.

The root should be used. It is white, long and thick, of an insipid taste and full of a mucilaginous juice; boiled in water and the water made strong, it is excellent to promote urine and to bring away gravel and small stones; it is also good for coughs.

The root of this plant is also of great use as an outward application in poultices, fomentations for allaying the pains arising from inflammatory tumors; it is also good for burns, festers and all other local affections; its virtues as a cough medicine are much increased by the addition of Licorice, Coltsfoot, Horehound and other pectoral herbs.

There is no substance entitled to so much confidence and which has proved so pre-eminently useful for the above purposes; the poultice of the root is prepared by first cutting the root, fresh if possible, into very small pieces, bruising them as finely as possible, and then boiling the mass in new milk, occasionally adding a small quantity of powdered Slippery Elm Bark until reduced to the proper constituency. The inflamed surface should be completely covered with this poultice spread moderately thick on linen for that purpose, and applied as warm as can be borne, renewing it as often as it becomes dry, especially in cases of an aggravated character, threatening to run into the gangrenous state. It is a soothing and powerful application, relieving the pain and removing the inflammation with promptness and certainty.

Its great anti-mortification properties have obtained for it in many parts of the country the popular name of Mortification Root.

In France, the powdered root is much used in forming pills, troches and electuraries. The following are a few handy methods of its use:—

Syrup

Marshmallow Root (bruised)...8 ounces
Refined Sugar........2 pounds
Water...............4 pints

Boil down the water with the root to one-half and press out the liquid when cold, put it by for twenty-four hours, that the dregs may subside, then drain off the liquid, and having added the sugar, boil down to a proper consistence.

Decoction

Marshmallow Root (bruised)...4 ounces
Raisins (stoned)......2 "
Water...............7 pints

Mix them and boil down to five pints, strain the liquor and set aside to allow the fecula to subside, and then decant. This is a most useful demulcent in the dose of a cupful taken frequently.

Lozenges

Marshmallow Root (powdered)...1½ ounces
White Sugar......4½ "
Mucilage of Tragacanth...sufficient

Make into Lozenges. Iris root or Orange Flower water may be used to give a pleasant taste and aroma. These Lozenges are very useful in hoarseness, coughs, etc.

It is interesting to note that when horticulture in former days was but little understood, and that of course the choice of esculent vegetables was extremely limited, the plants of the Mallow Family were admitted amongst the more common articles of diet, and we are told that even to this day the Chinese still eat the leaves either raw as a salad, or boiled as Spinach.

Other members of the same family are the Round Leaf Mallow (Malva Rotundifolia), Musk Mallow (Malva Moschata), Tree Mallow (Lavatera Arborea, not forgetting that beautiful garden variety the common Holly Hock (Althea Rosea); this last is a native of China, but has been so long naturalized in our gardens that it has become thoroughly acclimatised and thrives thoroughly well.

The Garden of the Lord—Cont.

CANCER—CARCINOMA

This terrible disease of the blood occurs in two stages; first, the occult or incipient stage, in which the ulcer is hard and sometimes movable, and with the slightest irritation sets up an amazing activity; and secondly, the ulcerative stage, in which the ulcer is involved in diseased action, enlarges and sloughs and emits an offensive and profuse discharge. The disease proceeds from a poison in the blood, which is carried forward by the blood stream among the glands and other vascular portions of the system, where the poison accumulates and obstructs circulation, hence a morbid change in the function and texture of the organ affected. The organs which are most frequently the seat of attack are the mammary glands, the womb, the pyloric end of the stomach and the lips.

The breast is often, or most commonly the seat of Cancer. A hard, movable tumour is felt, and frequently the breast diminishes in size owing to the absorption of the fat, showing large veins ramifying over the surface of the tumour. When ulceration begins, the surrounding tissue breaks down, revealing a sore which looks irritable, with greyish slough in the centre, and there is a thin discharge at first, the surrounding tissues are of a dusky-red. In the case of Cancer of the stomach, vomiting occurs, the vomit being reddish-brown in colour and often likened to coffee-grounds. The symptoms in all cases are debility, nervousness, darting and burning pain in the regions affected, increasing as the tumour enlarges. The discharge of the tumour is dark-coloured and offensive. There is not unfrequently bleeding from the ulcerations, when the constitution of the patient soon sinks beneath it and death comes as a relief from terrible sufferings.

Improve the general health and purify the blood by taking the following mixture:—

Fluid Extract Yellow Dock	½ oz.
" " Poke Root	2 dr.
" " Burdock	½ oz.
" " Barberry	½ "
" " Agrimony	½ "
Tincture of Capsicum	1 dr.
Camphor Water	8 oz.

Take a teaspoonful three times daily after meals.

Poultice the Cancer with the following:—

Fresh Common Daisy	2 oz.
" Red Clover Flowers	1 "
Witchazel Leaves	1 "
Lobelia Herb	½ "

Boil in a little water and place some of the herb between muslin and apply, keeping the poultice wet with the liquid. Renew every six hours. When the Cancer is emitting an offensive smell and is painful, bathe the part often with a solution containing half an ounce each of Tinctures of Myrrh, Blood Root and Celandine in a gill of water; indeed, this solution could be used advantageously with the above poultice.

1 oz. Narrow Dock Leaves to a pint of boiling water; simmer to half-pint, and add a dessertspoonful of pure honey.

Dose: ½ teaspoonful three or four times a day.

Treatment.—Do not delay in

seeking advice and treatment from a reliable physician, preferably, a specialist, if any of the symptoms afore mentioned are perceived and cancer is suspected. Early medical treatment has often been successful. The same may be said of any other serious ailment.

CARBUNCLE

Carbuncle is a specie of a boil, differing in its form and the severity of the constitutional symptoms which attend it. The disease attacks those people whose constitutions are broken down, either by long residence in tropical climates, by intemperance, or from disease, more particularly derangements of the digestive organs. It commences as a small pimple, which soon extends in depth and circumference, until it forms a large flattened tumour. The pain is severe and burning, and increases as ulceration proceeds, then a sieve-like appearance is seen, due to the ulceration at many points from which matter oozes; at first thin in character, but soon thick and in large quantity. If the wound is not treated, sloughing of deeper seated parts will be brought about with dangerous results, especially in the case of the head being affected.

The symptoms of this complaint are of a low and debilitated character. There are first shiverings, profuse sweats, sickness, loss of appetite and flatulence, pale white tongue, low pulse, headache and turbid urine, and in severe cases delirium follows.

In these cases prompt action should be taken to prevent sloughing, and alcoholic drinks avoided, as these irritate the complaint.

Treatment. — Constant bathing of the part with hottest water bearable allays pain and is essential in assisting the carbuncle to burst. Take internally:—

Fluid Ext. of Yellow
Dock ....1 ounce
Fluid Ext. of Burdock.1 "
" " Mandrake...2 drams
Infusion of Sarsaparilla 8 ounces

Two teaspoonsful in water after each meal.

Apply Olive Oil over the surface of the Carbuncle to soften the skin, and then use the undermentioned ointment, renewing often when the discharge is noticed:—

Powdered Marshmallow
Root ....½ oz.
" Slippery Elm ....½ "
" Lobelia ....½ "
Compound Resin Ointment 2 ozs.
Olive Oil ....1 oz.

Melt the last two named and thoroughly mix the other ingredients. Apply good quantity on lint or flannel as directed above, and when thoroughly drawn, take enough powdered Cinchona Bark to lie on a sixpence three times a day in water as a tonic.

CHICKEN-POX

Commonly called "Swine-Pox," this mild disease may be classed as a mild form of Small-Pox. The symptoms are drowsiness, loss of appetite, weariness, chilliness, headache and other febrile symptoms, for three or four days, when an eruption appears consisting of small reddish pimples. Usually the rash appears first on the back, then spreads over the neck and face and body. Now the pimples have a small vesicle in the centre and about the fourth day of the appearance of the rash the spots become red and globular, similar in appearance to that of a scald, which begins to dry up about the eighth day, forming a scab which peels off about the twelfth day. Avoid the scab being scratched off, otherwise a pox-mark will be left behind.

Treatment.—Confine patient to a warm room through which fresh air is allowed to circulate. No complication will arise if this medicine is taken freely:—

Senna Pods ....1 ounce
Elder Flowers ....1 "
Pleurisy Root ....1 "
Yarrow ....1 "
Ginger Root ....¼ "

Allow to boil slowly for half an hour in 3 pints of water down to one pint, add ½ lb. Honey, again boil and strain. Give to a child in teaspoonful doses often, taking care that the bowels are moved. Complications are sure to arise if the system is chilled during this form of fever; this must be avoided, and food must be light.

N.B.—See Children's Ailments Chart.

CHILBLAINS

These are inflammations or sores arising from exposure to cold, and are one of the results of a partially frostbitten state. There is much heat, itching and redness of the parts, and become blistered when not attended to, when the pain is most severe and commences to slough. They most frequently occur in delicate persons, and hence women and children, who are little habituated to sudden changes, are most liable to the attacks.

Paint the parts with:—

Tincture of Camphor ..2 drams
" " Myrrh ....2 "
Oil of Cajaput........1 drams
Fluid Ext. of Celandine 2 "

If Chilblains are broken, apply Boric Ointment.

CORNS

By this term is meant the ingrowing process of a piece of detached skin, which becomes hard, and increases in size and gradually becomes established in the deep layers of the epidermis. The practice of cutting corns is a most dangerous one, and may lead to blood poisoning. There are two methods of treatment.

By carefully scraping out the centre of the corn, the sides fall in, and by repeating this often the corn disappears. The more satisfactory method is to use the following paint and foot bath:—

Extract of Ivy Leaf....1 dram
Salicyclic Acid ....1 "
Collodion ....to 1 ounce

Paint on night and morning, and bathe the feet every night for four or five nights in a hot solution containing:—

Common Washing Soda....1 oz.
Borax ....1 "
Alum ....1 "
Hot Water enough for foot bath.

COLIC

There are many varieties of this trouble which are referable to different exciting causes. It is characterized by severe pain, with a sensation of twisting in the region of the naval and bowels—is accompanied with sickness, vomiting, obstinate costiveness, and often spasmodic contractions of the abdominal muscles. Pressure on the bowels gives temporary relief which distinguishes colic from inflammation of the bowels; furthermore, there is no fever connected with colic, another diagnostic mark in these two cases.

Flatulent Colic is the most common form, and is caused by indigestible food and costiveness. Apply a mustard plaster to the abdomen, and take

Tincture of Myrrh	½	oz.
" " Red Lavender	½	"
" " Ginger	½	"
Essence of Spearmint	½	"
Tincture of Rhubarb	½	"

20 drops to be given every half hour till relieved.

Bilious Colic is more obstinate than the former and produces fever, thirst, violent vomiting, leaving a bitter taste in the mouth, and costiveness. This is caused by partaking of varied foods.

Treatment:—

Fluid Ext. Barberry	1	oz.
" " Century	1	"
" " Dandelion	1	"
Tincture of Cayenne	½	"
" " Rhubarb	1	"

Take one teaspoonful every four hours in water.

In all cases of Colic where the bowels are costive injections are indispensable, and can recommend ½ ounce of Asafoetida dissolved in a pint of warm water and injected as early as possible. Hot fomentations of Chamomile Flowers are also beneficial; apply frequently to the stomach.

COMMON COLD OR CATARRH—INFLUENZA

Inflammation of the mucous membrane of the nose, frontal sinuses, accompanied with sore throat, constitutes this disorder. The cause of this affection is cold applied in any manner to the body, as by exposure to wet, draughts and sudden changes of weather. The symptoms are sudden shiverings, headache, fullness and stoppage of the nose, followed by increased secretion from the nostrils, sore throat and cough, and sneezing. Often the eyes "water" and become sore; the patient usually is constipated.

Treatment.—If one took heed of the first warning, namely, shivering, and took a hot drink of Composition Essence, much inconvenience and sickness would be avoided in every case of cold, or inflammatory condition. A sound and speedy cure is effected by taking:—

Yarrow	1	ounce
Red Sage	1	"
Cinchona Bark	1	"
Popular Bark	1	"

Boil in 2 pints of water down to 1 pint, and add when cool 2 drams of Essence of Cayenne and 1 dram of Essence of Cinnamon. Take one teaspoonful every three hours. A liver pill twice daily will remove the constipated condition, and Chillie Paste, if applied to the throat, will cure the sore throat and prevent the swelling of the glands of the throat.

CONVULSIONS, EPILEPSY AND FITS

may be described as a sudden discharge of nervous energy in the part known as the brain, and due usually to an exciting cause acting in other parts of the body. The common causes are irritations of teething, whooping cough, worms, and very often the high temperatures of fevers, measles, scarlatina, etc. Children in rickety condition are very liable to convulsions, as also those who have had a severe blow or knock. The feet should be placed in a warm mustard bath, and given any suitable stimulant which is at command. When the patient has recovered sufficiently, wrap in warm blanket to avoid chill and put to bed.

Take:—

Mistletoe	1	ounce
Motherwort	1	"
Wood Betony	1	"
Scullcap	1	"
Rue	½	"
Sugar	4	ounces

Simmer for half an hour in 2 pints of water, and add to the strained liquid ½ ounce Antispasmodic Tincture, and make up to 1 pint with water if necessary.

Give to children half a teaspoonful every five minutes while the fit continues.

It is our desire here to advise parents to desist from the dangerous practice of hitting the children on the head, as such violence is undoubtedly the cause of epilepsy, deafness and defective eyesight.

DIABETES (Excessive Flow of Urine).

This disease, unfortunately more common then generally imagined, is characterised by an excessive discharge of urine, which is altered in chemical composition. The most remarkable symptoms are: large flow of urine, large appetite, little or no cutaneous perspiration, thirst, and muscular debility. There are two forms of this disease, the one known as Diabetes Mellitus, the other is known as Diabetes Insipidus. In the former case, the urine contains sugar, in the latter the urine is practically unchanged in comparison, but the amount of urine passed is enormously increased.

Treatment.—Bring about perspiration by rubbing the body with Methylated Tincture of Cayenne, and have a hot bath every third night, and take:—

Stinging Nettles	1	ounce
Cranesbill	1	"
Agrimony	1	"
Yarrow	1	"
Ginger	1	"

Boil in 3 pints of water down to 1 pint and take a tablespoonful three times daily after meals.

Nettles. — A diet of Nettles (Stinging), which, it is claimed, will supercede Insulin as a cure for Sugar Diabetes, has been the means of reducing the weight of a Diabetic sufferer at Rotherham from 17st, 12 lbs. to 11st. 2 lbs., and vastly improving his condition. The treatment consisted of a two days' fast, followed by eating young Nettles and drinking the brew of them.

It is said that anyone can obtain relief from Sugar Diabetes in three days by this method.

Particular attention must be paid to diet, which regulate according to list below.

Items to Allow.—Meats of all kinds, **except liver,** poultry, game, fish, eggs, cheese, butter broths, watercress, celery, cabbage, cauliflower, sprouts, lettuce, tea and coffee sweetened with saccharine, mineral waters, plain chocolate, and fats.

Articles Not to Allow.—Preparations of flour, starch, rice, potatoes, barley, peas, grapes, pears, prunes, cherries, onions, radishes, melons, and no alcoholic drinks.

Vary the food as much as possible, and give plenty of water or mineral waters, as its prohibition may cause death. Gluten Bread or Diabetic Bread can be obtained quite readily, and is advised, and for a change occasionally use brown bread.

DIARRHŒA.

This term is used to express looseness of the bowels, and is a symptom rather than a disease, for it depends upon some irritation of the stomach or bowels, which may arise from many causes—cold, indigestible foods, acid fruits or drinks, inflammatory conditions of the intestines, etc., unchewed foods surely will bring about this painful and uncomfortable trouble. Since everyone knows this form of trouble, we will not enlarge upon the subject, but give the treatment as below. Take:—

Fluid Ext. of Bayberry..	½	oz.
Fluid Ext. of Tormentil	½	"
Tincture of Catechu.....	½	"
Infusion of Gentian to....	8	ozs.

One tablespoonful to be given after each liquid motion till relieved.

Give cool food and drinks during the attack. Milk, sago and rice are good, and when the diarrhœa has ceased, give the following tonic:—

Tincture of Chiretta.....	½	oz.
Tincture of Gentian.....	½	"
Tincture of Calumba....	½	"
Tincture of Ginger......	¼	"
Cinnamon Water to	8	ozs.

Children's Diarrhœa. — Meadowsweet tea is a specific for the disorder. Infuse 1 oz. of the herb in a pint of boiling water. Dose: A wineglassful after each motion.

DROPSY

A collection of water or serum in certain parts of the body is called a Dropsy of the part in which it occurs. For instance, when a watery fluid accumulates in the cellular membrane, it is called Anasarca or General Dropsy; if in the abdomen, the disease is called Ascites or Dropsy of the abdomen or belly; in the head, Hydrocephalus. General Dropsy is the most common. It commences with a swelling of the feet and ankles, the swelling disappearing on resting. Slowly the swelling extends and occupies the trunk of the body. The skin becomes pale, dry and glossy, and often the water oozes out of the pores or glands, especially those of the lower regions, and brings about a low erysipelas inflammation. Breathing becomes difficult, the bowels are tardy and the stools assume a clay-like appearance, whilst the kidneys are still inactive, the urine scanty and high coloured and deposits a red sediment. There is a great thirst, drowsiness and aversion to motion.

Give a hot bath every day, taking while in the bath a good dose of Yarrow and Cayenne tea. After well rubbing the body with the Compound Capsicum, Liniment, give the following mixture:—

Agrimony	1	ounce
Broom	1	"
Juniper Berries	1	"
Mountain Flax	1	"
Mandrake	¼	"
Lily of the Valley.....	¼	"

Add 3 pints of water, and boil down to 1 pint, add 1 ounce of Spirit of Nitre, ½ ounce Tincture of Lobelia, and 2 ounces of Glycerine. Take one tablespoonful three times a day. Massage the abdomen daily, and give nourishing and stimulating food.

ECZEMA

Of all skin disorders, Eczema is one of the most troublesome. It is an eruption of the small vesicles, preceded by redness, heat, and itching of the part. It is an inflammatory condition of the skin, and is due to retention and accumulation in the blood of poisonous matter which should naturally be removed by the kidneys and bowels as fast as they are formed.

Treatment.—In all cases the general condition of the patient must be attended to. It is useless applying poisonous ointments, which may remove the Eczema but simply driving more poison into the blood and cause grave diseases internally. Constipation is invariably present, whilst the liver and kidneys are often at fault. The following alterative mixture is most useful. Take:—

Yellow Dock	1	ounce
Burdock	1	"
Poke Root	½	"
Sarsaparilla	1	‚,

Boil in 2 pints of water down to 1 pint, and when cool add 2 drams of Potassium Iodide. Take a tablespoonful three times daily, an hour after meals. Apply the following lotion twice or thrice daily to the parts affected:—

Tincture of Blood Root. .	1	oz.
Witchazel Ext. (Distilled)	2	"
Liquid Ext. of Marigold	½	"
Glycerine	1	oz.
Lime Water to..........	1	pint

EPILEPSY OR FALLING SICKNESS

This may be defined as convulsion with torpor. It is a sudden deprivation of sense, accompanied by unusual emotions and violent convulsions of the whole body. The eyes become fixed, the teeth gnash against each other, and the mouth foams. It takes place more frequently among young children than adults. The exciting causes are various. Malformation of the skull, injury to the spine, worms, blows to the spine or head and violent mental emotions are the most obvious, and lastly, a hereditary tendency in the constitution, which is not easily explained, but of the existence of which there is abundant proof. After an attack there is generally much languor, debility, stupor and drowsiness.

Treatment.—Restore the circulation by bathing the feet in mustard and water, and apply heat to the feet straightway. Give:—

Tincture of Scullcap....	1	ounce
" " Valerian ...	1	"
" " Wood Sage..	1	"
" " Cayenne ...	1	"
" " Cinchona ..	1	"
Syrup of Senna.........	3	"

Give two teaspoonful every three hours till relieved.

ERYSIPELAS (St. Anthony's Fire)

This is an acute inflammation of the skin, originating for the most part in the neighbourhood of wounds or sores, attended with redness and infiltration; the most common seat of attack is the face. At first it commences with a small spot, but soon spreads, and the surface is often studded with blebs. Usually, the disease sets in with the conditions of a cold, pulse is rapid, the breathing rapid, the tongue coated and dry, and if the face is attacked the symptoms are violent, often the eyes are closed. Usually, between 7 and 10 days the terrible heat, swelling and redness begin to subside, when the blebs burst, dry, and the skin peels off in scales. If the inflammation continues after this period, control is lost over the evacuation and muscular powers, and delirium sets in. The disease is produced by living in damp places, sudden changes from heat to cold, intemperance, application of irritating substances, gunshot wounds, stings and insect bites.

Treatment.—If the symptoms are severe, a vapour bath is good. In case of restlessness and delirium and insomnia, give Hops and Ladies' Slipper tea. Should blistering occur, or ulceration set in, apply a poultice of Slippery Elm and Witchazel leaves, and follow with this application, applying hot:—

Solution of Witchazel	1 ounce
Glycerine	½ "
Camphor	1 dram
Chickweed Tea	1 pint

Take the following mixture immediately:

Elder Flowers	1 ounce
Yarrow	1 "
Holy Thistle	1 "
Peppermint	1 "
Senna Pods	1 "

Boil in 2 pints of water and simmer down to 1 pint. Take a tablespoonful every four hours.

GANGLION

A small reddish gray knot found generally on the wrist or some other part of the nervous system of the hand. Usually the swelling is globular, when if enlarged is rendered irregular by the pressure of the tendons. They arise from twists, over-exertion or sprains. The treatment consists in rupturing the cyst and allowing the fluid to be absorbed by the cellular tissue. The best method of rupturing is either by compression with the thumb, or by striking the swelling sharply with, say, the back of a book. By applying a lotion of Fluid Extract of Witchazel and bandaging the hand, the cyst will have disappeared completely within three days.

GANGRENE

This may be defined incipient mortification, or that degree of mortification where feeling to motion and warmth are present. It is attended with a sudden diminution of pain in the part of the body affected, a livid brown discolouration, a detachment of the skin under which a turbid fluid is effused; lastly swelling and hardness of the inflammation subside, and on touching the part, a rattling sound is noted, owing to the generation of air in the gangrenous parts. If the part turns black and no feeling of heat or circulation is felt, it is said to have mortified.

Treatment.—Apply a poultice containing equal parts of Myrrh, Lobelia Seed, Golden Seal and Linseed, and renew every six hours, and keep the poultice moist by pouring over the poultice a hot decoction of Cayenne Pepper. Keep the bowels open with a decoction of Mountain Flax, and drink often Composition Essence. Food should be invigorating, as highly seasoned broths, egg and milk, milk puddings. Fresh air is also essential.

Where the gangrene is sloughy (or attended with much pus), wash well the part with a weak solution of Lysol before applying the above poultice.

GASTRIC ULCER OF THE STOMACH

Fluid Ext. Golden Seal.	4 drams
Fluid Ext. Mountain Grape....	4 "
Fluid Ext. Sanicle....	1 "
Infusion of Peach Leaves....	12 "

Dose: One tablespoonful after food. As food, use Malted Slippery Elm, or the powdered Slippery Elm Bark mixed with boiling milk and sugar to sweeten.

GOUT—PODAGRA

Gout is the result of excessive feeding, more particularly alcoholic drinking, causing the blood to be charged with impurities which are deposited in some debilitated portion of the body. Naturally, these deposits set up inflammation, generally in the joints, causing great pain, coldness of the parts, and stiffening of the muscle or ligaments.

The inflammation usually extends to many parts of the body, as the hands, feet, elbows, knees and wrists. If it attacks the heart, palpitations and faintings are produced; when it occupies the joints, it does not terminate in suppuration but an effusion of thick dry matter, which causes the swelling and difficulty of movement.

Treatment. — Here a Turkish bath is most useful; a bath every third night will soon bring about circulation, thus throwing off much of this waste matter.

Now take the following:—

Tincture of Guaiacum..	½ ounce
Tincture of Colchicum..	¼ "
Fluid Ext. Yellow Dock..	½ "
Fluid Ext. Mezereon..	½ "
Fluid Ext. Wood Sage..	½ "
Decoction of Sarsaparilla..	6 ounces

Take a dessertspoonful every four hours and a dose of Senna tea at bedtime; rub the parts with the undermentioned Liniment often:—

Oil of Wintergreen.....	1 ounce
" Origanum	1 "
" Turpentine	1 "
Tincture of Cayenne...	1 "

Dr. Good says in his book that he tried the effect of cold water on his own person for several years, and is anxious that others should participate in the benefit which he himself has derived. In the paroxysms of pain he plunged his foot into cold water, and found the application refreshing, while the fiery heat, pain, and inflammatory symptoms diminished instantly. He repeated the cold bathing every two hours during the whole of the day.

FOR THE CHILDREN

By AUNT JENNIE

HELLO! CHILDREN. Each of you must, I feel sure, be observant of Nature in its varied spheres. Animals, birds, fishes, insects, plants, all are interesting. It is life, movement and change that attract. Country scenery may not impress you, yet the life and movement there abounding arrests your attention and wonderment. A bird flying from branch to branch, the tiny bee visiting one flower after another delights even the baby at its first moment of observation. This we always encourage, for it fills our own heart with delight, and keeps we "Aunties" and "Uncles" youthful.

In my own home is a dear girl now eleven years of age. During creeping days the antics of a kitten provided a chase. When she could toddle, a Yorkshire Terrier puppy gave joy, and "Peggie" is still her guardian friend and romping companion. A goldfish in a bowl resulted in a garden fishpond. More life and movement was produced by the introduction of spawn, from which issued tadpoles to develop into frogs, those amphibious animals which delight one by their agility in swimming and leaping when in search of insects and vegetation as food.

Keen observation in seed sowing and plant cultivation early sought request for "Jean's own garden, all to herself," and of great interest it has been. Even Scarlet Pimpernel, Wood Betony, Celandine, and other pretty wild plants have appeared, the seeds probably carried by wind or birds. But, dear "Nephews and Nieces" you are all alike. You will make a pet of any moving creature, even tame mice, that will respond to affectionate attention; from the Buttercup and Daisy upwards you have loving adoration for God's wonderful handiwork in plant-life.

An even more strange pet arrived—a tortoise! What a queer creature! So shy at first that the slightest sound of footstep or voice caused rapid withdrawal of head and claws into the shell. It soon became tame, freely moving about with peculiar crawl in search of food vegetation. Instinct seemed to direct its movements to tasty morsels—such as young Clover growing among the lawn grass. It is a true vegetarian and selects only the best. On one occasion we observed it travelling faster than usual, and curiosity was aroused. It had been attracted a distance of several yards by a brilliant golden bloom of Dandelion. First

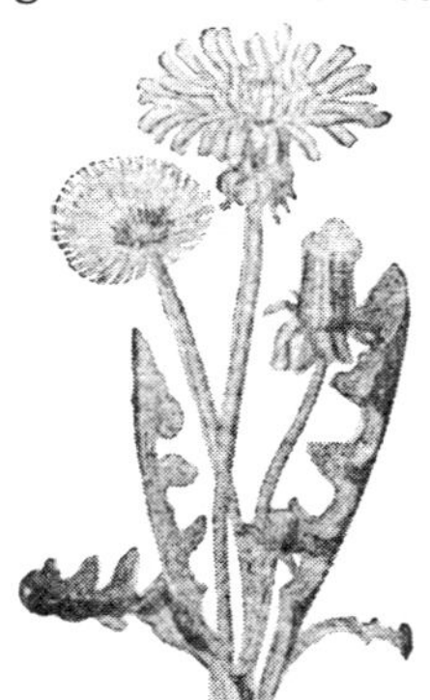

DANDELION

it ate the florets, which perhaps you call the petals, then the receptacle portion of the flower, then off again to another golden head, finishing the meal with a few tender leaves.

Did the tortoise know by instinct as we know by tuition that Dandelion is a liver stimulant, gentle laxative and general tonic? The young succulent leaves improve a salad, and in France they are eaten between bread and butter. Dried roots, after being roasted and ground, provide a stimulating coffee more delicious than coffee prepared from the bean (seed) of **Coffea Arabica,** which contains the drug Caffeine.

The name Dandelion makes an appeal to children, who imagine a fine dandy lion as having derived strength and beauty from the plant. If you carefully observe the formation of the leaves, you will note that the tooth-like margins agree with the old generic name **Leontodon,** derived from two Greek words meaning "a lion" and "a tooth." Our own word "dent" means "something resembling a tooth," and makes it clear that Dandelion is a corruption of the old specific name **Densleonis,** and the French **Dent-de-lion. Taraxacum,** the official botanical name, comes from an Arabian alteration of a Greek word denoting "edible." You will all have found pleasure in the white downy ball which arises after the yellow florets have fallen. Probably tried how many breathblows are required to move the "little angels" (winged seeds), and then noticed the bald appearance of the receptacle, like the shaven head of monks you see in pictures. That explains another common name for the plant—Monk's-hood **(Caupt monachi).** The Editor says "Stop!" so good-bye, dear little friends. Look out for your page next month. Don't forget your letter to "Auntie Jennie."

"FOUNTAIN OF YOUTH" HERB

The article below was sent to me by a correspondent in Ceylon. It is reprinted here word for word, exactly as it appeared in the *Celyon, India, Daily News, December, 22, 1932.*

We want it understood that we have made no analysis of this plant and do not vouch for its medicinal value—which appears to be greatly exaggerated. The plant undoubtedly contains the organic minerals and vitamins common to all green vegetation; but whether or not it contains some undefined therapeutic element we cannot say until we hear from some of the laboratories to whom we have sent samples of this plant. The only property we can attribute to this plant is that it is harmless in an infusion of one teaspoonful to a cup of boiling water and drank during the day. Our own experiments have shown no marked change for the better in the general health of the user. We had a very hard time to secure a quantity of this plant, but we finally have it for sale at 25c a box, with no guarantee as to its virtues, except that it is harmless. Address your request to "The Herbalist," Hammond, Ind.

Because of the unbelievable miraculous claims made for this plant, we believe it should have the attention of the scientific world, and we will furnish a reasonable amount, free of cost to any university or scientific laboratory, on condition that the results and findings will be revealed to us without charge.

We believe we would be neglecting our duty to mankind to ignore this plant because of the apparently ridiculous claims made for it.

(See page 159)

CURE BY SIMPLES

Medical Man Proclaims the Efficacy of Herbs

The efficacy of wayside herbs in the treatment of the common ills to which flesh is heir is attested by the number of letters which the London "Daily Express" has received on the subject.

One of the best known medical men in the West End said to an "Express" representative on the night of Friday, November 24th:—"You have opened up a subject which I have felt particular interest in for years. Undoubtedly there is a wide field of usefulness in the neglected herbs of the field. My idea is that, when gathered and dried and used as a decoction, they may be very potent agents in the alleviation of disease.

"Their effect, however, is to a great extent lost when the herbs are kept too long. Their chief virtue is in their freshness.

"The Marshmallow is invaluable for wounds, and the common Mullein is still much used in Ireland as a remedy for consumption. The Cuckoo-pint is efficacious for fits, and Mistletoe possesses properties for the cure of epilepsy.

"The Yarrow is a common English plant, which can be used with effect in cases of external and internal bleeding, and the Dandelion is most useful in liver troubles. The Mugwort is indispensable in cases of hysteria.

"The monks of old distilled simples from the herbs, and as a medical man, I can say that if the chemists of the present day would revive their old recipes, sufferers would benefit enormously."

GRAVEL ROOT

(Eupatorium purpureum)

Properties.—A valuable diuretic-stimulant, and mildly tonic.

Useful in all urinary diseases, gout, and rheumatism. It is an American plant known as Trumpet Weed, Joe Pie, Queen of the Meadow, but must not be confounded with the English plant of the same name, Spiræ Ulmaria, Queen of the Meadow or Meadow Sweet.

FOR RHEUMATISM

Burdock	½ oz.
Dandelion	½ oz.
Dock Root	½ oz.
Dwarf Elder	½ oz.
Sassafras Bark	½ oz.
Guaiacum Raspings	½ oz.

Boil in 2 quarts of water down to 1 quart. Dose: One wineglassful three times a day an hour before meals.

"PUBLIC HEALTH ENEMY NO. 1."

By MARRE ISRAEL

THE COMMON COLD

To understand the nature of this simple ailment is to understand the cause of all disease. To know how to prevent a cold is to have found the secret of health itself.

The common cold is caused by the closing of the pores of the skin, of which there are, in the human body, about 7,000,000. Every one of these pores should be acting as a sewer to throw off waste matter from the system. It has been estimated that five out of every eight pounds of substance taken into the system pass out of it again by the skin, leaving only three pounds to pass off by the bowels, lungs and kidneys. Not only do solid and fluid matters escape through the skin, but gaseous matters also, which, being retained in the system, are as poisonous as either solids or fluids. For this reason, loosely-woven cotton or linen underwear is better than that made from other materials, as it allows the skin to **breathe.** When in health the deleterious matter expelled from the body by means of the skin will amount daily to one or two pounds. When the functions of the skin are imperfectly performed, the whole body suffers; thus it can readily be seen that checked perspiration is the primary cause of the common cold, of serious disorders, and of death itself.

This explains the prevalence of colds among office workers. These and brain workers in general are more likely to develop colds than the agricultural toiler, who subsists by "the sweat of his brow." In this connection it is interesting to recall that the handkerchief was not originally used as it is to-day, but was carried merely in order to mop the brow, etc., when perspiratory moisture had gathered. When the medico of the future visits his patient, perhaps his first question will be: "Do you perspire freely?"

The question now resolves itself into four parts:—

(1) What causes the pores to close;
(2) What evil consequences would naturally follow;
(3) How to prevent these evil consequences;
(4) How to cure, within a few hours, the cold which has been allowed to develop.

(1) Cold suddenly applied, perhaps over a long period, will bring about an inactive state of the capillary vessels, by which the pores are closed. Sometimes a very slight degree of cold suddenly encountered will cause the great quantity of blood in the small vessels of the skin to recede, and thus destroy the balance of the circulation. Prolonged grief will produce the same effect. Sudden fright or fear will produce a puckered condition of the skin, sometimes described as "goose-flesh," i.e., flesh like that

of a plucked goose. This is referred to in the Scriptures' "Terror and trembling seized me, till my limbs all shuddered; . . . till my hair was bristling" (Job iv. 14, 15). The sudden closing of the pores literally makes the hair stand on end, the familiar phrase indicative of intense mental distress and astonishment.

(2) The ordinary cold, in common with almost all forms of disease, arises from one general cause, i.e., OBSTRUCTION.

The life is in the blood, and if the blood becomes obstructed in the vessels of the skin, it is withdrawn from the general circulation and driven back or forced upon the vital organs. The blood soon becomes charged with impurities to an almost incredible degree, and the natural sequence would be the usual early symptoms of the common cold, which is Nature's initial effort to dispose of the accumulated impurities.

(3) The prevention of the common cold consists in maintaining the equal diffusion of blood over the whole body by means of internal heat. Never allow yourself to feel cold. It is necessary that there must be a certain temperature of the body to maintain a healthy state of the system, but a greater degree of heat or cold can be borne by the human body if applied thereto gradually; if it is suddenly applied, a cold often follows. A great heat can be better borne than a great degree of cold; the latter plays the most important part in the production of disease. From a physical point of view, one thing is necessary to prevent a cold from developing:—**Maintain the heat of the body so that it will continually keep the blood-stream circulating freely throughout the system.** Fresh air, good food and drink, suitable clothing, sufficient work, and the divinely-ordained rest every seventh day, will go far towards maintaining the normal ninety-eight degrees. The determining factor will be, however, a freedom from fear and trouble: "Thou wilt keep him in perfect peace whose mind is stayed on Thee."

When the imminence of a cold is suspected, or the early symptoms have appeared, take a hot drink of a cordial nature. A non-alcoholic beverage is best, and may be prepared in the following way:—To a half-pint of freshly boiled water, add a little honey (the incomparable healing energiser) and stir in, according to taste, a small quantity of one of the following stimulants: Cayenne, powdered cinnamon, ginger, or cloves, or "composition powder." After this, rub the body briskly with some good oil or ointment or even with the bare hands —using both hands at once—and baring only a part of the body at a time, beginning with the feet (soles especially) and legs. The friction, combined with the exercise and the stimulating drink, will produce a warm, comforting glow, and all signs of "The Public Health Enemy No. 1" will disappear.

Attention is directed here to several Scriptures which have bearing on this subject:—"The leaves of the tree are for the cure of the nations" (Revelations xxii. 2; Ezekiel xlvii. 12). The word "cure" here is translated from a Greek word meaning WARM-FROM, literally, **the result of warmth and care.**

The same word occurs in Mark vi. 13; " . . . And they rubbed many of the ailing with olive oil, and they were cured."

(4) A fully-developed cold should not, of course, be suppressed, but it may be perfectly cured, within a period varying from six to twelve hours, by the following method:—

Put half an ounce of Elder Blossom into a jug, pour over it half a pint of boiling water and cover closely; put half an ounce of Peppermint leaves and a quarter of an ounce of Yarrow into a saucepan (not aluminum) containing a pint of boiling water, cover closely and stand the saucepan over a low heat for fifteen minutes, whilst the jug of Elder tea stands in the oven or under a cosy for the same period. The two liquids should then be strained, added together, sweetened with honey if liked, and a large cupful (half a pint) given to the patient in bed, as hot as possible; a hot-water bottle should be applied to the feet. The dose may be repeated, if necessary, a few hours later. Following this, the patient should "nurse himself up" with COMPOSITION TEA, which can be taken at any time. Composition Powder is probably the most useful preparation in the home medicine chest. It is not a proprietary article, and anybody could make it up. The ingredients can be obtained from any herbal store, also the powder ready mixed, if preferred:—

Composition Powder

Bayberry (Powder) . . . 8 ounces
Ginger (Powder . . . . . . 4 "
Cloves (Powder) . . . . . 1 "
Cinnamon (Powder) . . . 1 "
Pinus Canadensis . . . . . . 4 ounces
Cayenne . . . . ¼ "

Mix well and pass through a sieve. Dose: Take a quarter of an ounce of the Powder to a pint of boiling water poured over it; sweeten with honey or brown sugar to taste, and take a wineglassful every two hours or as required.

Note.—In acute cases of pneumonia, bronchitis and influenza, in any inflammatory or acutely feverish condition, or in any case where the sufferer is disinclined to drink the large dose at one time, give the Elder-Peppermint-Yarrow medicine (hot) in small doses every ten or fifteen minutes; a tablespoonful for an adult, less for children according to age, until the complete dose has been taken. In fact, whenever the attendant can spare the time (of which, by the way, there is an eternity before us) and energy, this method is by far the best. The patient greatly appreciates the minute dose and the frequent visits of the nurse, especially if the latter is of a cheerful disposition, which is usually the case where the true healer is concerned. Indeed, they themselves, the true healers, are part of the cure. God has arranged it that way.

The Lemon (Citrus Limonium)

ERNEST GRUNDY, M.N.A.M.H.

The Lemon is looked on generally as something that will make us a nice soothing drink, quench our thirst. Mother makes the real Lemon Cheese from the peel, and if there is someone sick in the home it may be used as a drink. It is also used as a flavoring agent.

On extensive enquiry into the virtues, food and medicinal values of this fruit, we find that it is something which ought to enter our daily diet. Confound that word diet (so we introduce the words, a natural method of living), and I, personally, like to look upon all foods as medicines, and am convinced from a knowledge of the human body and its make-up, its requirements in health and disease, that we must obtain thorough understanding of all food values, and make all foods medicines and all medicines foods.

We find the Lemon contains certain elements which will go to build up a healthy system and keep that system healthy and well. A system which will be able to withstand so-called attacks of the terrible germ and bacteria, which are really not the causes of disease, but are the result of malnutrition, a fancy word for starvation. We find the germ infested areas where unhygenic conditions and under-nourishment exist, and we find very few medical men who have the courage to denounce the foul conditions in which they find men, women and children existing under. A body well armoured with all the requisite elements will not be so susceptible to disease.

Now the Lemon and the elements it contains, Potassium, 48.3, Calcium 29.9, Phosphorous 11.1, Magnesium 4.4 As a food we find owing to its potassium content, it will nourish the brain and nerve cells. Its calcium builds up the bony structure and makes healthy teeth. Combined with iron (natural) to keep the blood corpuscles red and to keep the digestive organs healthy. Calcium gives firmness to the arteries and vitalises the cells. Its magnesium, in conjunction with calcium, has an important part to play in the formation of albumen in the blood. Magnesium is a vitaliser, the muscular tissues and the brain and nerves must be supplied with it. Magnesium is a cell-builder to the nervous system and the lungs, etc.

The medicinal value of the Lemon is as follows: It is an antiseptic. By antiseptic, I mean an agent which will prevent sepsis or putrefaction. It is also antiscorbutic, the term meaning a remedy which will prevent disease or assist cleansing the system of impurities. It is known as the anti-malarial remedy, and it has produced several cures.

Suffers from chronic rheumatism and gout will benefit by Lemon Juice. It is useful in: Hoarseness in singers and speakers, sore throats and irritable coughs. The following troubles will certainly benefit by its use: Tendencies to bleeding; uterine hæmorrhage; rickets; tuberculosis; softening of the bone; broken bones; in pregnancy it will help to build bone in the child, sores; asthma; hay fever; scurvy, and wherever there is tendency to the formation of pus.

For a whilow, cut the top off a Lemon, and place the affected finger in the Lemon. For a bunion, put a slice on the joint each night and secure on going to bed. Freckles if rubbed with some Lemon, will disappear. If the face is rubbed with some Lemon, it will produce a clear skin.

So do not forget your drink of homemade lemonade every day!

MENTAL AND PHYSICAL REGENERATION

By J. MAXWELL, N.D.

THE OUTDOOR LIFE

Get out in the sunlight whenever possible. Court the great outdoors. Be a child of Nature. Plants thrive best in sunlight. So do we. Sweat and sweat again; let us earn our bread by the sweat of our brow, by honest toil. Nature has provided us with four major outlets for the disposal of waste. The bowels, from which there should be an evacuation after every meal. The kidneys, which should not be congested by the end-products of high protein foods, or by the use of salt, pepper, mustard, vinegar or other condiments. The lungs, with which we should breathe deeply, and, in the reaction, throw out a full volume of the waste carbon dioxide at each respiration. Fourthly, the whole skin is intended among its other functions, to be an eliminatory organ. Exercise, regular exercise and activity in general are absolutely necessary to health and long life.

Use the machinery of the body sensibly; never overtax it. Be temperate in all things. Avoid over-tensing; relax frequently.

Buy With Care

Many dried fruits are bleached, sulphured, chemically treated and surface poisoned. Avoid them, and aim to secure those which are natural, sun-dried. There are dealers who specialise in these.

Food concentrates are not so good as foods in their natural order. Always prefer fresh fruits and vegetables to that which is canned. Throw away the frying pan, and you can generally dispense with the can-opener.

Don't peel potatoes, carrots, turnips, peaches, pears, apples. Wash and brush them clean.

Some day we will get away from sprayed fruits and vegetables, from bleached nuts. There would be no need and no excuse for the use of poisonous arsenical or other spraying of trees if the soil were healthy, and sufficiently supplied with clean humus, decayed vegetable matter, and minerals from finely comminuted basic rocks, pulverised granite, gneiss, porphry, marl, limestone and phosphate rock.

Body Drainage Important

Proper and regular drainage of the body is essential. The blood stream is our transport system, to carry nourishment to the millions of cells on the outward journey from the heart; to pick up waste materials on the return journey. When we clog it with excess wastes from an unnecessary amount of food or incompatible mixtures, we slow up the works in general, create congestions here and there, suffer from poor circulation.

Avoid Operations

Let no one stampede you into an operation, or scare you to consent to the removal of an organ, because some part of your anatomy has become congested. It shows the bankruptcy of a doctor's skill in caring for and protecting the body as a whole, if he counsels the removal of an organ, because he can suggest nothing to bring about its restoration to health. The body can never again work in natural rhythm if any organ is removed. If you have to go to the grave later, if possible go with a whole body, and not like the doctor's daughter described by my acquaintance Edmund Vance Cook, in his inimitable

Serum Comic Tragedy

She was a doctor's child and he
Embraced the opportunity
From all disease to make her free
With absolute immunity.

"And first," said he, "as I endorse
Prevention of diphtheria,
This anti-toxin from a horse
Should kill some bad bacteria.

"This vaccine virus from a cow
(And I endorse it fully)
Should help along, and anyhow
'Twill make the child feel 'bully.'

"Of snake-bite serum just a touch;
We get it from a rabbit
Which we have bitten up so much,
It really likes the habit.

"Some meningitis toxin, too,
Would better be injected;
A guinea pig we strain it through
To get it disinfected.

"Some various serums of my own
I'm rather sure will answer;
I make them for all troubles known,
From freckles up to cancer.

"Alas! Alas! For all his pains
The end was scarce desirous;
She soon had nothing in her veins
But various kinds of virus.

"Part horse, part cow, part sheep, part goat,
Her laugh was half a whinney;
"Dear me," said he, "she's half a shoat,
And badly mixed with guinea.

"A girl who bleats and chews a cud
Will never make a woman;
I'd better get some good clean blood
And make her partly human."

A tumor, or an inflamed appendix, an enlarged gland, are only effects of malnutrition, of intestinal stasis, of toxins accumulated in the system, of imperfect drainage; and if they are cut out, one may, sometimes, feel temporary relief until the poisoned condition of the body fastens on some other organ or seeks an outlet through some other channel. Then one will find that cutting is no remedy. Study Nature Cure!

COUGHS AND INFLUENZA

Yarrow	¾ oz.
Horehound	½ oz.
Boneset	½ oz.
Coltsfoot	½ oz.
Hyssop	½ oz.
Cayenne	10 grs.

Infuse in 1 quart of boiling water and sweeten with sugar.

Dose: One wineglassful three or four times a day one hour before meals. Or a little may be taken when the cough is troublesome.

FOR THE CHILDREN

By AUNT JENNIE

HELLO! CHILDREN. First, my sincere thanks to those who so thoughtfully sent me New Year greetings. This page is certainly proving to be of real worth, Children, always exhibiting interest in the wonders of botany and its general application to life and health of all living creatures. With the packet of "greeting cards" the Editor enclosed a note reading: "The Children will desire an inspiration for the dawn of Spring." As I write, we are experiencing the dark, wet and dreary days of early January, a month ere this letter

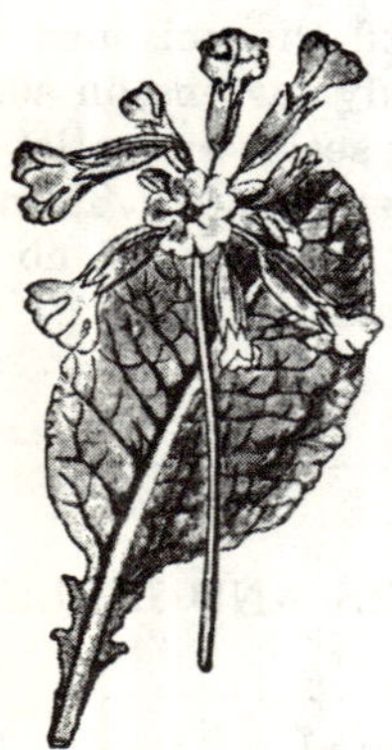

PRIMROSE

will be in your hands, yet we must look ahead and join the Editor in his joyous outlook for Spring, sunny days and life-renewal.

Searching for a theme, I turned to page 102 of this Magazine, and under "The Garden of the Lord" found mention of the "Primrose." What a delightful subject for the dawn of Spring! May I interpose a request that our "Nephews and Nieces," particularly the elder ones, carefully read "The Garden of the Lord" now appearing in serial. The writer—Rev. T. Gwernogle Evans—is a saintly pastor, who combines with his spiritual work a deep interest in the healing of the body. He is truly the children's friend. Round, cheery countenance, with an appealing smile for everyone. A wealth of hair and thick beard, now white with age, combine to create a veritable "Father Christmas," graciously abounding in good works throughout the year. To him every buttercup and daisy, every blade of grass is the Lord's and part of His mighty Garden.

Of our Spring token—the Primrose. The County from where I write abounds with the little plant—from the crown of which spring up dozens of cream-coloured flowers. Thousands of the star-like blooms adorn every hedge-bank of fields and country lanes, even beautifying the railway cuttings. It is noticeable that where shelter is afforded from bleak winds and mid-day sun, growth is more abundant.

The Primrose has made appeal to every poet. Milton describes it as "The rathe Primrose," the word "rathe" being the origination of the word "rather," or sooner, justly alluding to its appearince sooner than other Spring flowers. Under trees and on sheltered rockery of our garden we usually have a few blooms from Christmas onward, to be followed by thick masses of golden flowers. It is always welcome, ever cheering and inspiring.

"The humble Primrose's bonnie face,
I meet it everywhere;
Where other flowers disdain to bloom,
It comes and nestles there;
Like God's own light—on every place,
In glory it doth fall,
And wheresoe'er its dwelling-place,
It straightway hallows all.

"Wher'er the green-wing'd linnet sings,
The Primrose bloometh lone;
And love it wins, deep love from all,
Who gaze its sweetness on;
On field-paths narrow, and in woods,
We meet thee far and near;
'Till thou becomest prized and loved,
As things familiar are."

Certain characteristics you should be told. The Primrose is of the **Primulaceæ** family, which includes the Cowslip, Oxlip and even the Pimpernel, together with the Primula and Auricula of the garden. To casual observation, the leaf of the Primrose and Cowslip appear alike, yet I would ask you to gather and compare a leaf from each. You will perceive the difference between the two in the gradual narrowing of the Primrose leaf toward the base, while that of the Cowslip suddenly narrows below the middle, forming a footstalk. No one can say how or why the pretty flower became internationally known as the Primrose. In no manner is it like the rose so much loved in the summer. The bloom is not even formed of petals, it is a monopetalus corolla, or, in simple language, a flower all in one piece ending in a long tube which encloses the seed-vessel. As the flower fades the seed matures and gradually ripens, eventually bursting the vessel, the action throwing out the seed, probably to fall in a suitable spot to germinate into another adorable Primrose plant.

SENECIO CINERARIA

Dear Mr. Editor,—There has been much written of late about the new plant that is supposed to be a new species, and I think it will be of some help if I settled up this misunderstanding which been caused.

Senecio Cineraria **N.O. Compositæ** synonyms with **Cineraria** maritima.

Habitat: Found growing in the Mediterranean region, and most parts of Southern Europe.

Description: Perennial, leaves greyish white, pinnately divided, with a coating of hairs beneath, segment three-lobed, very downy.

Flowers: Yellow.

Found July and September.

Parts used: Fresh juice, said to be of great use in removing cataract.

This plant is no new discovery. It has been known to grow along the South Coast for a great many years, extending as far east as Broadstairs.

The only difference lies in the fact that the plant found in Southern Europe is known under a different botanical name.

It is interesting to know that this same plant is cultivated as an annual, and used as a bedding plant in most public parks.

J. PASKE.

HAEMOPTYSIS AND SPITTING OF BLOOD

The symptoms of this disease are a redness and flushing of the cheeks, pain, and a sense of uneasiness, heat in the chest, a hacking cough, followed by the ejection of blood from the mouth, often frothy. There is also a sense of oppression of the heart and difficulty of breathing. This must be distinguished from "vomiting of blood" by the blood being more florid and frothy, and not of so dark a colour as that vomited from the stomach and which comes in greater quantity than that merely brought up by coughing, and further, that from the stomach is usually mixed with undigested food.

The disease is more frequent in youth than advanced age, and is caused by the debilitated state of the lungs, or may be symptomatic of some other disease, as consumption.

Treatment.—Food must be light, acidulated gruel, barley or rice water, with toast, should be given. The bowels should be opened with an injection of Asafoetida and heat applied to the feet and take:—

Ipecacuanha Root	1	ounce
Comfrey Root	1	"
Bistort Root	1	"
Marshmallow Root	1	"
Tansy Herb	½	"

Boil for half an hour in three pints of water and make one pint of mixture. Give a tablespoonful every half-hour until the bleeding ceases, and give two Compound Asafoetida pills at bedtime every night.

HEADACHE

This is one of the most common affections, and quite as difficult to treat as any other disease. The dyspeptic or sick headache and the nervous headache are complaints among the sedentary and those deprived of exercise. There is sickness and chillness felt particularly after a meal, dizziness and confusion attends the headache.

Treatment. — Outdoor exercise must be resorted to; walking, or any active outdoor employment will assist circulation materially. Take a teaspoonful of Compound Rhubarb powder every night for the bowels, and the following mixture:—

Chamomile Flowers	1	ounce
Barberry Bark	1	"
Peppermint Herb	1	"
Scullcap	1	"
Peruvian Bark	1	"

Add four pints of water, boil, and simmer down to one pint. Take a tablespoonful three times a day or every three hours until relieved.

Nervous headache is promptly relieved by infusion of Garden Sage and Cayenne.

HEARTBURN

A hot burning sensation at the pit of the stomach, attended with belching and discharge of sour fluid into the mouth. It is caused by acidity of the stomach, and is a symptom in dyspeptic cases and also during pregnancy.

Treatment.—Give a teaspoonful of Antacid powder immediately after meals until burning sensation ceases, and follow with the indigestion pills, which take three times daily.

HEART DISEASE, OR WEAKNESS

Motherwort ½ oz., Lily of the Valley leaves 1 oz.; infuse in a quart of boiling water. Strain when cold.

Dose.—Half a teacupful frequently.

HEART—PALPITATION OF

One of Scullcap, ½ oz. each of Valerian and Tansy, boiled 20 minutes in a quart of water. Strain when cold.

Dose.—Wineglassful three times a day.

DILATATION OF THE HEART

The Bugleweed (Lycopus) is one of the best. It relieves the difficult and oppressed breathing. It is also good for all chest troubles. Infuse one oz. of the plant in a pint of boiling water for 20 minutes.

Dose.—Wineglassful four times a day. Fl. Ext. 10 to 60 drops.

INDIGESTION

Columbia Root, Peruvian Bark, and Cascara Bark, one ounce of each, and Ginger Root ½ ounce. Boil 3 pints of water half-hour. When cold, strain. Dose: A tablespoonful three times a day. Take an aperient before commencing this.

ITCHING OF RECTUM AND ORGANS OF GENERATION

Known as Pruritis, it gives rise to intolerable itching of those parts, attacking both male and female, most often between ages 40 and 50.

Treatment. — Attend to the bowels and wash the parts often. Food should be light; broths and soups with vegetables are good. Take the following: — Dandelion Root, Burdock Root, Yellow Dock Root, Barberry and Juniper Berries, 2 ounces of each.

Boil in two quarts of water for 20 minutes, and simmer down to one quart. Take a tablespoonful after each meal.

Dust the parts with the following powder:—

Golden Seal (in powder) . . 1 oz.
Gum Myrrh . . . . 1 "
Slippery Elm . . . . 1 "
Blood Root . . . . 1 "
Lobelia Leaf . . . . 1 "
Oak Bark . . . . 1 "
Starch (Maize) . . . . 4 ozs.

Mix thoroughly and pass through sieve. Apply two or three times daily.

INFLAMMATION OF THE LIVER—HEPATITIS

There is, perhaps, with the exception of nervous affections, no other class of diseases so fruitful a source of uneasiness as those various shades of complexion which troubles of the liver assume. There is the usual chilly feeling as noticed in all inflammatory conditions, stabbing pains in the right side like those of pleurisy, irregularity of the biliary secretion, producing jaundice, and particularly affecting the stomach and bowels; the tongue is coated. Chronic inflammation is accompanied with loss of appetite and other conditions of acute form, but the pain is less severe. In the acute form the membrane of the liver is the part affected, whilst in the chronic it is the glandular part diseased. The urine is high coloured, and the two symptoms which may be regarded as characteristic of this disease are, difficulty of lying down on the left side, and a pain in the right shoulder.

Treatment.—As in all inflammatory conditions of the internal organs, we must restore the equilibrium to the circulation. A hot bath is essential, and water bottles applied to the feet and side. If the pain is very severe, apply the Compound Capsicum Liniment and cover the body with a warmed flannel; repeat the rubbing every eight hours till relieved, and take:—

Yarrow	1	ounce
Liverwort	1	"
Barberry	1	"
Centuary	1	"
Dandelion	1	"
Lobelia	1	"

Boil in 3 pints of water and simmer down to 1 pint, and add 1 ounce Tincture of Rhubarb. Dose: One tablespoonful every four hours. If the bowels are not moved, give two Liver Pills, and repeat daily if required. Indeed, it is advisable to give an injection straightway, the Asafoetida Milk being the most efficacious.

INFLAMMATION OF THE PERITONEUM—PERITONITIS

The symptoms of this form of disease are a dull pain and weight over the abdomen; the skin is hot and dry; the tongue foul and red along the edges; short and laborious breathing; and appetite impaired. The patient has restless nights through the sudden attacks of pain, lies still on the back, every motion being attended with pain. The pain shoots round the navel in a twisting manner, and often the knees are drawn up for relief; there is frequent distressing vomiting; the bowels are constipated; the urine is high coloured. Give an injection every four hours and foment the bowels often with Cayenne, Marshmallow and Hops. Take the following medicine:—

Marshallow Root	1	ounce
Slippery Elm Root	1	"
Sweet Flag Root	1	"
Dandelion Root	1	"

Boil in 3 pints of water and simmer down to 1 pint, and strain. Carefully mix one ounce of Gum Myrrh, and take a teaspoonful every hour. The diet must be very low, and the patient requires to be careful of himself for a long time after the attack.

INFLAMMATION OF THE STOMACH—STOMATITIS

Stomatitis is common in infancy, and is caused by general debility, sudden chill, improper food, etc. There is pain and twisting of the muscles of the face, contraction of the limbs, spasmodic movement of the fingers, rejection of the breast, inflammation of the tongue and mouth, and the gums are coated and the breath foul.

Treatment.—Apply a warm Slippery Elm poultice to the stomach, and keep it there for ten hours until the symptoms are removed.

Give six drops of Lobelia Syrup every ten minutes, until the stomach is freely vomited. Then give the following mixture:—

Tincture of Ginger....	1 dram
Tincture of Podophyllin.	1 "
Fluid Ext. of Peppermint..	1 "
Fluid Ext. of Elder Flowers..	1 "
Honey	4 ounces
Water ....to make	10 "

Give half a teaspoonful every 4 hours.

Slippery Elm Food, sago, Arrowroot and custards all have the tendency to reduce inflammation; on no account give wines or spirit, or meat.

INFLUENZA

Give the following infusion:— Yarrow and Boneset, ½ oz. of each; Pleurisy Root and Lobelia Herb, ¼ oz. of each; Cayenne Pods, 2 or 3. Boil in a quart of water for half-hour. Strain on to 2 tablespoonfuls of Black Treacle. Drink freely until perspiration begins, then reduce quantity sufficient to maintain the circulation to perspiring degree. Keep the bowels in action, and watch the urine. Food should be of light nature, such as Slippery Elm Powder, flavoured with Cinnamon and a teaspoonful of Composition Powder or Essence.

In mild form of 'Flu:—Elder Blossom and Peppermint, ½ oz. of each; Lobelia Herb, ¼ oz. Infuse 20 minutes in a pint of boiling water. Dose: Half a teacupful every hour.

ITCH—SCABIES

Of all skin diseases, this one is the most troublesome, irritating and contagious. Although the disease never proves fatal, it is sufficiently troublesome, and it is pitiful to see infants suffering from its tormenting itch without being able to know what to do. The disease attacks every joint, between the fingers, arms, legs and toes; scratching only spreads the disease to other parts. It generally commences between the fingers, where small spots or vesicles are noticed, in the centre of which a black speck can be seen. Heat causes the insect which is the cause of the trouble to "work," and at night-time there is no rest or peace for the abominable scratching and itching. So contagious is this, that by the simple shaking of hands with an infected person it can be contracted. On first noticing these spots, which spread rapidly, immediately wash the part in Lysol lotion; and apply the following ointment often:—

Black Hellabore (in powder)....	1 oz.
Black Root (in powder)..	½ "
Witchazel Extract	½ "
Hog's Lard	4 "

JAUNDICE OR ICTERUS

This disease is characterised by a yellowness of the skin and eyes, whitish fæces, and dark-red urine which tinges linen of a yellow colour. The most remarkable symptoms depend upon the absorption of bile into the circulation after it had been previously secreted; upon this depends the colour of the skin. Individuals subject to indigestion and diarrhœa are most liable to attack. Jaundice comes on in a slow insidious manner; the patient shivers and experiences sickness, thirst, fever, and often severe pain in the pit of the stomach and no desire for food. One is indisposed for three days before the Jaundice appears, then the tongue is found to be heavily coated, the bowels costive, the urine loaded, there is great prostration in strength and lowness of spirits, and tenderness on pressure over the region of the stomach.

Great advantage will be derived by an enema every morning, composed of half a pint of thin gruel and half a pint of Asafoetida Milk. Take:—

Fluid Ext. Barberry Bark....½ oz.
Fluid Ext. Agrimony....½ "
Fluid Ext. Dandelion....½ "
Tincture of Rhubarb....½ "
Tincture of Mandrake...½ "
Peppermint Water to....10 ozs.

One tablespoonful to be taken in water three times a day about an hour after meals.

A suitable drink is lemon water.

LUMBAGO—MYOSITIS LUMBAGO

A painful rheumatic affection of the loins or lumbar region. Sometimes it is ushered in with general fever, and the patient thinks he has strained the back. Soon the pains become excessive and of a gnawing kind, being similar to rheumatism, and settles or progresses into the hips, causing difficulty of stooping or walking.

Treatment. — Rub the painful parts with this liniment:—

Oil of Wintergreen....1 ounce
Violate Oil of Mustard ½ dram
Oil of Peppermint.....1 "
Tincture of Cayenne...1 ounce
Oil of Turpentine to....4 ounces

And take:—

Tincture of Guiaicum. ½ ounce
Tincture of Benzoin...½ "
Tincture of Gelsemium ½ "
Oil of Juniper........½ "
Fluid Ext. of Yarrow to 3 ounces

20 drops to be taken on sugar or in water every four hours.

MEASLES OR RUBEOLA

This is a disease which few escape in childhood; it is infectious but is not a dangerous fever under favourable conditions; neglect will most certainly bring about complications. During Measles, there is always a tendency to irritation of the lungs, hence any draughts or chills will cause Pneumonia or Bronchitis. About the fourth day, a small eruption appears, very similar in appearance to flea bites, over the neck and breast; soon these spots run into each other and form red streaks. The disease begins with drowsiness, sore throat, sickness, redness of the eyes, and inability to bear light without pain; there is a dry cough and fullness of the chest, and a slight discharge from the nose. About the sixth or seventh day from the time of sickness, the spots turn pale, until the tenth day the skin becomes natural. This period is the most dangerous since, if there is a relapse through chilling or other carelessness, the symptoms return with violence, delirium, inflammation of the lung and other serious illness setting in. When purple or black spots appear among the measles the case is serious, as also when the patient is very restless, extremely weak and experiences great difficulty in breathing. At this point apply the pneumonia oils and give Saffron and Marigold Flower tea.

When the disease shows itself, bathe the patient in warm water and mustard and put to bed, keep the fire burning daily, and as far as possible the air of the room at a constant temperature, and then give the following mixture:—

Pleurisy Root	1	ounce
Vervian	1	"
Marigold Flowers	1	"
Pennyroyal	1	"
Ginger Root	1	"

Simmer these ingredients in 3 pints of water to 1 pint, and sweeten with treacle. Dose: One tablespoonful every two hours; children, according to age. Give Syrup of Figs if the bowels are not regular. If the cough is troublesome, give No. 1 Cough Syrup as directed in formula.

Note: See Children's Ailments Chart, page.

It is essential to keep the eyes shaded, otherwise shade the lights and windows; endless trouble to the eyes in brought if this point is ignored.

MENSES OR MENSTRUATION

This female function is sometimes called the monthly discharge or the courses. It consists in a monthly discharge of blood from the womb of every healthy woman who is not pregnant from the time of puberty to the approach of old age. In this country, girls begin to menstruate from the fourteenth year, this, of course, is the average period of commencement, and from the forty-fourth that of cessation. The discharge should return every four weeks, lasting about four days; constitution and mode of living greatly depends this and its effect upon the system.

Late hours, little exercise, rich food, and the softest couch brings about profuse and painful dis-discharge, and often for a longer period than the robust, hardy peasant girl. Mother Nature is sufficient to produce the new functional formation the healthy girl, but in the case of the delicate girls at the time of this epoch, it is necessary that the mother should pay the keenest attention to the girl, giving good and wholesome food, exercise especially on horseback, laxative for the bowels and tonics, and local remedies such as immersing the legs in a hot bath as far as the knees frequently. The addition of Rue and Mustard in the bath is good, and when the patient feels anything like the symptoms of commencement, a decoction of Mugwort and Raspberry Leaves will assist the flow and give strength to the body.

We are convinced, from an extensive experience in case of the ailing and delicate girl, that outdoor exercise, diverting the mind by a change of scene, and course of moral and intellectual discipline suited to the disposition of the patient, will overcome the various peculiarities of Nature. In cases where menstruation does not commence until the age of eighteen or even later, one is safe is assuming that such calm serves to disguise some serious disease, that will make its appearance at a later period, such as disease of the heart or some chronic lung trouble.

As mentioned above, menstruation ceases at the age of 44, causing little pain or inconvenience.

Naturally, this depends upon the state of health and the consideration given the wonderful frame or body, for God has given us the faculty of thought, and we know that "what we sow, so we shall reap." If we treat Nature with impunity, then we must suffer. Let us consider the great changes brought about in the natural course only; think of the immense pressure upon the vascular system which must produce an alarming change of structure. It is unreasonable to expect that such an epoch in the life of woman should be at least of temporary disturbances and of partial storms? Just as it is necessary for the young girl to a certain amount of rest and judicious exercise, fresh air, etc., so it is necessary for the woman at this period, for much depends upon the future health from the time of cessation of the menses, also known as the change of life or menopause.

If the following mixture is taken during this "change of life," health will soon be restored:—

Essence of Pennyroyal . .	½	ounce
Rhubarb Root Powder . .	1	"
Cinchona Bark Powder .	½	"
Manna	1	"
Holland's Gin	4	ounces
Water . . . . to make	10	"

Mix thoroughly, and take one tablespoonful 3 times daily.

OBSTRUCTION OF THE MENSES —AMENORRHŒA

Absence of the menses, from other causes than pregnancy, is a very frequent complaint, even the robust are not exempt from irregularity. The most common causes are exposure at an improper period to a sudden change of temperature, standing in cold, wet places, or being subjected to frequent exposures to bad weather, whilst grief and great mental anxiety are fruitful sources of the disease.

This disease must not be confounded with other cases of protracted menstruation (See Chlorosis, etc.)

Treatment. — When suppression exists in the previously healthy female, give a hot mustard bath every third night—retiring to bed immediately. The bowels should be thoroughly opened by a draught of Compound Senna Mixture, folfollowed with the following pills:—

Oil of Pennyroyal
Cayenne Pepper
Extract of Peppermint
" Elder Flowers
" Gentian
of each 1 dram

Beat into a uniform mass, and divide into 60 pills. One pill to be taken three times daily until the flow commences.

FLUOR ALBUS OR WHITES— LEUCORRHŒA

This distressing complaint consists in an increased secretion from the mucous glands of the uterus, the discharge being of a white, cream or brown hue, mostly at the commencement white and pellucid. So acrid is the discharge, that often the parts are excoriated, and may even communicate the same symptoms by contact, to a second person. The appearances are accompanied by pain in the loins, loss of appetite, general debility and wasting of the flesh.

Treatments.—The external parts should be kept as clean as possible, owing to the irritating and caustic effect of the discharge. Food should be light, such as chicken broth, beef tea, sago and rice, etc., and much rest and quietude are essential, since violent exercise and violent mental emotions aggravate the disease. Fresh air is indispensable. Give an injection of the following herbs every night:—

Oak Bark	1	ounce
Witchazel Leaves	1	"
Blackcurrant Leaves	1	"
Raspberry Leaves	1	"
Cranesbill	1	"

Boil in two quarts of water for 20 minutes, strain and inject into the vagina with a female syringe or enema.

Take the following mixture:—

Fl. Ext. of Gentian	1	ounce
" " Comfrey	1	"
" " Tansy	1	"
" " Raspberry	1	"
" " Barberry	1	"

Cinnamon Water to make 10 oz. Two teaspoonfuls in water to be given 3 times daily after meals. The bowels should be moved with liver pills or Senna Pods, since constipation is always in attendance with this disease.

PAINFUL MENSTRUATION—DYSMENORRHŒA

This is one of those deviations from the healthy action of the functions, and to those who are afflicted with it, a most painful and harassing one it is. Usually, severe pains are felt in the loins, back and pelvis hours before the appearance of the menses, and is attended with a distressing sensation of bearing down, recurring at intervals not unlike the pains of labour, and immediately the discharge makes its appearance, the pain ceases. Extreme irritability of the uterus is the immediate cause of this complaint, and is generally caused by severe chills, rheumatism, colds, etc.

Treatment.—Apply hot fomentations of Hops, Mugwort and Tansy to the abdomen or immerse the body in a hot bath containing the above herbs for ten minutes.

Now take the following:—

Tansy	1	ounce
Valerian Root	1	"
Rhubarb Root	1	"
Ground Pine	1	"

Boil in a covered vessel in 2 pints of water down to 1 pint, and when cool add a teaspoonful of Essence of Cayenne and half an ounce of Tincture of Gelsemium. Take a tablespoonful three times a day. By commencing to take the above mixture four days before the due period and for four days after the discharge has ceased, Nature will be greatly assisted and a cure effected.

PROFUSE MENSTRUATION—MENORRHAGIA

This disease is known as flooding, and has or gives no periodical regularity which distinguishes the menstrual discharge. Sometimes the menses will make their appearance for two days and then the flooding continues about ten days, or will of itself cease for many hours and soon afterwards continue the accustomed course.

If the disease is not attended to,

it becomes constitutional, and the lungs, whose sympathies are so intimately connected with the genital organs, will become diseased.

The causes of menorrhagia are various. It will result from the presence of Polypi, from inflammation of the uterus, and occurs in plethoric habits. Violent exercise, sedentary, indolent life, and general debility are other causes.

Treatment:—

Poke Root
Tormentil Root
Cudweed
Marshmallow Root
Mandrake Root

Add two pints of water and boil down to one pint. Take a tablespoonful every four hours. It is absolutely essential to keep the bowels regular, either with liver pills or asafœtida pills (see formulæ).

SCALING AWAY MILK

℞

Olive Oil	4 ounces
Malt Vinegar	4 "
Table Salt	½ ounce

Dissolve the salt in the vinegar and mix with the oil. Shake well before using and apply night and morning to the breasts. Now sling the breasts high and keep in position with a triangular bandage. The mother should take about one teaspoonful of Pure Magnesium Sulphate in water an hour before breakfast and at bedtime, when the milk will disappear in 7 or 8 days.

OVARIAN CYSTS

Take one ounce of Witchazel Leaves, Blackcurrent Leaves, Raspberry Leaves, and Powdered Myrrh, and boil in a quart of water in a covered vessel for 5 minutes, then simmer for half an hour, and filter.

Mix one gill with a pint of boiled and cooled water, and inject gently with a syringe at night.

Take also the folowing medicine, regulate the bowels with Senna:—

Liquorice Root	2 ounces
Yarrow	1 ounce
Comfrey	1 "
Yellow Dock	1 "
Dandelion	1 "

Boil in a pin't of boiling water for an hour, strain and take one tablespoonful three times daily.

MUMPS

This term is used to denote inflammation of the parotid glands situated immediately in front of the ear. When these glands become inflamed, there is general fever; there is a swelling of the side of the face and is most painful to touch, the pain is increased when attempting to chew. Soon the whole side of the face protrudes, and though the swelling is elastic, it is hard in the centre. Generally there is deafness and humming of the ears; the tongue is coated and the bowels are constipated.

Treatment. — Move the bowels gently, and apply to the swollen parts Oil of Lobelia 1, Tincture of Myrrh 1, Camphor Oil 3, Mustard Oil 1, and cover with a warm flannel.

Yarrow tea with Ginger taken often will promote gentle perspiration, and Senna Tea will move the bowels as necessary. If there are any nervous symptoms noticeable, give Scullcap in addition to the tea as above.

NEURASTHENIA

It is necessary in this nerve and brain trouble not only to give nervines and brain tonics, but to use your strongest persuasive powers, and create new cheer and vim in the patient who allows himself or herself to sink and worry over trivial matters, indeed mountains are made out of mole heaps; the patient generally sinks into such a demented and listless condition that no interest is taken in life or anything else, it is a case of SELF. Find the most cheerful company for these unfortunates, keep the mind occupied in matters of interest. Convince them that their health and power has much to do with the regulation of their own mind. Kindness and persuasive power has much to do with the dispensation of those wild talks of the patient and the irregular sensations, nervous irritability and unfounded uneasiness and restlessness accustomary with this disease.

Diet for Neurasthenia. — When the nerves are in a run-down condition, it is surprising the effect that diet has upon them. On no account must heavy meats, such as pork, veal, beef, or rabbit be taken, but the patient must endeavor to keep to lean mutton, lamb, poultry, and fish. Milky puddings should enter the diet. Dandelion Coffee is a splendid nerve and liver stimulant, and if tea is desired, only use the non-tannic brands as Typhoo Tea, etc. Fruit is allowable, but sweets, cream, chocolate, pastry and sweet cakes are detrimental. Slippery Elm Food and Scotch Oat flour are nourishing and strengthening. We advise the following drinks: Sarsaparilla Wine, Herb Beer or Ginger Beer, Barley Water, Dandelion Wine or Coffee. If the bowels are constipated, use the constipation powder.

Take the following medicine:—

Lady's Slipper	1	ounce
Vervain	1	"
Valerian	1	"
Scullcap	1	"
Saw Palmetto	1	"
Raspberry Leaves	1	"
Peruvian Bark	1	"
Liverwort	1	"
Kola Nuts	1	"
Barberry Bark	1	"
Mistletoe	1	"

Add 5 pints of water and simmer down to 2 pints, and add ½ ounce of Essence of Cayenne, and take one tablespoonful three times daily after meals.

NETTLERASH OR HIVES

An eruption similar to that produced on the skin by the Stinging Nettle, hence its name. The rash is often preceded by sickness, symptoms of cold and headache, which symptoms are generally relieved on the appearance of the rash. In other cases the rash disappears almost as soon as it appears, re-appearing on some other part of the body.

The eruption commences generally between the shoulders or over the breast, and is attended with an intolerable heat and itching. It is symptomatic of disorder of the digestive organs, and articles of food which often produce this trouble are: Shell-fish, unripe fruits, pastry, nuts (especially when not chewed), and sour fats.

Treatment—

Stinging Nettles	1	ounce
Yarrow	1	"
Golden Seal	¼	"
Dandelion Root	2	"

Simmer for 20 minutes in 2 pints of water, and take a tablespoonful every four hours. A tepid bath is very soothing to the irritable skin.

FOR THE NERVES, AND SEXUAL DEBILITY

Kola, Damiana, and Saw Palmetto, 1 ounce of each of the Fluid Extract, mixed. Dose: Small teaspoonful three times a day. Before meals, in water, a wineglassful. Good for all kinds of nervous ailments. Take the Constipation Herbs daily, if required. Let the diet be light, easily digested, such as Malted Slippery Elm, and Composition Essence; boiled fish and mutton as much as possible.

NERVOUS HEADACHE

Pour a quart of boiling water on ½ ounce each of Scullcap and Chamomile Flowers. Dose: Teacupful often.

HYDROCOTYLE

Hydrocotyle Asiatica, Linn

A small umbelliferous plant found in India and other tropical countries. It is claimed that Hydrocotyle possesses marked diuretic qualities. Has been given in fevers, bowel complaints, and for syphilitic and scrofulous conditions.

"Oh! Doctor, is my husband better?"

"Unquestionably, Madam; he has just tried to blow the froth off his medicine."

OBESITY

Corpulency, an excessive development of fat in the body. There are two varieties: First, general obesity, extending over the whole body, being an increased deposition of animal oil into the cellular tissue; second, abdominal or visceral obesity, where the fat is confined to the abdomen, giving that roundness of the abdomen vulgarly called pot belly. When corpulency becomes so great as to cause inconvenience, the best remedies are active exercise, purges and fruit diet. Take the following:—

Bladderwrack	2	ounces
Mandrake Root	½	ounce
Gentian Root	1	"
Calumba Root	1	"

Boil slowly in 3 pints of water and allow to simmer down to 1 pint. When cold, add 2 drams of Potassium Iodide and 2 drams of Spearmint, and take a tablespoonful three times daily after meals.

PILES—HAEMORRHOIDS

These are small purple coloured tumours, situated around the anus, or rather disposed in a circle either within or without the anus. When there is a discharge of blood on going to stool, they are then termed Bleeding Piles; in the case where there is much swelling, pain and itching, without bleeding, they are known as the Blind Piles. Piles are brought about by constipation, and sudden chills to the region of the rectum, and irregular diet; wines and spirits taken in excess is one of the surest causes.

The treatment consists in first moving the bowels and watching that they are moved daily; if one has to strain while at stool, serious consequences will follow, such as rupture of intestine or veins. If there is much swelling and pain, apply often a poultice containing Elder Flowers, Hops, Marshmallow, and Pilewort. Now use the Pilewort Ointment night and morning and take the following medicine:

Pilewort	1 ounce
Yarrow	1 "
Senna Pods	1 "
Guaiacum Chips	2 ounces
Poplar Bark	1 ounce
Raisins	2 ounces

Boil in 4 pints of water and simmer down to 1 pint; take a tablespoonful three times a day.

Bleeding Piles.—Boil 2 ounces Silver Weed and 1 ounce of Tormentil Root in 2 pints of water, and take a tablespoonful three times a day. By applying a lotion containing Distilled Extract of Witchazel 1 ounce, Spirit of Camphor 1 ounce, and Tincture of Myrrh ½ ounce, in 10 ounces of water, the part will soon be cleansed and rendered healthy, but it must be applied often and lukewarm.

GLAND EXTRACT FOR WOMEN

It is now well established that timely use of glandular extracts will lessen the rigors and mitigate ailments that so generally attend the meneopausal stage, during which the system undergoes organic changes and adjustments.

As comparatively few people are familiar with gland facts, irregularities in organic functioning are seldom thought of in this connection. They were considered and treated as purely local disturbances. It is now known that the endocrine glands actuate such primary functions as heart action, breathing, digestion, elimination and other familiar phenomena.

While ovarian disorders such as dysmenorrhea may be caused by shock, worry or infection, they are often due to constitutional derangement, with the underlying cause found in deficiency of glandular secretions. Normal cyclic rhythm should follow restoration of endocrine balance, induced by such hormonic stimulation as is contained in this Hormone Extract for Women.

Application of this testicle hormonic solution is usually followed by a prompt and favorable reaction that allows no doubt of its quick absorption, through this pleasanter method of treatment. The patient experiences a new sense of well-being; of elation and energy, indicating response of the nervous system to its help.

Restoration of glandular balance, with functional regularity, frequently improves skin texture and color, tending to clear blemishes and other faults. New vivacity and clearer thinking follow such improvement.

The external application of Hormone Extract has not been officially recognized. Therefore, it must be subjected to further extensive experimentation before it can be presented to the general public for practical use.

HAVE WE A TRI-UNE BODY?

By *E. B.*

"Never heard such a preposterous suggestion before," I suppose you say!

Below the arched base of the large brain or the Cerebrum there is a cavity which contains apparently nothing. I especially say "apparently" nothing, because there is no such thing as nothing as the word itself implies.

If I was to ask you what is nothing, you would desperately try to find an answer, and the answer would depend on your frame of mind!

If you are a Froth Blower, you would say: "It is a bung-hole without a barrel round"; but where the barrel and the bung-hole should be there is air. If you are a poultry enthusiast, you will say: "It is wire netting without the wire round." There again there's air, and that's more than what a bald man can truthfully say! And yet! and yet! when I come to think more deeply about it, that's exactly what he can say. What he cannot truthfully say is "There's hair!" Pooh! that's a bald-headed joke, anyhow.

If in your desperation you say, "It's an enclosed space with nothing in it." Well! well! that's a vacuum, and it's explosive of compressed. What will you want to play with next—a bomb?

Now let me think. Whatever was I going to write on before I wrote on nothing? Oh! yes, I was writing on apparently nothing. I thought it was paper I was writing on, but one gets so used to things not being what they seem to be that I'll take your word for it.

I think the best illustration is the boy who asked his father: "What is nothing?" The parent did not seem to take much notice, but said: "What's that you have in your hand? An acorn! Cut it open and let's see what is inside it. There's a lot of little seeds in it! Well, cut one of the seeds open and what do you see in it?" "Nothing," said the lad. "Well! my boy, where you see nothing, there is an oak tree!"

It's just the same with this cavity where you see apparently nothing; we know there must be something even though we cannot see it, with a microscope, and that something, in the form of a very fine transparent gaseous substance, is in all probability the spiritual brain or the brain of a spiritual body. This brain we call the mind. I am not writing dogmatically, because we cannot prove anything to the Sceptic who thinks on the natural plane, as we are not dealing with a natural substance. It is spiritual; it is Spirit. My readers must not take any references to a spiritual body from a religious point of view; that is the Celestial body or Soul that our religious friends refer to usually. Animals have a spiritual body, or they could not live.

You might say: "Is not spirit

a transparent fluid? Take petrol, for instance. That is spirit; it is a fluid, and I can see it!" There again what you see is not true spirit; it is condensed spirit. It is not true spirit until it is evaporated and become mixed with air, which it does at atmospheric temperature. Does this statement fit in with the rest of our statements? First natural, then spiritual? Yes, it does. In its descent into the natural it became so material as to become an asphaltic rock. This is quarried, ground up, heated, the solid mineral separated from the fluid which is a thick tar-like substance. This is the first stage of the ascent and corresponds to our body changes; for as the natural body descends, for dust we are and unto dust shall we return, the spiritual body develops or ascends, commencing on the return journey from whence it came. You might wonder why I am labouring so much on the spiritual; but natural without the spiritual is dead. The spirit is vitality, and vitality is Life. How can we keep healthy and prevent disease, insanity, immorality and crime, if we don't try and understand life from its very foundations? The time for prevention is at the time of conception nine months before the time of birth. Nay! I am wrong. The right time is before marriage, by the development of proper thoughts and the very discreet choice of your matrimonial mate. Subsequent contributions will deal more fully with this subject.

Now this tarry substance is refined, casts off more earthy matter, becomes an amber coloured oil; one or two more stages of refinement gives us petrol. This petrol evaporates at atmospheric temperature, mixes with air, and becomes a gaseous spirit. Now can you see it? You cannot! Well! strike a match; you may possibly see it then, or you may possibly feel it, or possibly you may both see and feel it. "Gosh! that's a vacuum that was," said he, sinking into unconsciousness. Maybe this spiritual brain or mind is the evaporated gaseous substance derived from the fluid of the solar plexus, and this is where we must admit ourselves beaten to the wide world; though the solar plexus is known as the abdominal brain, and it is an ancient statement that some people can think with their solar plexus. We have also an astral body, but how this is connected with the spiritual body I do not know; but it would appear that we have three or more bodies, definitely—two plus! that is, the natural, the spiritual, and the embryo of the Celestial to which the conscience and higher intelligence belong. So we have a tri-une body, and the suggestion of the telescopic principles we mentioned last month gives us a fairly reasonable conception of it

And so for the present—so long. Adieu.

Health Brevities

WE can't see any difference between doctors who treat "imaginary ailments" and doctors who give "imaginary treatment." They both keep the patient "coming back." Then there is the class of doctor who gives serums for disease that they "imagine" a person might contract. Preventive Medicine is based upon a "vivid imagination," which pays big money. No one ever proved a prevention.—*The Truth Teller.*

MILK
FOOD FOR THOUGHT

By MARRE ISRAEL

The question is asked by J. G. Frazer, in his book, "Folk-lore in the Old Testament" (p. 363): "Why was the precept not to seethe a kid in its mother's milk deemed of such vital importance that it was assigned a place in the primitive code of the Hebrews, while precepts which seem to us more important, . . . were excluded from it?" (Compare Exodus xxxvi. 26, 27, with Exodus xx. 1-17).

Among pastoral tribes in Africa at the present time there appears to be a wide-spread and deeply-rooted aversion to boil the milk of their cattle, the aversion being founded on a belief that even after the milk has been drawn from the cow, it is supposed to remain in such vital connection with the animal that any injury done to the milk will be sympathetically felt by the cow. This belief is shared by the Mohammedans of Morocco, the Mohammedan natives of Sierra Leone, the natives of Ukani, the Wahuma (Bahima) women, the Masai of East Africa, a Baganda, of Central Africa, the Thonga, a Bantu tribe of South-Eastern Africa, the Banyore, of Central Africa, the Nandi of British East Africa, and the Wagogo, the Wamegi, and the Wahumba, three tribes of what till lately was German East Africa.

Dismiss this superstition if you will, but not so easily disposed of is the following from the pen of Dr. Josiah Oldfield:—

BOILED MILK OR FRESH?

Should milk be boiled? When milk is taken from the cow it may be looked upon as a living food, and if kept clean under clean and healthy conditions, it may remain as a living food for many days and then be gradually transformed into other forms of extremely valuable nutrition, but once milk is boiled, it become like dead meat—it is a dead food, fit only for decomposition processes if digestion is delayed.

A piece of dead meat rapidly decays, it goes rotten and smells most foully, whether kept outside the body or whether put into the body and not forthwith digested.

A glass of boiled milk decomposes, goes rotten, and develops similar repulsively odoured gases, whether put on a shelf in the larder, or whether drunk and not digested.

A glass of fresh milk, on the other hand, does not decay or decompose; it passes through processes of souring, by which it becomes a victim to the spores and bacteria which are ever present in the atmosphere, and so eventually, but after a long interval, does it pass into the condition of putrefaction.

For people whose intestines are already a hive of bacteria, fresh milk or already soured milk is far superior to boiled milk. And in many cases where boiled milk is used, it is better to mix it with other foods, e.g., with cereal flours, like groats, arrowroot, or cornflour.—("Milk and Growth": Best Food Series No. 7, The Fruitarian Society, 155, Brompton Road, S.W.).

MILK—SEPARATENESS FROM MEAT ADVISABLE

There is good reason to believe that the Divine law quoted at the beginning of this article may actually be a prohibition of two things, i.e. (1) The boiling of milk. It is not suggested here that this law is directed against the use of milk in cooking. In the preparation of cornflour and similar cereals, it is necessary, of course, to bring the milk to boiling point; and, in many cases, to allow the milk to cook with cereal for some time. Milk is a perfect food in itself, and when taken as such, should be taken in its natural state. (2) Its use together with flesh-food.

Many of the pastoral tribes already referred to are careful not to bring milk into contact with animal flesh, either in a pot, or in the stomach. A considerable interval is allowed to elapse between a meal of milk and a meal of meat. It is known, of course, that similar rules are observed by the Israelites to this day.

Many ills, to-day, are attributed to errors in diet, and there is a tendency among some leaders in the so-called Food Reform movement to discourage the use of milk, one of the arguments being that as milk is the provision of Nature for the young of the cow it is, therefore, unsuitable to be used as a food for man. But this theory cannot be reconciled with what the Bible says about milk—and the Scriptures are the true guide in all the important matters of life. One phrase in particular comes readily to the mind—the symbol of a peaceful prosperity and satisfying goodness—"A land flowing with milk and honey."

WINE AND MILK

Comparing certain Scriptures with some ancient "wisdom" sayings or proverbs, one is able to piece together a valuable health secret. The proverbs and the Scriptures are quoted below and the reader may draw his own conclusions.

"Milk says to wine, Welcome friend."—"Outlandish Proverbs," selected by G.H., 1639.

"Wine washes off the daub."

"If you would live for ever

You must wash milk from your liver."—Scottish proverbs from Ray's collection.

"Wine on milk is desirable; milk on wine is poison."—(French).

Dr. Morris Fishbein, editor of "The Journal of the American Medical Association," announces: "Milk is not a cure for a 'hang-over.' "—"Daily Express," November 21, 1935.

"Come, buy wine and milk without money and without price."—(Isaiah lv. 1).

" . . . Use a little wine for thy stomach's sake and thine often infirmities."—(1 Timothy v. 23).

"I have drunk my wine with my milk."—(Song of Songs v. 1).

"And it come to pass in that day that the mountains shall drop down new wine, and the hills shall flow with milk . . ."—(Joel iii. 18).

MENTAL AND PHYSICAL REGENERATION

By J. MAXWELL, N.D.

THE VITAMIN THEORY

To-day we hear much about Vitamins A, B, C, D and E. They claim to have discovered still more. Those who are scared lest they get an insufficient supply may be comforted by such an "authority" as the "Joint Committee of Lister Institute and Medical Research Committee of London, England," which made the following announcement:—

"The vitamins are ALWAYS present in NATURAL foodstuffs instinctively consumed by men and animals."

We may compare vitamins to the spark of life which ignites the charge of nutritive materials, which releases their latent energy. Doubtless they are associated with the activities of the organic minerals which are taken into the system. Let there be a deficiency of organic minerals and there will be vitamin deficiency.

Vitamin A is said to be anti-opthalmic. A lack of it leads to eye troubles. It is also said to be growth promoting and anti-rachitic (preventing rickets).

Vitamin A is found in spinach, watercress, lettuce, celery leaves, turnip tops, beet tops, carrots, sweet potatoes, cabbage, cauliflower, peas, tomatoes, Swiss chard, oranges, almond nuts. Also, many pin their faith to the supplies found in liver and fish liver oil, but we can find sufficient elsewhere and in a more agreeable form.

A lack of VITAMIN B is said to produce Beri-Beri, a form of paralysis. It is deficient in white flour, degerminated corn meal, polished rice, starch, sugar, glucose, the muscle of meats and fats and oils.

It is abundant in many of our common foods, leafy vegetables, tuber and root vegetables, fruit, whole cereals, egg yolk, milk, beans and peas.

VITAMIN C is said to be anti-scorbutic, preventing scurvy. Found in fresh citrus fruits, tomatoes, celery, carrots, raw cabbage, lettuce, watercress, fresh milk.

VITAMIN D is also anti-scorbutic, preventing rickets, which is essentially a disease brought about by nutritional disturbance. One of its chief manifestations is abnormalities in growth of the bones.

Butter and egg yolk are the only common foods which have been shown to contain the principle most needed to cope with that disease. Cod liver oil is recommended, but I do not see any need for its use and am opposed to it on principle. Here is a case where sunlight is very helpful.

VITAMIN E has properties which assist women who are pregnant in bringing forth their young. It is contained in the germ of wheat and in lettuce.

To be quite sure of adequate nutrition, we may see from the table appended what might be considered protective foods, which should always include one meal of fresh fruit, four ounces of nuts per day, or two ounces of nuts and two ounces of cottage cheese, and a liberal supply of green leafy vegetables at one or two meals, preferably eaten raw, in salad form. For the portion that may be cooked, steaming will be better than boiling. Whole wheat bread or whole grain cereals, with sweet butter, can be added, and if milk is used, it should not be pasteurized.

If one takes some of each fruit and each vegetable as it·comes into season, there is a measure of safety in that.

One should insist that every food taken is a whole food. Take a firm stand against denatured foods.

Calcium foods are needed where there is evidence of tooth decay or tuberculosis.

Lime foods play a very useful part where there is anæmia.

Foods rich in potassium are valuable when there is arthritis stiffness in the joints.

Foods with a fair content of sodium are useful to correct gall bladder trouble.

We need every one of the twelve organic mineral elements, and the following table should be helpful in enabling one to place a well-balanced ration. It is well to use fruit at one meal, vegetables, at another. Better if they are not mixed at the same meal.

Generally, desserts at the end of a meal are not to be recommended.

MASTICATE THOROUGHLY

Nature placed a mill just inside our mouths, ready for grinding food directly it enters the system. By thoroughly chewing and grinding the food we prepare its elements for ready contact with the various digestive juices. That is physiological necessity if we are to get the utmost out of our foods, and it is one safeguard against overeating, for the taste buds on the tongue convey their appreciation when we have need of food, and we should have no further desire, should feel satiated, when enough has been taken, leisurely, never rapidly. Never bolt a meal.

WATCH A SQUIRREL

It is a pity that so many people have the idea that a daily supply of meat is necessary to keep up one's strength. There is absolutely no physiological necessity for meat. See my article: "Why I am a Vegetarian." They are thinking of the need for proteins. Everybody eats too much protein. Man was intended to be a low protein feeder. They fear loss of strength. If one has a reasonable supply of fresh fruits, nuts, fresh green vegetable, a little butter, if you please, combined with fresh air, sunshine, exercise and sufficient sleep, there will be no loss of strength. If you crave milk in addition, refuse that which has been pasteurised, get raw milk just as it comes from the cow, or, better still, from a goat.

We get a very fine grade of protein in many vegetables and their seed pods, as in pease, beans and lentils, also in whole grain cereals, and if one wishes the proteins in a more concentrated form when called upon to do more strenuous labour, there is an excellent supply in nuts.

"But," says one, "we are not squirrels." True, but a valuable lesson can be learned from that clean, exceptionally active little animal. Watch him eat a nut.

Give him a pecan. First watch him balance and weigh the nut in his paw. He's a stickler for quality, and will reject a nut that is light weight, that is dried up, shrivelled or bad. Note the tiny hole he bores in that nut, and watch him use one of his long teeth as a chisel, scooping out just a particle of the nut at a time, and as he turns that over in his mouth, he seems to get satisfaction out of every atom. To him, eating is a delight.

Eat nuts slowly; chew, chew every atom. You need only two tablespoonsful at a meal. Never gluttonise. Nuts are a very concentrated food.

ELIMINATION DIET

The first need is to "clean house," cleanse the body of encumbrances, accumulated toxic material, putrid residues which may be lining the colon and other passages.

This chemical laboratory of ours has often indulged in many incompatible foods, and many have not understood, sometimes, why there have been violent explosions of gas.

Among the causes of body weakness we have the congested condition of tissues throughout the body, waste material between the muscular fibres, or accumulations of fat here and there.

Others have been so badly nourished, tissues starved, although they ate plenty. The proper combinations and quality of food were lacking, and they are thin as a rail. They will, temporarily, get a little thinner as the diet I suggest begins its cleansing work. But no need for alarm, for Nature will not allow a healthy tissue to leave the body; they will only dispose of waste poisonous material. Then watch the body recuperate when the rubbish has been disposed of.

The first few days of cleansing is a critical time. It will test the strength of one's will. So many raise the white flag and cry out in fear if they lose a pound or two every few days; imagine they are slipping, that the treatment is no good or a mistake. Their fears, however, are groundless. The fear, the emotional disturbance will harm them if persisted in, but no harm can possibly come from the use of the cleansing, vital foods prescribed. Clean house, then feed rejuvenating foods as suggested, and presently the cavernous hollows will disappear, or in the case of the stout ones, the bay window over the abdomen, layers of fat on the hips and elsewhere will gradually reduce, and the figure will begin to take on that rounded form and suppleness admired by all.

BLOOD CLEANSING; ALKALINE BROTH

Two carrots, and 1 turnip, unpeeled; 2 large stalks (bunches) of celery; 2 large handfuls of spinach; 4 onions, peeled; 1 handful of parsley, chopped fine; 3 beets, unpeeled.

Cut the carrots, turnip, beets, onions, celery into small pieces, then put whole of ingredients into pan. Put into a muslin or cheesecloth bag a handful of wheat bran and the peelings only of 4 potatoes. Tie up the sack and put in pan with other vegetables. Cover the whole with cold water and let simmer until vegetables are tender. Remove the bag of bran and potato peelings. Then add to the broth a teaspoonful of savita or Vegex, which should first be dissolved in a cupful of the clear hot soup. Take a cupful or two of this broth three times daily. Oftener, if desired.

HARMONIES AND INCOMPATABILITIES

Cereals, which should be from whole grains, and not have the bran or germ removed, and whole wheat or whole rye bread, will harmonise with green vegetables and can also be used with butter. BUT they do not digest so well when used with proteins, milk or any sweets or sugar. They should never be used with any acid foods as lemons, oranges, grapefruit, tomatoes or cranberries, or sub-acids such as strawberries, sour apples or pineapple.

Dried beans, dried peas and lentils will harmonise and can be served with green vegetables, BUT do not use them with other protein foods, milk, fruits of any kind, or any sweet foods.

Butter, cream, and any vegetable oils can be used with green vegetables and all starchy foods, and with all protein foods.

Eggs—take the yolk only—can be taken with any vegetable meal, but do not use them with other combinations.

Milk is best when taken alone, and should not be pasteurised. On occasions it can be used with fruit —but do not combine it with other proteins. Cereals are better eaten with butter instead of milk, and they should be well masticated before swallowing.

Cheese goes well with green vegetables; not so well with other foods.

Nuts make a good combination with green vegetables and acid fruits. Always use them in that way or alone.

Green vegetables are at home with all protein and starch foods. Do not use them with fruits.

Acid fruits can be taken with milk and nuts. Not good with sweet foods or starches.

Sweet fruits should be taken alone as a meal, or in combination with milk.

One cannot go far wrong if foods are combined after the above order. Test the matter out for yourself Read these instructions several times until they are well fixed in the mind.

The saliva has a powerful effect on starches, and further aid is given later to these foods by the pancreatic and intestinal juices.

The pepsin in the gastric juices accomplishes much in the digestion of proteins.

The bile does much in the digestion of fats and acid foods.

THE PREPARATION OF FOODS. LAYING OUT A REGULAR RATIONAL DIET

Salads

Green vegetable salads are among the finest foods for alkalinising the blood, neutralising acidity, supplying the invaluable alkaline elements, potassium, sodium, calcium, magnesium and iron.

They are best eaten in a crisp condition, without any dressing.

Never use vinegar or salt in preparing a salad. Some, however, never relish them without a dressing. In such cases one may mix a teaspoonful of Olive Oil, and teaspoonful each of lemon juice and honey.

Most salads can be laid on foundation of lettuce leaves.

When tomatoes are used, do not serve them with any starchy food. Acids and starches do not harmonise.

. . . .

(1) Quarter head of lettuce. Sliced tomatoes, chopped celery and chopped parsley.

. . . .

(2) Raw spinach and watercress, finely chopped; Romaine or cos lettuce, grated carrot, dressed with cottage cheese.

. . . .

(3) Radishes served with the green tops finely chopped, sliced (unpeeled) cucumber, ½ head of lettuce, young green onions. Few chopped dates.

. . . .

(4) Quarter head of lettuce, finely chopped celery and **onion**, raw sweet corn cut off cob, two tablespoonfuls flaked nuts or finely chopped walnuts or pecans.

. . . .

(5) Grated raw beets, shredded raw cabbage, finely chopped celery, grated carrot, ½ head lettuce.

. . . .

(6) One cup steamed diced carrots, one cup cooked green peas, one-fourth head of lettuce, chopped watercress.

. . . .

(7) Mix two tablespoonfuls of cottage cheese with half a teaspoonful of vegex or savita. Serve with finely chopped green onions or chives, stalks of celery, chopped raw spinch and one-fourth head of lettuce.

. . . .

(8) Chopped endive and Romaine lettuce, radishes, celery, chopped green peppers, slices of Avocado pear, cottage cheese mixed with vegex as above.

. . . .

(9) Grated raw rutabaga turnip, finely chopped parsley and celery, Romaine lettuce, two tablespoonful of flaked nuts.

. . . .

(10) Make a bed of finely chopped lettuce. Place on it grated raw carrot and turnip, and tomatoes cut in quarters. Two tablespoonfuls of cottage cheese.

. . . .

(11) Large combination salad, sufficient for a meal in itself. Bed of lettuce, with chopped Romaine lettuce on top. Shredded carrots, radishes, including their fresh, green tops, celery, sliced, unpeeled cucumbers, young green onions, sliced tomatoes. Two tablespoonfuls of vegex or savita.

. . . .

(12) Grated raw parsnip, grated carrot, chopped celery, chopped Romaine or leaf lettuce, laid on a foundation of lettuce leaves.

. . . .

Other combinations of green vegetables, with or without grated cauliflower, carrots, beets or raw asparagus tips, may be used as desired.

DISEASES OF WOMEN AND CHILDREN

SARAH A. WEBB, M.D. (U.S.A.)

The centre of speech may be inactive and show no signs of development until the end of the second year. If the child is otherwise healthy no alarm need be felt. Children will study the movements of the mouths of adults and learn to note the difference in sounds, and remember the meaning of words especially when brought into use in connection with certain objects or places. Words will be uttered in accordance with no distinct rule. The "memory" of a child will be noticed about the thirtieth week. The child will notice the absence of its mother about the fourth month, also notice the difference in voices. Tears when crying and laughing are often noticed about the eighth or tenth week.

Sight.—This is present from birth, but the eyes are very sensitive to light, and not till the fourth month do they seem to be used voluntarily.

Hearing.—Deafness is present for a few days. This is probably due to the absence of air from the tympanum (or drum), but when respiration is well established the hearing begins, and later becomes quite sharp. The baby does not seem to locate sounds before the fourth month.

Touch.—Sensation is present, but is dull for three months. It is highly developed in the tongue and lips, where the "temperature sense" is also acute.

Taste.—This sense is highly developed from birth.

Development of the Normal Infant.—During the first year the child should be weighed every week, and during the second year every other week. The gain or loss in weight from one weighing to another is the very best indication we have of the welfare of the child. Often the signal of commencing trouble, is the absence of a regular weekly gain or the presence of a slight loss.

At six months the birth-weight should be about doubled, and at the end of a year about trebled. During the first six months the gain should average four to eight ounces per week, and from two to four ounces during the second six months. From four to six pounds per year is an average gain for the next ten years. Sickness of any kind, and particularly digestive disturbances, stop the normal gain, and usually substitute a loss. Even the physiological process of dentitions is accompanied by a diminished weekly gain.

Height.—During the first year the growth is about eight inches, an average of two-thirds of an inch per month, the increase being somewhat greater during the first quarter. During the second year the growth is about four inches, and during the next ten years it averages about two inches per year. This growth, in infancy, takes place more rapidly in the extremities than in the trunk, although at birth the trunk is relatively longer than the limbs. The average height of a new-born male is from 19½ to 20 inches, and of a female from 19¼ to 19¾ inches.

Weight.—Boys average 7½ lbs., and girls about 7 lbs. If below 5½ lbs., a very low vitality is indicated, and suggests prematurity.

Dentition.—At birth the teeth are enclosed in the dental sac in the alveoli of the jaws, and their growth is upward by calcification of their roots, this growth beginning at birth. The milk or deciduous teeth are twenty in number, and are cut in the following order, although quite wide variations are frequent:—

1. Two lower central incisors, at six to nine months.
2. Four upper incisors, at eight to twelve months.
3. Two lower lateral incisors and four anterior molars, at 12 to 15 months.
4. Four canine, at 12 to 15 months.
5. Four posterior molars, at 24 to 30 months.

Early teething usually means early ossification of the chanial bones; and late teething usually indicates rickets or other forms of malnutrition.

Poison

"More important still, it is necessary to break down the adhesive wall and this is extremely likely to spread the poison throughout the system and give the patient general peritonitis.

"Most of the acute cases, however, will yield to treatment designed to reduce the inflammation.

"When months have passed, not only is the difficulty of the operation and the danger of general infection removed, but the patient is in a stronger state to stand the operation and has more reserves of strength to help him recover.

"By no means all doctors and surgeons have yet adopted the new theory, but in time they will all have to come round.

"There is no longer any doubt that meat has a great deal to do with appendicitis. The disease is known almost exclusively among meat-eating people.

"The old idea that appendicitis is caused by such things as fish-bones, grape-pips, and other such is exploded. Foreign bodies are exceptional causes."

We have often wondered why the sudden rush for surgical interference in these cases of appendical and supposed appendical troubles. The cases of acute and chronic appendicitis we have been called upon to treat have responded to natural treatment. Personally, we doubt if the disease itself is spreading; but while we table every case suffering from pain in the right iliac region as appendicitis, we shall certainly keep up a high rate for statistical purposes. We are of the opinion that many of these cases are really due to coli-sepsis, and a treatment based on clearing the colon and keeping it clean would not only reduce our appendix cases, but render incalculable service in the general health of the people.

We know of many physicians who have, for the last fifteen years, been working on this method, and have never had a death. It is a simple treatment; clear up, clear out, and keep clear. But you need to know your job, and then do it thoroughly.

While we were writing the above, it suddenly came to our mind of a question and answer given in "The Chicago Medical Observer," April, 1898. At that time it was edited by W. H. Cook, M.D., M.A., author of "The Science and Practice of Medicine" and "Woman's Book of Health." We give the question and reply below:—

"Dear Editor,—Will you do me the favour of giving me some suggestions on appendicitis? It has become a professional 'fad,' and every time a man gets a pain in the right groin he concludes he has it. The knife is the one resort; and I notice by the papers that a Chicago surgeon has operated on fifty cases in three months at $1,000 a head. No wonder he can give a grand supper costing $5,000, and get free advertising in the papers for both his suppers and his operations. Is advertising a professional crime when you pay for it, but a great gift to humanity when you get columns of it without paying? Really I would like to know just where the quack and the fake come in on this advertising business; for there is any quantity of free advertising done in the appendicitis, anti-toxin and similar lines. But more particularly would I like to know if anything can be done to cure appendicitis without using the knife; and what is the outcome of the operation, anyhow?—J. L. Miller, M.D."

"(Like to many other operations, glowing reports are made too soon after the procedure, and before the patient has fully recovered from the ether. What the final result is in appendicitis is not always made public. There is ground for fearing that the real recoveries from an operation are very few. Three years ago, in this city, we were treating an elderly man for pain and swelling in the right groin, located a little above and inward from Poupart's ligament, following a slip and fall. A brief rheumatic seizure laid us up, and a famous surgeon was called in. He pronounced it appendicitis requiring an immediate operation to save life. The man refused. The case proved to be an abscess of the inguinal glands, in due time requiring lancing and nothing else.

"Several cases of acute appendicitis have come under our treatment, and all have recovered. We empty the bowel by a large enema of nepeta infusion, carefully filling the fluid around the colon to the cæcum. A little Lobelia may be added. By this the cæcum and appendix are both relaxed; and the appendix is then in condition to discharge its contents when encouraged by the peristalsis of the bowel. A large dose of Leptandra has a peculiar and an invaluable influence in relaxing the appendix and opening its mouth, and may precede the enema by a few hours. Sometimes a second or third enema will be necessary, at intervals of four to eight hours, according to conditions.

"Our treatment will not bring in $1,000 to a case, but it will save human life, which operations will not always do. It is based upon the physiology of the structures as all truly curative means must ever be. Soften and loosen out the appendix, which has spasmodically closed upon some foreign substance getting into it. This done, the intruding materials will be ejected and inflammation prevented.—Ed. Obe.)."

Many years have elapsed since the above was written; the good doctor has gone to his long rest. He was a true student of Nature, basing his treatment on physiological lines. Since his day, much water has run "under the bridge." Surgery has advanced; opinions have changed; new anæsthetics have been discovered; new technique for producing anæsthetisation has developed. We believe the Physio-Medical treatment for appendicitis in the acute or chronic state to be the best medical treatment yet discovered.

We advise our students to keep in mind the above treatment. Do not forget to use Leptandra in these cases, which has, apart from its relaxing effect on the appendix, an invaluable influence on the liver causing the elimination of bile, this acting as a purgative and antiseptic.

Check Bad Habits Early

Thoughts and habits travel by certain nerve routes, and the same thoughts and habits always by the same routes. These get in time actually well trodden, like a footpath, and a nerve current will flow more readily along them than through an unaccustomed channel. To prove it, try and write, or use a knife or spoon with the left hand. A physiological reason why habits are so easy to check at first, so difficult afterwards, is thus shown. Never, then, let a child acquire bad habits, however trivial. An immense amount of life education may be done between two and six years of age with far less difficulty than afterwards.

Diagnosis

Swelling under the eyes, greyish white or waxy colour of the skin denote granular disease of the kidneys.

Swelling of the labia, one or both sides, will accompany inflammation of the kidneys.

Carbuncles on the shoulders, or scapular region, are frequent accompaniments of diabetes.

Pain referred to the meatus urinarius is sure to be the result of cystitis, prostatis or nephritis.

Pruritus of the anus will be the only evidence, often, of disease of the prostrate.

Sciatic neuralgia often depends, in females, on inflammation of the ovary; in men, on irritation of lumbar or sacral nerves.

Pain in the heels, in females, may be the only evidence of ovarian abscess, while pain and swelling in the mammæ will evince some trouble in the same side of the uterus of fallopian tube.

Severe occipital headache is almost invariably accompanied with an extreme output of phosphates in the urine.

FOR THE CHILDREN

By AUNTY BEC.

TUSSILAGO FARFARA

Class 19, Syngenesia. Order 2, Polygamia

Dear Children,—Have you noticed anything lately? After the dark days of winter everything is changing. We hardly notice it at first, then all at once we know something has happened.

I took my dog for a walk the other day along the street, down the bank, across the field and away past the old pit. When we left the street I began to notice things—the grass on the bank side was greener, new shoots peeping through. In the field, what a change! My doggie started to race

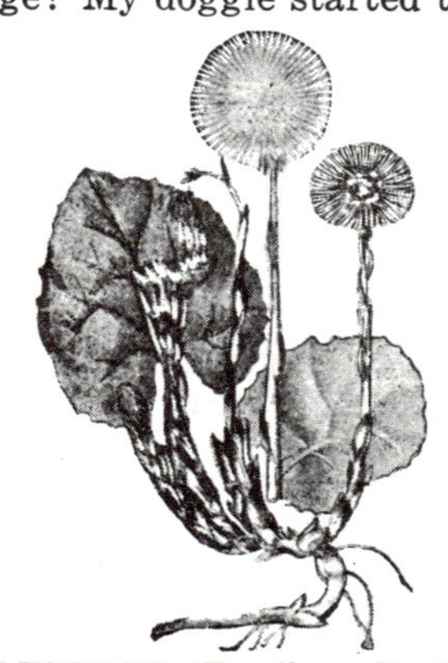

COLTSFOOT (Tussilago Farfara)

about and jump high over little tufts of grass. Oh my! she was excited. Her nose started to quiver and she gave a little yelp (which in dog language means "Rabbits!"), and off she went.

Left alone, I stood and took deep breaths of lovely pure fresh air, even the air was changed. All around I saw changes: little leaves uncurling among the grass, buds on the hedgerows swelling out to bursting point. Oh! yes, there was a change in everything. Now I wondered why? Then the thought came to me in a flash—Prosperina is leaving Pluto and the dark regions and coming to earth to delight us all with her beauty, and all things growing are heralding her coming and preparing the way for her feet, for everywhere she steps flowers spring up to greet her. Yes, Spring is coming, and in a few more days we shall be able to say: "Spring is here!"

Everyone loves the Spring. It is a new beginning in life—green grass, fresh flowers, leafy trees, little lambs, baby birds, calves, and all the rest of the new life. Isn't it wonderful? Let us always remember and praise the Giver.

My doggie came back to me, tired and disappointed; the rabbits had been too quick for her. So we continued our walk until we came to the old pit. There were little yellow flowers peeping up everywhere, but not a leaf to accompany them. Dozens of these flowers ranged up the side of the disused pit-heap. The name of this flower is Coltsfoot; in some places it is known as Foalsfoot and Bullsfoot, but these names are often misleading, as each district has a dialect and so name the flowers in that dialect. To be sure of the names of all plants we must know the Latin name, and then, of course, we must know the Class and Order that each plant comes under. If we know this, then we shall make no mistake in knowing one plant from another, and also know each virtue of the various plants. For this system of learning we are grateful to a man named Linnæus, who lived years and years ago.

Now, to continue about Coltsfoot, or, to give it the Latin name, Tussilago Farfara; it comes under the 19th Class and the 2nd Order. The flowers appear at the end of February, but the leaves come much later, and by that time the flowers have withered away. You will note the shape of the leaf, and it is covered with a layer of downy substance. This plant is famous for its medical properties, and is used in affections of the lungs. The leaves are used as a smoking mixture by many who suffer from Asthma. In some counties it has the name of "Old Man's Baccy." Country people gather the leaves, dry them, then rub them until they are broken up, and this is used instead of tobacco. Now, I do not wish any of you boys to try out this smoking mixture, for smoking is a bad habit, and I want both boys and girls to cultivate good habits. One good habit I want you to have is the habit of good breathing. Breathe always through your nose—the most intelligent people are "nose-breathers"; "mouth-breathers" are usually dull, stupid people. Each morning, go outside and fill your lungs with fresh air, breathe in slowly and raise your arms as high as your shoulders, then lower them to your side as you breathe out. Do this twelve times each morning of your life, all of you, whether you live in town or country. This will give the boys broad shoulders and healthy lungs, and the girls will develop a good figure of smart appearance. Your blood will circulate better, and instead of white faces, we shall see roses blooming in every cheek.

Cold Cures Still Wanted

"Some time ago I made an offer of a great reward to the doctor who found a cure for the common cold," said Sir Kingsley Wood, Minister of Health, at Foyles Literary luncheon in London yesterday

"That offer still remains open," he added.

(Press cutting,)

It seems obvious that the Medical Fraternity has no cure for a common cold as yet; if they had, this great reward which is pending would have been captured.

In the "Daily Herald," October 16th, 1934, there was a cartoon of a boxing match, Science versus Common Cold. At that time the Medical Scientists admitted that the common cold had got them beaten.

If Sir Kingsley Wood, "Minister of Health," is so interested in the public Health regarding a Cure for this distressing condition, why not extend his reward to some other school of medicine? Surely there is a cure.

We, as Herbal (or Nature) Practitioners, as one school, can prove to Sir Kingsley Wood that we have a Cure, if he would only make himself acquainted with the members of the N.A.M.H., who treat and cure thousands of cases during the winter months, and why?

We would be glad, yes, glad indeed to prove this, with or without the great reward he is offering, if only he would give us the chance; but I am afraid he will not do this because we are Unregistered. He has to do what he is told. What he wants is a cure;

but before that there should be the preventive.

Of course, there is no need to emphasise the symptoms, etc., as these are known by the general public.

The Medical Fraternity say that the cause of this trouble is germs, which enter the body; but our way of thinking is, that the diseased condition was there before the germs entered the body, brought about by the kidneys, bowels, lungs, liver and the skin not functioning, or not eliminating the waste matter from the body.

Persons are more susceptible to suffer from a common cold when their bodies are in this run-down condition during the cold and damp wintry months, following chills after chills, thus causing the blood to be driven inward, which soon sets up a fever, scanty urine, constipation, etc. The whole secretory organs become disordered by this destructive poisonous waste matter.

Nature along with the germs sets to work to eliminate this waste matter, which usually has been accumulating for weeks, sometimes months, also accelerated by the chills, and when all the waste matter has been cleared out of the system, the fever will subside, the germs die off, because there will be nothing for them to live on. Germs only live on unhealthy matter; healthy bodies will destroy them.

THE CURE

Regarding the cure, you will have to apply Nature's Remedies. How can one expect to get better from a cold, when all their blood stream is thick with waste matter, by taking a powder which only gives relief, but impossible to expel all the waste matter, leaving the patient liable to another attack, Or by taking from one to two teaspoonsful of cold medicine every four hours, when the fever is high and the congestion wants breaking up, and worse still if the medicine contains drugs (or poisons) which cannot co-operate with the vital force in its efforts to remove the cause of disease, but only impair its powers. Herbal (or Nature's) remedy will help Nature to eliminate the poisonous waste which has been allowed to develop and accumulate in the body.

If Sir Kingsley Wood wishes for a cure, here it is. First put the patient to bed with a hot-water bottle to his feet. Take ¾ oz. each Peppermint, Elder Flowers, ½ oz. each Marsh Mallow, Hyssop, Black Horehound, Raspberry Leaves, and Pleurisy Root, and 1 to 2 teaspoonsful of best Composition Powder.

Pour on them 2 quarts of boiling water, stand in the oven for 20 minutes, then strain through a fine cloth.

Dose.—Adults, ¾ teacupful, children 1 wineglassful, every half-hour for the first six doses as hot as can be taken; after, the same dose every hour for six doses. By this time the hot, dry skin will become moist and relaxed, and the patient will be in a gentle perspiration; the poisonous waste that has caused the cold will soon find its way through the skin, Lungs, kidneys and bladder.

There is only one way to treat a common cold, and that is to eliminate the waste, see to the diet; also see that the essential organs of the body are working perfectly, and you need have no fear of germs. F.W.

Diseases of Women and Children—Cont.

SARAH A. WEBB, M.D., (U.S.A.).

The second or permanent teeth are cut as follows.—1, First four molars, at six years, 2, right incisors, at seven years; 3, right tricuspids, at nine to ten years; 4, four canines at twelve to fourteen years; 5, second four molars, at twelve to fifteen years; 6, third four molars, at seventeen to twenty-five years. Except for the first four molars, the order is about the same as for the first set. In growing, the second set cause atrophy of the roots of the first set until they loosen and fall out. Particular attention should be paid to the teeth of children. Their regularity and soundness are of great importance to health, as well as being ornamental.

Exercise and Amusements. — Leaving children in their cribs without proper exercises has been the means of producing a marasmic or atrophic condition, due to faulty hygiene. A child of six months old should be placed on a large rug and permitted to roll or crawl at will. When infants are seven to eight months old and desire to stand, they should be encouraged to do so. This grasping and other muscular efforts stimulates the circulation, besides giving tone to the muscles. Older children should be permitted to exercise, so that there is a symmetrical development of the body.

Let the amusements of the children be outdoors as much as possible as they grow older, and let them exert themselves as much as they please. Their feelings will tell them when to rest and when to begin again. Let them be happy, joyous, and laughing—what Nature intended them to be. They ought to be encouraged to engage in those sports where the greatest number of muscles are brought into play, and let them shout, romp, and riot about as much as they please. Their lungs and muscles want development, and their nerves strengthening. As soon as children can run, let them race for half an hour through the rooms before going to bed. Regularity should be observed, as it is very essential to health. A young child should be put to bed at 6 p. m. in the winter and 7 p. m. in the summer. An old adage and a good rule is, "Early to bed and early to rise, brings good health and happiness." During storms children should be kept indoors. It is necessary to regulate the amount of exercise to the strength of the child. If fatigue or over-exhaustion are brought on by excessive exercise, it will be found to be just as productive of harm as under-exercise. As the child grows older sponge bath every morning chills the surface and causes the infant to draw long breaths; this expands the lungs and is the best form of pulmonary gymnastics.

Disorders of Infancy.—Injuries often occur during birth, when labour has been tedious, or where instruments have been used, such as elongation of the head, swelling upon the scalp, and distorted features. Usually no treatment is necessary other than gentle massage. The natural shape will be regained in one or two weeks.

Disease of the Umbilicus. — Bleeding from the navel cord sometimes occurs after birth, through carelessness in dressing, which is very dangerous. This should be watched by the nurse and a new ligature applied tightly, or fatal hæmorrhage may result. The neglect of such a condition, improper bandaging, or uncleanliness in this region is liable to cause not only convulsions, but blood-poisoning and death. Great care must be used to prevent the child from crying, as crying aggravates the abdomen and irritates the umbilicus.

Ulceration of the umbilicus sometimes occurs after the cord is separated. If so, dust it with equal parts of Slippery Elm Powder and Fuller's Earth, cover with a few layers of sterilised gauze, and keep in place with an abdominal binder.

Sometime granular tissue or fungus forms after separation of the cord, resembling a red bead; a discharge usually oozes, and it bleeds easily. Dust the granular tissue with a little Blood Root Powder and over this place Slippery Elm Powder, and cover with sterilised gauze.

Umbilical Hernia.—This varies in size from a simple convexity of the navel to a tumour large enough to become strangulated. A mechanical application is usually all that is required, the main care being to prevent the formation of a rupture by using an abdominal band during the first four months. I always make a pad with a large wooden button or a slice of a large cork, covered well with cotton. Place this securely over the navel, cover with a pad and bandage. This should be worn continually until the hernia is cured.

Icterus. Infantile Jaundice.—This is a common affection of the newly-born. There are two varieties, mild and severe. The mild is due to bile forming in the liver and then being carried into the circulation, the re-absorption being either due to congestion or to œdema of the hepatic tissue. The intense congestion of the skin observed during the first few hours of life often produces a yellowish colour that cannot be considered jaundice. The yellow tint is at first seen only on deep pressure, but as the erythema fades the colour increases. The conjunctivæ are not coloured, and the urine appears normal. Icterus is usually first noticed on the second day, and may continue a few days or a week. All the treatment needed for this is a laxative for the bowels.

The second form is fortunately rare, and may be produced by several different conditions such as defects in the bile ducts gall bladder, and liver. The yellowish discolouration of the skin may vary from day to day, at times being much more intense than at others. The conjunctivæ are yellow. The fœcal discharges lose colour and have an offensive odour, while the urine stains the napkin a yellowish or greenish brown. The spleen, as well as the liver, is usually enlarged, which accounts for the increase in the size of the abdomen. A very good laxative is made by steeping a few Senna pods in a little cold water over night, add a little simple syrup next morning, giving 1 teaspoonful every hour for three or four doses.

Conjunctivitis.—The eyes of a newly-born infant are very sensitive, and frequently the seat of inflammation. A mild inflammation is often seen, unattended by swelling, the lids and the inner surface being reddened, and covered with a slight viscous secretion, due to some infection, or soapy water getting into the eyes. The eyes must be kept cleansed by bathing them frequently in an infusion of Purple Loose-strife herb. A little vaseline may be applied to the lids at night to prevent retention of the secretion by adhesions to their edges.

MASTITIS (inflammation of the mammary glands).—The breasts of the new-born infant often secrete a milk-like substance, which appears between the fourth and tenth days after birth. During this time there may be a swelling of the glands, which generally abates with the subsidence of the secretion. In some cases the glands may remain engorged and tender and suppuration ensues. Massage with camphorated oil and apply hot applications to the breasts, covering with a breast binder. With care, this condition will pass away in a few days.

It is by no means easy for a mother to tell exactly when or how an infant begins to be ill, and a close observation of symptoms and their proper interpretation becomes highly important. Slight causes often produce very marked and sudden effects at this time of life. This is explained by the active growth of infants, and especially by the rapid development and irritability of the nervous system. In the absence of speech, the infant shows discomfort or suffering principally by cries and restlessness. If watched closely, it may by certain signs indicate to some extent the seat of the trouble. In headache, the hand will be frequently raised and held beside the head; in ear-ache, the hand will be held to the ear, and often pull upon that organ, or the child will keep rolling its head from side to side, or upon pressing in front and behind the ear, the baby will wince or cry.

The Power of Habit

"I trust everything to habit—habit, upon which in all ages the law-giver as well as the school-master has mainly placed his reliance; habit, which makes everything easy and casts all difficulties upon the deviation from the wonted course. Make sobriety a habit, and intemperance will be hateful and hard; make prudence a habit, and reckless profligacy will be as contrary to the nature of the child grown an adult as the most atrocious crimes are to any of your Lordships. Give a child the habit of sacredly regarding truth; of carefully respecting the property of others; of scrupulously abstaining from all acts of improvidence which can involve him in stress and he will just as little think of lying, or cheating, or stealing, or running into debt, as of rushing into an element in which he cannot breathe."—Lord Brougham.

HEALERS OUSTING DOCTORS.

Twenty-two million Germans, or one-third of the nation, are claimed as 'devotees' of the new 'Nature-Healing Movement,' in an interview published by the 'Voelkischer Beobachter.'

"The head of the 'Nature Doctors' League,' which now numbers 5,800 members, and enjoys Government recognition as a scientific organization, announces that 'there is today a great crisis in German medicine.'

300,000 Patients

"Statistics of the Society show that in February Nature-Doctors and Faith-Healers treated 300,000 patients—despite the fact that about 200,000 of these were 'State-insurance' cases.

"This is hailed as striking evidence of the popularity of Nature-healing, since a visit to an ordinary physician is paid by Government insurance, while treatment by a Nature-Doctor must still be paid for out of the patient's own pocket.—Reuter."

Acute Articular Rheumatism or Rheumatic Fever

By J. R. YEMM, F.N.A., D.O.

I have been requested by a subscriber to contribute a short article on this particular form of rheumatism (which is undoubtedly the most dangerous form), from the fact that it is often followed by permanent heart weakness. It is a disorder most common in males from 10 to 30 years of age, occurring most frequently in spring and autumn.

As to the cause there are numerous theories; some claim it being due to lactic acid in the blood, while others think it is of bacterial (Streptococcus) origin; many cases are apparently hereditary. The onset is generally abrupt after an ordinary chill, sore throat, feverishness with slight pains in the wrists, elbows or knees. Soon one of the larger joints become enlarged, hot, reddened and painful; the pains pass from joint to joint, disappearing from one to quickly appear in another, until most of the larger joints have in turn been attacked. The temperature rapidly rises 102 degrees F. to 105 degrees F., declining just a little to rise again with each access of joint symptoms. Hyperpyrexia, that is, an excessive high temperature of sometimes 110 degrees F., may occur at any stage of the disease; this is a very dangerous feature, but there is not much fear of this happening if you can get the secretions working. The pulse is often disproportionately frequent, full and bounding. The tongue is covered with a thick white coating, the bowels constipated, urine scanty, highly coloured and freely deposits uric acid. Another feature is copious acid prespirations, after a spell of which the temperature falls a little for a time.

Among the numerous complications of rheumatic fever is endocarditis. This is an inflammation of the membranes lining the heart, and occurs most frequently in the young rather than the older persons. Chorea or St. Vitus' Dance also frequently follow the fever in the young.

Treatment

The patient should be put to bed and lie between blankets, and wear a flannel night shirt. Complete rest is one of the first essentials, and it is a wise plan for the patient to rest a week or so in bed after the temperature becomes normal. I always advise this, especially in the case of young children, relapses and recurrences are thus offtimes averted. As soon as the patient is in bed, make an infusion of Meadowsweet 3 parts, Angelica 2 parts, Pleurisy Root (pulv.) 2 parts, Ginger 1 part. Use 2 ozs. of this compound to make a pint of medicine, and give warm in doses according to age of patient. This warm herb tea should be given frequently every ½ to 1 hour until the patient is in good perspiration, then give every 2 to 3 hours, keeping the patient gently perspiring all the while. Keep the bowels open with Herbal Liver Pills. The bowels should be opened at least once a day. At the onset of the attack it is sometimes useful to give a good brisk purge; this, of course, is determined by the condition of the patient. Keep the kidneys gently stimulated with Gravel Root or Clivers; these may be added to the infusion first mentioned. If the pains are very bad, add a few drops of Anti-Spasmodic Tincture to each dose of medicine, or give a pill composed of equal parts of Valerian, Wild Yam and Lobelia 2—5 grains, according to age of patient, 2 to 3 times a day. It is rare I use any treatment to the joints, but in bad cases I use a liniment compounded of Tinct. Blue Cohosh 2 parts, Tinct. Lobelia 1 part, Tinct. Capsicum 3 parts; shake well together, rub a little on the joints very lightly and cover up warm. When the fever is declining massage the joints very gently. The diet should be light. Slippery Elm Food is a good article for use. Milk and sugar I have found harmful. Good vegetable soups will be found far more nourishing. Fruit can be used freely; a baked apple makes a nice change for the patient, white fish, steamed, can be given. Drinks should be lemonade or orangeade, unsweetened, and given ad lib. Tea and coffee are best avoided, but good drinking water can be given at all times. The patient should be wiped down daily to keep the skin clean. There is no fear of the patient "getting chilled" if a reasonable amount of care is taken; just do one limb at a time so as not to expose the whole body at once.

"This 'Samson' Lives on Oranges, Bread and Milk

"By TERRENCE HORSLEY

"I have found a young giant in Ashton-under-Lyne who, after eating two oranges for breakfast, can bend half-inch mild steel bars, snap chains, and remain calm while motor cars run over him.

"Lunching on bread and milk, and eating another two oranges with a little brown bread and butter for tea, he will absent-mindedly twist the poker round his middle finger while he is talking to you.

"In between times he stokes a furnace for 10 hours every day, and keep his mother in their little house on his wages.

"Jimmy de Looze was not impressed by the B.M.A. menus which have recently been given publicity in the 'Daily Dispatch,' and wrote to tell us what he could do on a diet of oranges, bread and milk, an occasional onion, and brown bread and butter, washed down with barley water. I went to see him.

"To show that he wasn't joking, he tossed me a steel bar and invited me to make it look like a hairpin. I tried, but as far as I was concerned it was clear that the bar would remain straight for ever.

"Then Jimmy took it. He made it ring with a flick of his finger nails to show that it was good steel, and then politely folded it up. After that he wrapped a chain which had a breaking strain of 600-lb. round his chest and took a deep breath. The chain snapped with a noise like a pistol shot.

"The exhibition was interrupted by the little old lady by the fireside. 'Your tea's waiting for you Jimmy,' she said, and thereupon Jimmy sat down and made a hearty meal of two oranges and three slices of brown bread.

"A Furnace Stoker

"'Wouldn't you like some nice roast beef,' I asked him.

"'I couldn't stand it,' he replied. 'I've been living on this for years now, and feel so fit that 10 hours stoking a furnace just seems to loosen my muscles.'

"The only training that Jimmy does is 15 minutes' exercise in his bedroom every night, contracting and expanding his muscles. After that he has a bath and goes to sleep.

"'Are all your family as strong as you,' I asked him.

"'Not quite,' he smilingly replied.

"A delightful fellow, with a charming smile, he has a chest which grows from 35 inches to 45 inches when he breathes. I'm going to try oranges for breakfast myself now!"

From the "Daily Dispatch," September 27th, 1935.

Diseases of Women and Children—Cont.

SARAH WEBB, M.D. (U.S.A.)

In painful dentition, the fingers will be constantly inserted in the mouth, as if to pull out the cause of the distress. Irritation of the stomach and bowels may be accompanied by a continual rubbing of the nose. During an attack of colic, the legs are drawn up over the abdomen, which feels hard; there is likewise a withering motion of the body, the hand is tightly shut, with the thumb thrust deeply into the palms, and the toes strongly bent, and there is much nervous irritation, which may end in convulsions.

A mother will soon learn where the trouble lies by the kind and style of cry. It is laboured, as if the child were half-suffocated, or as if a door were shut between the child and the hearer, in pneumonia and capillary bronchitis; it is hoarse in croup; brassy and metallic, with crowing inspirations, in cerebral diseases; in marasmus and tubercular peritonitis it is moaning and wailing. Continual and obstinate crying is usually due to earache or hunger. A louder shriller cry, sometimes with coughing when the child is moved, is pleuritic. A cry with wriggling and writhing and preceding defecation denotes intestinal trouble. Moaning is especially characteristic of an alimentary canal trouble.

Changes of the Features.—When illness is present it is quickly shown in the countenance of the infant, which, during health is in a condition of easy repose. In general, it can be stated that the upper part of the face is involved in diseases of the head, the middle part of the face in affections of the chest, and the lower part in disturbance involving the abdominal organs. Thus, in diseases of the brain, the forehead and eyebrows will be sharply contracted, and the eyes sensitive to light, with various changes in the pupils. Puffiness and swelling about the eyelids point to dropsy, which is usually caused by diseases of the kidneys, following scarlet fever or other infectous processes, but occasionally by severe anæmia. In pneumonia and pleurisy the nostrils are sharply defined, they dilate and contract with the movements of respiration, which will appear more or less laboured. The mouth is the feature most affected in abdominal diseases, shown by a drawing up of the upper lip, and other movements indicating pain.

Discharges.—These are very important, and a careful examination of all the organs opening upon the surface of the body must be made to detect any abnormal discharges, including the eyes, ears, nose, mouth, urinary, and rectal regions. The upright position of the stomach during infancy renders vomiting a frequent and easy symptom when this organ is distended, or if there be a regurgitation of some curdled milk after each feed. The infant shows no distress from this act when in good health, the stomach simply rejecting any excess of food which it cannot readily hold. But sudden and profuse vomiting, without any error in diet, may indicate the approach of severe illness, such as scarlet fever, diphtheria, or some brain disease. Or vomiting may be simply a sign of local disturbance in the stomach, as when mucus is ejected in cases of gastric irritation. Where tough curds are vomited, with the milk very sour, there is evidence of fermentation of the milk and an over-acid condition of the stomach. If this persists, the mouth will become red and sore from continued irritation.

Much will be learned by investigating the number and character of the discharges from the bowels, and in observing urine. During the first two months there are usually three or four stools in twenty-four hours, and during the first two years, two stools a day on an average. The stools are homogeneous, of a soft, semi-solid consistency, and of yellowish colour. In cases of diarrhœa or inflammation they may be green, or contain hard, lumpy curds, or have an admixture of mucus and blood, or be of a very watery consistency.

"THE COMMON COLD

"Doctor Claims He Has Found A Cure

"What is claimed to be a cure for the common cold is given by a naval surgeon commander in a letter to 'The Times.'

"He writes, 'A heaped teaspoonful of ordinary soda bicarbonate (baking soda) taken in an ordinary (half-pint) tumblerful of hot water four times in 24 hours will speedily dispel an existing cold or ward off an incipient one.'

"The writer adds that he has tested it repeatedly on his naval patients and found it to 'work like magic.' "

We have also read of an equally

effective cure with lemon juice. In fact, its advocates—and there are many—claim that unsweetened lemon juice to be **the** remedy. To a person of an enquiring mind, these two "cures" do not seem to reconcile, because one is an alkali and the other an acid (although it is argued that the acid in the lemon is converted into alkali within the body; primarily it is an acid). To our mind, there are times when lemon juice is contra-indicated; there are also occasions when Sodi Bicarb "works like magic"—the black kind.

In our eagerness to find "cures," we are apt to forget the rudiments of our science, which really is the foundation on which we build. Occasionally our circulating fluids get into an acid state, "Acidosis"; it also can become excessive alkaline, "Alkalosis." When we can recognise these states, then we can employ an acid or an alkaline agent with sure results, because we supply a physiological deficiency, and it "works like magic."

Our old Eclectic Masters knew these different states: the colour of the tongue was their indication. At that time physicians were observant men; they studied their patients; the name of a disease was of secondary consideration. It was their endeavour to ascertain the deficiencies within the circulating fluids; they studied drug action at the bedside. For the harvest which we now gather in the form of a wonderfully replete Materia Medica, our thanks are due to those intellectual giants—the Fathers of the Botanic and Eclectic systems of medicine.

Shakespeare wrote: "For nought so vile that on the earth doth live, But to the earth some special doth give." We have often thought over those two lines. In our study of the marvellous economy of Nature, of the various changes and interchanges which are continually taking place in the wonderful phenomena of Life; everything seems to have a relationship: it serves its purpose and then dies. Or take another form. The mineral feeds the plant, the plant the animal, and the animal man, who again dissolves into the mineral state. To our mind, man is the head of creation, and whilst most things are for his use, or subservient to his will, there are certain things of which he has no direct use for but are part of the great plan whereby they have certain work to do. But with the advancement, (?) of Science, we must modify or change our viewpoint, as witness the following:—

"WOUNDS CURED BY MAGGOTS

"A use has at last been found for the universally condemned housefly. Its maggots can be used to clean up wounds.

"Hospitals can now purchase supplies of clean living maggots for the treatment of infected wounds. They can even obtain extract of ground-up maggots.

"Injections of this extract have been found useful in the treatment of certain bone disease, such as mastoid infections."

God help Medicine if we shall have to stoop to such a practice, or become so destitute of medicinal agents that we must resort to such filth.

To our way of thinking, the "universally condemned housefly" is one of Nature's scavengers. Take a piece of putrid meat, place it out of doors, and flies are attracted. They blow on the meat and maggots appear, which eat up the mass of putrefying matter. Then the birds of the air eat up the maggots—Nature's method of cleansing.

CATTLE AND TUBERCULOSIS

"Dear Sir,—I was amazed to read in your issue of June 29th the full page report concerning the campaign against the Tuberculosis scourge. The state of affairs, as at present exist, is not much of a compliment for the medical system which has been operating all these years. To allow Tuberculosis to run rampant amongst the cattle and human beings, as is now admitted, is a woeful position. Moreover than this, it seems ludicrous that the medical profession should still endeavour to formulate vaccines to cure people from the dreaded disease, or if not to cure them, to prevent contracting them.

"A logical person, which, of course, is not usually a doctor, would consider the best way to prevent the disease by obviating the use of foods which cause it. There is no difficulty in anyone living comfortable and in perfect health without utilising either flesh or milk which often comes from diseased cattle.

"Bovine Tuberculosis has increased since the commercialisation of cows, and the mass production of milk by pouring Cotton Seed Oil down their mouth, and allowing the body to churn it up, which is afterwards sucked away by an apparatus which breaks down the cells and draws blood, manure, bacteria and pus away with the milk. If more investigations were made in this respect, a successful issue could be eventually anticipated.

"This method of inoculation which the doctors adopt, of putting the cart before the horse, will only fill hospitals and continually increase the living costs and the general burden of the people.

"Health is our birthright, and if the Ministry of Health and the medical fraternity cannot produce a healthy race in this country, it is time they got out and let someone else to get on with the work.

"It was proved during the War that we are a C.3. nation, and since then, Cancer has jumped up in leaps and bounds; Bovine Tuberculosis has increased, while the last epidemic of Diphtheria was a disgrace to the authorities. If only we could revert to the more natural and rational laws of living as laid down in the Book of Moses, utilise the vegetable kingdom as it was intended to be utilised, and avoid the inoculation and vaccination craze, life would be worth living for those who are at present destined to perish from some of these abominable and unnecessary diseases.—Yours,

"C. C. ABBOTT."

"The Nature-Doctors use herbs and other old-fashioned remedies. One of their aims is the abolition of medicaments."

RHEUMATISM

By F. WORTHINGTON

Rheumatism is a term applied to an inflamed and congested part of the body, having various names according to the part affected—in the joints, muscles, tendons, nerves, etc. Rheumatism is brought about by certain organs of the body such as the kidneys, lungs, bowels, liver, and skin not functioning, or in other words, not eliminating the waste (or poisonous) matter from the body, which gradually becomes overloaded.

This waste is absorbed and carried to different parts of the body by the blood vessels, and is finally deposited in the joints, muscles, etc., causing an obstruction in the system.

In all cases of Rheumatism, we find an excess of acids in the body, and it is often said that the presence of uric acid in the blood is a contributory factor, but there are, however, other acids formed in the body which are also absorbed into the blood stream (they are not caused by eating acid fruits, but by the result of fermentation and putrefaction of foods taking place in the alimentary (bowel) canal, thus causing a toxæmic (a poisoned state) condition of the blood.

Rheumatism is a diseased condition, and can only develop in the human body when the blood stream is in an impaired or unhealthy state.

We must, then, remove the cause that has produced this condition (whether it be faulty kidney, liver, bowels, etc., and excess of starchy foods, decayed teeth, or by the presence of some injurious poisons circulating in the blood, which is present in certain diseases when there is a toxæmic state of the blood), and live in harmony with Nature's laws, to build and keep up the vital forces within the body, then this condition (or any other disease) will go, and we need have no fear of the so-called streptococci germ, or any other germs entering the body.

Healthy bodies will destroy germs—they only become dangerous when suitable soil or culture is found for their habitation.

There are many other factors which cause Rheumatism, but space will not permit me to enlarge upon it.

ACUTE RHEUMATISM (Rheumatic Fever or Inflammatory Rheumatism)

Symptoms.—This condition may develop suddenly, though commonly the onset is gradual for several days when the patient will complain of general illness, or feeling uncomfortable, with a slight soreness of the throat, and soreness or pain in the limbs, usually the knees.

About the third or fourth day, the pains increase, and fever quickly follows; within 24 hours the fever may be fully established, the temperature rising rapidly to about 103 or 104 degrees, which in the course of the disease may rise and fall; the latter may be expected after a good sweating.

The pulse is rapid, full and soft,

and somewhat unsteady. The urine becomes scanty, and of a high colour, often loaded with urates (acid). The face is flushed and puffy, especially under the eyes.

There is constipation, loss of appetite, and they suffer from great thirst, usually the tongue is larger, flat, and covered with an extremely thick fur, which gets the name of "blanket tongue."

The patients get tender to touch all over the body, with a desire to lie on their back, with limbs in various positions so as to give relief; they will lie very quiet, afraid to make any attempt to move, on account of the agonising pain they are in, lying there prostrated and completely helpless, which is usually worse during the night.

Inflammation and congestion have now rapidly subsided in a joint becoming involved before the shiny, and very painful, and often changes suddenly from one joint to another (metastasis), another joint becoming in volved before the recovery of the first one. It generally takes from three to four days for a joint to rise and subside, and the same joint may return again.

The joints most commonly affected are the knees, wrists, elbows, and ankles. In milder cases the small joints, such as the fingers and toes, are usually affected, but in severe cases the larger joints, such as the shoulders and hips, also suffer.

With the severe pain and high fever, the patient perspires profusely (poisonous waste being expelled from the body, which should have been passed through the natural source, the kidneys, bowels, etc.), causing a decidedly sour (acid) smell in character, increasing the weakness of the patient without relieving the pain, and often by the excess of this sweating, the follicles of the skin, and other cutaneous glands, become inflamed and painful in consequence, causing unpleasant eruptions, such as sudamina miliaria (small besicles or blisters on the skin), pelioses (small red spots like fleabites around the ankles), and purura (purple spots on the legs).

Sometimes there are subcutaneous fibrous nodules develop over the bone ridges, and an enlargement of the lymph glands. As the disease advances, the poisonous waste in the body causes a rapid destruction of the red blood corpuscles (leucocytosis), and the patient becomes very pale and anæmic.

Complications may intervene with or after the attack if not attended to and rightly treated.

The most serious affected is the heart, when the commonest trouble develops endocarditis (inflammation of the inner lining membrane), which may lead to injury of the valves, pericarditis (inflammation of the membrane which envelops the heart), and myocarditis (inflammation of its muscular substance).

Other complications on some occasions are pneumonia, bronchitis, and pleurisy, etc.

TREATMENT

The patient should go to bed as soon as the pains and fever appear, the bed should be soft and level, in a well-ventilated room, but care should be taken to keep up an even and moderate temperature, by having a fire in, preventing draughts by means of a screen round the bed.

A hot-water bottle should be placed at the feet, and one on each side of the body.

A flannel night-gown should be worn, made to open all the way down, with sleeves loose or slit down from the shoulders to the wrist, fastened with buttons. Two or three of these should be made to allow frequent changing.

The patient should lie between soft, light, but warm blankets, instead of sheets, and when the pains are very severe, these should be supported by a cradle over the body.

Medicine.—Get from any Herbalist of repute the following:—Meadowsweet Herb, ¾ oz.; Yarrow Herb, ¾ oz.; Clivers Herb, ½ oz.; Broom Herb, ½ oz.; Bittersweet Herb, ½ oz.; Sassafras Bark, ¼ oz.; Prickley Ash Berries, ¼ oz.; Celery Seeds, ¼ oz.; Ginger Root, ¼ oz.; Spanish, ½ oz.; Senna Leaves, as required for the bowels.

To the above pour on one quart of boiling water, stand in the oven for 20 minutes, then strain through a fine cloth.

Dose.—Adults, ½ to ¾ teacupful, children ½ to ¾ wineglassful (hot), every two hours for the first two days, so as to produce free perspiration, thereby assisting Nature to throw the toxic material out of the body through the pores of the skin, also through the kidneys. Also, get an Herbal Practitioner to make up for you:—

Fluid Ext. Passiflora Incarnata. . ¾ ounce
Fluid Ext. Cypripedium Pubescens. . 1¼ "

Take from 10 to 15 drops in a tablespoonful of warm water, in between the medicine. This will soothe and relieve the excited or irritated nervous system.

If you should find any difficulty, consult a Herbal Practitioner as soon as possible.

Herbal (or Nature's) remedy will help Nature to eliminate the poisonous waste which has developed in the body. Drugs cannot co-operate with the vital force in its efforts to remove the cause of disease—they tend to impair its powers.

After the medicine has been taken two days, the same dose can be taken every four hours (warm).

(Note.—Don't keep all the medicine warm, as it will not keep—just add a little hot water to each dose).

An injection to the bowels should be given every night, made from Peppermint Herb, ½ oz. to about 1 or 2 quarts of boiling water. Strain through a fine cloth, and when blood heat, inject into the bowels what can be taken.

The patient should be sponged down twice or three times a day to prevent the waste (or sweat) being absorbed into the body again, with warm water and a few drops of pure malt vinegar added.

The joints should be gently rubbed with Methyl Salicylate (fort) B.P.C. ointment.

Diet.—Generally, at the first onset, the patient does not want any food—this will not do them any harm for a few days—it will help Nature to get rid of the waste in system; if they desire a drink, they should have orange or lemon juice mixed with warm water (unsweetened), or a drink of Slippery Elm food.

All sugar and starchy foods should be avoided.

The herbal medicine being taken acts as food as well as medicine.

If the patient desires any food, the fruit should be taken raw, and vegetables fresh.

Fruits that can be taken are apples, pears, oranges, grapes, cherries, plums, dates, and figs.

Vegetables.—Cabbage, cauliflower, carrots, celery, turnips, watercress, and vegetable soup made from some of the above (if in season), with addition of parsley and sage, and a little crumbled wholemeal bread added.

Any of the white fish may be taken, but should be fried in best olive oil.

Diseases of Women and Children—Cont.

SARAH A. WEBB, M.D. (U.S.A.)

In a new-born baby the urine sometimes causes worry to the nurse. The baby nearly always passes urine when born, due to pressure on the parts. When the baby does not pass water in reasonable time, great pain and screaming soon take take place, due to stoppage of the bladder. If twelve hours pass without evacuation from the bladder and bowels, place the baby in warm water for 10 minutes, and apply a flannel dipped in warm water over the bladder or lower organs. In some cases where the urine is highly acid it may be expelled when a few drops collect in the bladder, and as this amount quickly dries in the diaper, there is no evidence from wetting that urine has been passed. A dark, smoke-coloured urine, loaded with uric acid and urates, may leave a red deposit upon the napkin simulating blood. Make a tea from water melon or marrow seeds and give the child the warm tea to drink every half-hour, in teaspoon doses. This generally relieves the condition.

Thrush, or Nursing Sore Mouth. —This is an inflammation and ulceration of the mucous membrane of the mouth, occurring within the first year of life, due to improperly prepared food, and general lack of cleanliness. The babe refuses to take its nourishment, and is very irritable. The mouth is tender and hot. First there is marked drooling and then redness of the surface of the tongue and all around the gums. The tongue may be coated. Soon whitish spots appear arising above the surface of the mucous membrane which do not rub off easily, and leave a bleeding surface. They appear first on the tongue, spreading to the cheeks, and may spread to the lips, palate, tonsils, and pharynx, and at times to the œsophagus and stomach. Each spot has the appearance of a little lump of coagulated milk. These cases usually have diarrhœa, and acrid, irritating stools, followed by pain, emaciation, and often death.

The trouble can be prevented through cleanliness of nipples, bottles, and mouth, and moderating the food. Wash the mouth out after each feed with Sage Tea, applying it with a soft rag, or make a decoction of Hydrastis (or Golden Seal) Powder and wash the mouth; this is found to be very good.

Follicular Stomatitis, or Sore Mouth, is an inflammation with the formation of small vesicles, the latter forming superficial ulcers.

These ulcers are at first discrete, but may coalesce into larger ones, always, however, remaining superficial. At first isolated yellowish-spots on the lips, mouth, or palate are noticed, surrounded by a reddened mucous membrane, due to uncleanliness, dentition, or gastro-intestinal disorders. With proper treatment and care the period of this condition can be considerably shortened. But if improperly managed it may lead to ulcerative stomatitis, which is more serious. Cleanliness is very important. Wash the mouth every two or three hours with an infusion of Golden Seal Powder, made by pouring one pint of boiling water on one teaspoonful of the powder, or make a weak solution of the Compound Tincture of Myrrh.

Ulcerative Stomatitis, or Sore Mouth.—This may be a continuation of the follicular sore mouth, and it may be due to decayed teeth, improper food, bad hygiene, taking of mercury, exhausting diseases, scurvy, or infectious diseases. It is generally found in the second year of life. Attention may be attracted to the child because food is refused and pain is caused by attempts at eating. The breath is foul and the tongue is coated. Children with this condition are irritable and sleep badly. They become weak and depressed from lack of food. Examination of the mouth shows the gums at first to be swollen and red. The lower jaw is commonly involved at some point situation on the edge of the gums. A purulent exudate is then formed, leading to necrosis and ulceration on the gum margin, which spreads all over the mouth.

Risking Death For Flowers

By PETER DAVIS

" 'Death Flower—Kills Climber —300 ft. Fall in Alps—Trying to Get Edelweiss.'

"So said a recent headline. There followed a story of an intrepid sparetime explorer, a plant enthusiast, who had crashed to his doom while striving to get one more blossom.

"Thus it is all too often. Behind the tranquility of every Flower Show there frequently lies a tale of death faced in forgotten valley, on dangerous mountain slopes, in perilous marshes—somewhere on the other side of the earth.

"Men at this moment are fighting the demon altitude or warring against hostile natives, daring flood and fever for the sake of flowers.

Heroine of the Arctic

"A dwarf plant climbs to a height of eight inches because men fought and wrestled for it in the perilous hills on the Tibet-Assam frontier. A mere slip of a leaf tells of a woman's fight against Arctic cold. This carnation, much sought after by growers from Iceland, Norway and Sweden, is the result of 20 years of work for its perfection.

"As a result, England will be further beautified for our children. Already Britain has been changed into a country of strange flowers.

"We have wrested roses from India and China; pinks, carnations, and daffodils from Asia Minor; nasturtiums, dahlias, and cosmos from Mexico; rhododendrons and crocuses from the warm lands bordering the Mediterranean. Lilacs, laburnums, chrysanthemums, Michaelmas daises and horse-chestnut flowers are but a few of the 12,000 exotic plants we have made grow upon our island against all Nature's plain first intentions.

"Still the search proceeds for new seeds which horticulturists and botanists may breed by selection and acclimatise until you and I shall be able to buy a packet of new seeds. In the most inaccessible places, more and more inaccessible as the process of robbing the world for our gardeners goes on, plant-hunting is proving one of the most adventurous professions left to a sombre modern world.

"A short time ago Isobel Hutchinson, a young Scotswoman, set out for the Arctic Circle in search of rare flower and plant specimens. No sooner had she started her adventure than she encountered blizzards and was forced to charter an Eskimo vessel to help her on her way.

Dog-Team Journey

"This craft, however, became frozen-in 350 miles from her destination. It took courage—the plant-hunter's courage—to set out alone as Miss Hutchinson did, to complete the trip with borrowed dog teams, despite a temperature that was sometimes 60 below zero.

"The King of the botanist-explorers Captain Kingdon Ward, recently returned to this country successful in the discovery of more than 40 new kinds of trees, shrubs, and Alpine plants. Now he is off again to comb Pome and Poyou, two of the least known provinces of Tibet.

"He is the hero of a hundred adventures in China, Burma, India, and the Himalayas. He has climbed peaks untrodden by white men, floated down torrential rivers on shaky rafts, has discovered an unknown race of people, as well as many unknown varieties of flowers.

"He discovered the lost source of the Irrawaddy, but felt far more pleased when he brought home the seeds of the blue poppy of Tibet.

"Plant hunters brought back broad beans from America. In a decade intensive cultivation reduced the plant to a stature so small that it can be grown successfully in a frame, much earlier than when it was in the open garden.

"Garden peas were discovered to be too small to be worth the labour of shelling. So we have managed to double their size.

"We have turned weeds into glorious cinerarias. We have turned useless roots into staple food for man and beast.

"Can you wonder that Nature occasionally attempts to get her own back?"

From the "Daily Dispatch," August 29, 1935.

Botulism Case at Hammersmith

"Doctor's Experiments
"Special Serum's Efficacy

"Experiments on mice were described at an inquest held at Hammersmith yesterday on David Rees Edwards (55), a commercial traveller, of Nascot Street, Wood Lane, Hammersmith, who died in hospital on August 22.

"The jury returned a verdict of death by misadventure due to the toxic poisoning of botulism.

"Food poisoning had been suspected, and Dr. Edwin Smith, the coroner, had adjourned the proceedings so that there could be an analysis of the contents of the stomach.

"Mrs. Mabel Edwards said that she made a meat pie for her husband on Wednesday, August 14, and on the following Sunday he said: 'There's a little left. Do you think it will be all right,' She replied: 'Do not eat it because the weather is so hot.' 'As far as I knew it was all right,' she added, 'but the weather was so hot that I should not have liked to eat it. I should think he did eat some that day.'

"Dr. B. Barling, senior medical officer at Hammersmith Hospital, said that he came to the conclusion that Edward's case was definitely one of botulism. 'We obtained a special serum from the Ministry of Health,' added Dr. Barling, 'as soon as we could, but he gradually became weaker and died seven and a half hours later.'

"Dr. A. Ashley Miles, assistant pathologist at Hammersmith Hospital, said that Mrs. Edwards brought him eight or nine ounces of gravy, some cooked sausages, and some cooked chops. He took two sets of mice, three in each set. Into one of the first set he injected some of the gravy, into another an extract of the sausages, and into the third an extract of the chops. Into the second set he injected similar substances, but they also received some of the specific serum against botulism. The mice receiving the sausages and chops were perfectly well the next day, as was the mouse which received the gravy plus the specific anti-serum, but the mouse which had received gravy was dead within fifteen hours.

"Sir Bernard Spilsbury said that from the experiments described he thought it was clearly established that botulism was the cause of death. Poisoning was more likely to occur in vegetable food.

" 'Vegetables are likely to be contaminated if they have been insufficiently cooked and then left in very hot weather. The organism may have time to develop. That is why in very hot weather these cases occasionally occur.'

"Sir Bernard added that the infecting bacillus would not grow in the body. It was only when the poison had already developed in the food that it was dangerous. Botulism was fortunately, rare in this country.

"Replying to the corner, Dr. J. B. Howell, Medical Officer of Health for Hammersmith, said that there was no evidence that there had been any other cases connected with this one."

From the "Manchester Guardian," September 10th, 1935.

BEES AND HONEY

Does the food which the Bees feed on, affect the Honey in any way, If so, please explain in what way? If not, why does C. C. Abbott say in the "Herbalist," March, 1936, "that honey is not the food that some would have us believe, from the fact that bee-keepers feed their Bees entirely on white sugar, as the Bees refuse to partake of natural brown sugar!" Many of the readers, besides T. Gwernogle Evans, will appreciate an explanation of the point.

Diseases of Women and Children—Cont.

SARAH A. WEBB, M.D. (U.S.A.)

In aggravated cases the teeth are exposed and loosened in their sockets. The submaxillary lymphatic glands are badly swollen and painful. The tongue is swollen, thickly coated, and shows the indentation of the teeth on the edges. Drooling is pronounced. The odour is distinctly fetid. Cleanliness is the first essential, keeping the mouth scrupulously clean by frequent washing with Golden Seal or Myrrh decoction. Remove the cause, whatever it may be, and give light, nourishing diet. Slippery Elm food is excellent. Also regulate the bowels.

Elongated Uvula.—Although rarely observed, this condition has led to much improper medication for persistent cough. The elongated uvula irritates the pharynx and causes a cough, which is especially marked when the prone position is assumed, or when the child is over-tired. If the chest symptoms are negative, this condition should be thought of. The elongation should be snipped off, or an astringent used such as Bayberry or Golden Seal Powder.

Tongue-tie consists of an abnormally short frænum. It may interfere with suckling, and later may possibly affect the speech, but it is not nearly so important as is commonly supposed. Snip the frænum near its attachment to the tongue with a pair of scissors, or with a dull instrument, or, better, with a **sharp point on the finger nail.**

Pharyngitis, or Inflammation of the Pharynx.—The pharynx and tonsils are inflamed and red. It may be, and frequently is, a primary disease; or it may be part of one of the infectious diseases, such as scarlet fever, measles, diphtheria, or influenza. There is pain in swallowing, and dryness in the throat, later an increase in the secretion, and an irritating cough. On examination, the soft palate, uvula, tonsils, and pharynx are seen to be red and inflamed. There is a rise of temperature. Headache and vomiting may be present. A stimulating emetic should be given, by giving the child warm Composition and broken doses of Lobelia. Wash the tonsils three or four times daily with Tincture of Myrrh and water (equal parts). For the bowels give one teaspoonful of Neutralising Cordial every two hours.

Nasal Catarrh. — Infants often sneeze normally during the first few days of life, the mechanical irritation of dust in the air being the cause. Children in many families have a predisposition to catarrh. It is most likely contagious. The handkerchief can, no doubt, carry the contagion from one to another. There are two primary causes of Catarrh: (1) Children that are kept indoors and muffled up so that their bodies are over-heated and so sensitive to exposure, will have catarrh; (2) children who, in order to be "hardened," are over-exposed while they are still sensitive.

There is a hyperæmia in the nasal passage, causing obstruction. This will compel the infant to breathe through the mouth. It will also interfere with the feeding. The nose being stuffed, the infant must breathe through the mouth. The secretions at first are thin and mucous; later on they assume a mucco-purulent character. This latter discharge is thick and sticky, and while drying obstructs the nostrils.

Put the child to bed. If there is fever, keep the child warm. The body should be warmly clad. Make an infusion of White Pine Bark, 1-oz. to 1 pint. Give in teaspoonful doses, sweetened; increase dose according to age.

Tonsilitis, or Inflammation of the Tonsils.—The whole mucous membrane of the pharynx and tonsil is inflamed. The tonsils may be somewhat enlarged and are covered with very fine pinhead points of a whitish exudation. There is fever and restlessness, and difficult swallowing.

Give liquid diet, and keep the child warm. Where the tonsils are enlarged, poultice with a Linseed Meal poultice sprinkled with a little Lobelia, Capsicum, or Ginger. Make a syrup (4-oz.) with Xanthoxylum 2 drams, and give in teaspoonful doses every 3 hours.

HERBAL REMEDIES

Directions how to make the following remedies:—Pour on them one quart of boiling water, stand in the oven for 20 minutes, then strain through a fine cloth.

Dose. — Adults, ½ teacupful; Children, ½ to 1 wineglassful every three or four hours, after meals.

St. Vitus Dance

Scullcap .... ½ ounce
Mistletoe .... ½ "
Ground Ivy .... ½ "
Valerian Root .... ½ "
Senna Leaves ...... as required
Spanish Licorice ...... ½ ounce
Ginger Root .... ¼ "
Decoction of Sarsaparilla . . 6-ounces

Nerves in the Head, Headaches &c.

Wood Betony .... ½ ounce
Scullcap .... ½ "
Vervain .... ½ "
Hops .... ½ "
Senna Leaves ...... as required
Valerian Root .... ¼ ounce
Ginger Root .... ¼ "
Spanish Licorice ...... ½ "

GOTU KOLA

The Secret of Perpetual Youth

By VINCENT DE SILVA

From the Ceylon *Daily News* of Dec. 22, 1932

Man's dream has always been to discover the secret of perpetual youth, and many men have devoted all their lives to this problem.

We have heard of Ponce de Leon who sought restoration of youth from the waters of a charmed fountain in Florida, the Kintan of the Chinese, the Red Elixir of Geber and the Vital Essence of Augsbourg. The Bolivian Indians made an elixir out of a thornless cactus which, it is said, had the power of keeping men young right up to their death, while not so long ago a Swiss named Spalinger claimed to have found a serum which prolonged life to a hundred and fifty years.

Instead of believing that the secret of perpetual youth could be thus obtained, they should have tracked an elephant in the wilds of Ceylon and observed what the behemoth ate for his lunch. Ten chances to one it would have been

Gotu Kola (Hydrocotyle Asiatica). Had they done this, the world would be growing this life-giving plant as commonly as lettuce and there might not be on earth, today, any one with a body that could truthfully be termed senile.

Gotu Kola has a very ancient history behind it. It was known to writers of India hundreds of years ago, always as a longevity plant.

It is a small herb that creeps along the ground, having fan-shaped leaves of a pale green color. The taste is slightly pungent, but eaten with rice or bread it is delicious.

It is claimed that this vegetable will increase the vitality of 70 and 80 to that of 40. The leaves have a marked energizing effect on the cells of the brain, and can preserve it indefinitely.

The leaves are not a stimulant but a brain food.

A Germain scientist, Baron Gogern, tells us that an old elephant, in captivity at Deshapur, was once rejuventated and bore a calf after Gotu Kola was sent for and mixed in her diet. A few of the leaves eaten raw every day will strengthen and revitalize worn out bodies and brains to a remarkable degree and will prevent brain fag and nervous breakdown.

In cases of mental troubles, blood pressure, abscesses and rheumatism, the efficacy of Gotu Kola has been highly valued. In elphantiasis, bruises, swollen parts and rheumatic swellings the oil of the herb or the juice extracted from it will check the fever associated with the affections. The powder of the herb, taken by drying it in the sun, is sprinkled on ulcers with effective results. The Gotu Kola is also a good leprosy cure. For skin eruptions, supposed to arise from heat of blood, the juice, if applied as a lap, will have instant effects. For mental weakness and memory improvement, the powder of the leaves, in small doses, is given with cow milk, while the juice if given with milk will also completely cure skin diseases, nerve trouble and jaundice.

To realize the truth of these assertions, it is only necessary to look back a few hundred years the medical history of the East.

"Two leaves a day will keep old age away." This is the claim made by the ancient Sinhalese for Gotu Kola, this famous longevity plant, which grows profusely in Ceylon.

In India the leaves are extensively used by religious orders to develop spiritual power, and to prolong the existence of the brain.

Miss Mary E. Forbes of America, the tutor to Her Highness, the widowed Queen of Mandi State in the Punjab, in 1914, commenced eating it in her salads, and after few months she never knew what brain fatigue was, and felt so physically well that she could not find enough to do to use up her energy.

It is the belief of the Sinhalese and the Indians also, that only one or two of the leaves of this herb are necessary, daily to bring about a gradual return to health and strength, provided the body is exposed to the sun. If this is eaten daily, it is said, that disorders like rheumatism, neuritis and nervous breakdown could be banished entirely from the constitution, and would be an important factor in breeding a beter race. It is claimed that Gotu Kola will increase the span of life by 50 years, by developing a brain incapable of breaking down for a very long time.

It is a well-known fact that no skeleton or corpse of an elephant has ever been found that had died a natural death. The villagers of Ceylon assert that they keep their youth and strength for hundreds of years because they eat Gotu Kola.

Not only is it certain that the average span of human life could be considerably increased, if people eat Gotu Kola, but it will also be a fact that the proportion of human beings who die a natural death will be very small. It will then mean that monkey glands will be given the go-by for this new herb which makes grandpa act like his grandson and puts a girlish smile on the wrinkled face of grandma.

Diseases of Women and Children—Cont.

SARAH A. WEBB, M.D. (U.S.A.).

Milk Crust is a severe itching disease of children due to a nervous irritation of teething, and is very annoying and often gives a good of trouble. First small pimples break out around the ear and on the forehead and head, then vesicles form filled with water, which break and form into a dirty-looking yellowish, and sometimes greenish, scab, which gives out a disagreeable odour. It spreads sometimes over a scalp and face. The eruption causes great irritation and itching; the child is constantly clawing himself and crying, and is prevented from sleeping.

Observe strict cleanliness. As a dusting powder use Slippery Elm Powder; as an ointment, Chickweed. Regulate the bowels.

Diarrhœa means too frequent stools. This increased peristalis is usually due to some specific cause. Infants fed on a liquid diet are more prone to loose evacuations than older children fed on solid or semi-solid diet. The active causes are excessive feeding and the use of foods unsuitable to the age of the child. We frequently meet with people who think it wise to give their children, regardless of age, a bit of anything from the table. This is very wrong. Diarrhœa is often Nature's method of eliminating poison, so frequently seen when a diarrhœa commences in the course of an acute infectious disease. The toxic or poisonous product can best be eliminated by the emunctories, and the intestines are one of the most valuable agents for eliminating poison from the body.

First find out the cause of diarrhœa and remove it if possible. Regulate the diet. Give a baby whey and rice water, or the white of an egg, beaten up in water, or arrowroot, or flour boiled in milk. To older children give Slippery Elm Food. Give one teaspoonful of Neutralising Cordial every two hours until the bowels are cleansed, or give Blackberry or Raspberry Leaves made as a tea.

Cholera Infantum, or Summer Complaint.—This is an irritative diarrhœa. It is a hot weather disease caused by heat, bad air, or improper food. In bottle-fed children, especially among the poorer classes, acute milk poisoning is frequently seen during the summer months. This is due to the chemical or toxic products developed in the milk. Summer diseases will appear as readily in breast-fed children who are improperly managed as in bottle-fed children. A child apparently quite well or only ill from digestive disturbance suddenly begins to vomit, and has a rise of temperature. A profuse diarrhœa follows, possessing the characteristics of decomposition. The vomiting is frequent, and follows every attempt to introduce food or drink into the stomach. In this case the food should be stopped for a time. At first curdled milk is ejected, and later mucus and serum and bile. The stools are frequent, fifteen to twenty in a day, at first fæcal, of yellow, brown, or green colour, and later losing all colour, and consisting simply of large quantities of serous fluid. These are typical stools of the disease. They are acid at the beginning, but when they become serous are alkaline. Thirst is intense, the child eagerly taking any fluid given it. The abdomen is usually distended, with a great deal of flatulence, and is very tender to touch. The tongue is coated early, but soon becomes dry and red. The pulse is weak and rapid, the respirations shallow and fast. The child loses flesh and colour very rapidly, the eyes sink in their sockets, a marked pallor develops in the skin, the flesh seems to disappear very rapidly, and the skin becomes cold and clammy. The nervous symptoms are very marked, the child crying or moaning, and throwing itself about in a very restless way. Delirium and convulsions may follow. Cases of cholera either die or show marked changes for the better in two or three days. On recovery, the vomiting usually stops first, then the stools become less frequent, recovery being slow.

These are sad and pitiful cases to look at, but with treatment and care there is no reason why they should not recover. First stop all foods. If the infant is breast-fed, discontinue the breast for twenty-four hours. Give rice water to drink in very small doses. When there is vomiting, only give enough to wet the mouth. Give Neutralising Cordial in doses according to age. It is best in these cases to give very small doses on account of the vomiting. Apply warm fomentations over the stomach and bowels of oatmeal or of flax-seed meal. Keep the child warm. Camomile Tea is very good to drink, likewise tea made of Blackberry or Raspberry Leaves, or the following may be given:—

Wild Cherry Bark Powder
Prickly Ash Berries Powder
Culvers Root Powder
Asclepias Powder
Rhubarb Powder

Equal parts. Take one teaspoonful to a cup of boiling water, sweeten. Drink a small wineglassful warm after each operation of the bowels. I have found the following good in such cases:—

Geranium Maculatum
Sage
Elder Flowers
White Oak Bark

Equal parts. Take one teaspoonful according to the age of the child and condition. Give an injection of the bowels of an infusion of Red Sage.

Constipation should be regarded as a symptom and not a disease, and accordingly the underlying cause should be sought for and corrected. Artificially fed infants are the most frequent suffers because of badly-balanced food mixtures, either too large or too small an amount of one ingredient of the milk, or the boiling of milk itself, being the cause. Breast-fed infants are constipated from deficiency in the fat or total quantity of solids present in the mother's milk. In older children a badly-arranged dietary, especially a deficiency in the carbohydrates and fruit juices, will cause this symptom. Next to diet, the lack of training of the child is an important cause in producing constipation, and constitutional diseases. Other causes are deficiency of the intestinal and bilary secretions. Again, the condition may be caused by congenital anatomical abnormalities, by new growths, or by the disproportionate length of the sigmoid flexure. The babe should have two or three movements daily. Some will be quite normal with one evacuation daily, while others will have three or four movements daily and enjoy good health. There are decided peculiarities noted with reference to bowel movement in children. If it is a breast-fed baby, the mother must keep herself well or wean the baby. Give the baby lots of water to drink. Oatmeal water is good to give. With older children, regulate their diet teaching them to eat brown bread made from wheat-meal, with a vegetable diet. If a laxative is needed, give Syrup of Rhubarb one-half to one teaspoonful once or twice daily.

Convulsions, or Spasms.—This is a disease which is probably more dreaded by mothers and nurses than any other, on account of the appearance and suddenness of the attack of the spasms. Convulsions are a violent and involuntary contraction of the muscles of the whole or part of the body, and are due to some affection of the spinal nervous system and disturbance in the motor area of the brain due to various causes. The susceptible age is the first two years of life. Children of a susceptible, irritable, and nervous temperament are most liable. The most common causes are difficult teething, worms, irritation of the bowels due to indigestible foods, eruptive fevers, scalds, burns, foreign bodies in the nose or ears, improper feeding. Spasm has been caused by a mother breast-feeding the child when overheated, also after some mental emotion, shock or anger, or rachitis.

The attack begins without warning. It may be preceded by slight twitching of the face and rolling of the eyes. Unconsciousness succeeds. The head is drawn backward, and the eyes are fixed and staring or rolled up under the eyelids. Respiration is usually arrested, the muscles of the face become affected, and finally the whole body becomes rigid. Irregular and violent movement of different parts of the body begin. The teeth are firmly set. The colour of the face is dusky. There may be involuntary passage of urine and fæces. When the spasmodic action ceases the muscles gradually relax and consciousness returns. A fit may last a few moments or may continue for hours. A child will sometimes have several fits during the day, but there will always be a longer or shorter interval between each spasm. They are very exhausting to the vital forces, and whatever is to be done must be done quickly.

Treatment.—First overcome the attack of symptoms. Get the little one into a hot mustard bath as soon as possible. As the water cools keep adding more hot water until relaxation occurs. Put a cold ice cloth to the head. Then wrap the little one in a warm blanket. After the bath, give a copious rectum flushing of warm water, which relieves the lower bowel of all effete material and assist in recovery. If caused by an overloaded stomach, give an emetic of tepid water. Tickle the throat with a feather, and give small continued doses of Syrup of Lobelia until vomiting occurs, then follow by giving Re-animating Drops, doses 10 to 15 drops, in hot, sweetened water, every half-hour until relieved. Give nourishing food and hygienic treatment.

Marasmus, or Infantile Atrophy.

Marasmus is a very common functional disorder in infancy, characterised by extreme emaciation resulting from inability to assimilate food. It is really due to a deficient metabolism, and results in a gradual decline. It is usually seen in the first year of life. The greatest number of cases appear in institutions and in dispensary practice. Poor food given in great quantities, coupled with insanitary surroundings, have a distinct bearing on the development of marasmus. If the digestive secretions have not been sufficiently developed by proper food, or if they have been over-produced for some time in efforts to digest abnormal food constituents, then the disorder may insiduously appear with symptoms of acid intoxication. Improper development, premature birth, congenital defects, and inherited diseases are all causes.

The train of symptoms begins insidiously. There is loss of weight and emaciation, in spite of the fact that the food has been the same or even increased in amount. The muscles become soft and flabby, the skin loose and wrinkled. The facial appearance changes, due to the loss of fat, resulting in a wrinkled forehead and sunken cheeks. The abdomen grows prominent and distended. Finally, nothing seems left but the skeleton covered by skin. Temperature is usually subnormal, pulse rapid and feeble, and respirations inefficient. The tongue is coated, and the mouth frequently the seat of thrush. The appetite is usually voracious. The infant will take an enormous quantity of food and still cry as if unsatisfied, the call of the starved issues for nutriment being strong and constant. The taking of foods does not seem to satisfy this hunger; naturally so, as the tissues do not receive it. The child lies quietly dozing a good deal of the time, constantly sucking the fingers and hands. The disease advances steadily to a fatal issue.

Treatment.—Remove the cause. Pure air and hygienic surroundings are essential. The mildest and most non-irritating food must be selected. We must begin with a dilute milk and gradually increase the ingredients with the child's ability to digest them. In some children where milk foods are badly assimilated and gastric symptoms follow, it may be wise to discontinue milk for several weeks, so as to give foods that are more easily assimilated until such time when milk may be again tolerated. Whey and egg albumen, and light Slippery Elm Food may be given to suit the condition, alternately or separately. Tea made from Catnip or Raspberry Leaves or Peppermint will be found very valuable given two or three days without any other food. Keep the child warm,—giving daily bath, and follow with masage of olive oil.

Rickets is insufficient bony development of the system, due to prolonged feeding on a diet which does not contain all the proximate principles of milk in comparatively proper quantities, or because in quantity and character it overtaxes the digestive functions, prolonged nursing at the breast, or condensed milks.

Symptoms of rickets are slow, with very gradual onset and progression. The child becomes very fretful, and there is disturbed sleep, and excessive perspiration about the head. The muscles are generally soft and flabby; the abdomen is distended, tympanitic, and evidences of imperfect digestion are found in the fetid stools and in the constipation alternating with an occasional diarrhœa. In spite of this, the appetite is generally good, more food being taken than is digested. This complaint is also characterised by the beading of the ribs, large bones, big head, crooked spine and limbs, short stature.

To treat these cases pay strict attention to hygiene, ensure plenty of sunshine and outdoor life, and give cool bath daily. The diet should be made to conform as nearly as possible to the normal one for a child of the same age. Abundance of fats and proteids should be taken. Cream, beef juice, starchy foods, and sugars must be avoided, and lime-water used with strained boiled oatmeal or wheatmeal is very good. Children of eighteen months or over may be given broths, bean soup, fish, and whole-meal bread. To check the diarrhœa give Neutralising Cordial and Wild Cherry Syrup (equal parts), one teaspoonful every two hours, or dose according to the age of the child. Keep the child warm.

Prolapsus of the Bowel is due to either prolonged constipation or diarrhœa, or to straining or bearing down on the part of the child in order to evacuate the bowels, causing irritation and inflammation. The bowel, losing its elasticity, is forced through the opening. It becomes swollen and chafed and painful. To remedy this lay the child across the lap. With clean hands gently sponge and anoint parts with Witch Hazel Salve, and gently push the bowel into position. Keep the child lying quiet.2 Regulate the diet and give laxatives.

Health Brevities

CELERY was recommended as a preventive of rheumatism. The writer claimed if this agent was cooked and eaten freely with a little milk, the excess of acids in the system would be neutralized and rheumatism would be impossible.—*Australian Paper.*

MEDICAL HISTORY

By A. A. DAWSON, M.B.B.A., F.N.A.O.

Looking backwards, we find that the practice of medicine has been in the chaotic condition in which we find it today since its earliest known beginnings. We also find the cautious prescriber achieving success and the heroic prescriber failure.

For instance, during the warlike days of Rome, she was for 600 years without a Physician who made the healing art a profession; superstitions and ceremonies were used against plague and epidemics. 200 years before the Christian Era, Arcagathus established himself as a practitioner in Rome, but so severe was his practice and so unsuccessful its results that the citizens prohibited the practice by law. 100 years later, Asclepiades of Bithynia acquired great popularity by mild and cautious practice; he was the first to classify diseases into acute and chronic. Themison of Laodicea, a pupil of Asclepiades, was the founder of that system of medicine now called Eclectic and Physio-Botanical; he referred to diseases as states of contraction or relaxation, and divided his remedies into astringents and relaxants.

Half a century later we have Thessalus, who styled himself "the conqueror of Physicians." He introduced the method of medical treatment called metasynocrisis, which consisted in producing an entire change in the state of the body, instead of regulating, correcting and removing morbid actions and symptoms. The method of Thessalus is now the principal corner stone of present medical practice. Since his time, faith in the integrity of Nature has steadily declined, and the reliance on the power of art has steadily advanced until now, when we find doctors using the most deadly and destructive agents, heedless of the great truth that Nature is the true physician.

Celsus, a native Roman physician, wrote several books which show that surgery and pharmacy had by his time made considerable progress. The first pharmacopia was written in the reigns of Claudius and Nero by Siribonius Largus, and about this time we got a mixture of sixty-one ingredients by Andromachus. This mixture appeared in pharmacopias until the end of the 17th century.

Pliny and Dioscorides followed, and both added history, the latter writing a Materia Medica which was printed and translated for many ages.

Then comes Galen, probably the most familiar name in the whole list. Galen actually did study, to do which he had to travel, after which, at the request of the Emperor Aurelius, he settled in Rome. Galen wrote 200 treatises on all subjects connected in some way with medicine.

The Greek school of medicine terminated with the death of Paulus about the middle of the seventh century. The Arabians, who about this time came into power, destroyed the immense Alexandrian Library, yet they adopted the opinions of Galen. About this time comes the invention of Chemistry, and Rhases, the Arabian physician, born at Irak in the ninth century, wrote a treatise on Measles and Smallpox, in which he introduced chemical remedies.

After this we have Avicenna, who was born at Bokhara in 980 A.D., and was educated in the schools in Bagdad. He wrote an Encyclopædia of Medical Sciences, which was the text book in most of the Arabian schools for centuries.

Mesue the elder and Mesue the younger were among the last of the Arabian Medical Writers, and we still have their preparations in our pharmacopias; for instance, Syrup and Oxymel of Squills. With Averroes the Arabic school of medicine terminates.

From the twelfth to the fifteenth centuries the practice of medicine was principally in the hands of the monks, and their healing resources were mainly drawn from magical arts and astrology. The attempts about this time to transmute the baser metals into gold introduced many chemical preparations into medicine, and laid the foundation of the mineral drug system of today.

The Medical School at Salerno was the first to grant diplomas, and it maintained some reputation until eclipsed by the schools of Bologne and Paris in the thirteenth century.

The first English Physician of note was Anglicanus, who published "Medicinæ Compendium" in the early part of the fourteenth century. Then comes the invention of the art of printing, and with it the works of Hippocrates and Galen reprints and ideas, the establishment of Medical chairs in many of the universities in Europe; and LINACRE who, after Oxford, spent some time at the court of Florence, returned to England, and established medical professorships at Oxford and Cambridge, and laid the foundation of the London College of Physicians.

Then the Galenists and the Chemists became the rival sects of the Medical World, in which the Galenists predominated until they were overthrown by the greatest quack of all time—Paracelsus. Aureolus Phillippus Paracelsus Theophrastus Bombast de Hohenheim was born in Switzerland in 1493; an accident in early life made him an eunuch, and he became a hater of womankind. He lived a dissipated life, and died prematurely at the age of 48. His principal doctrine was copied from Valentine, and his panaceas were Mercury and Antimony.

In the rivalry which followed through the sixteenth century, the disciples of Paracelsus won. Each sect with much truth accused the other of killing their patients, and yet the medical use of Mercury and Antimony has developed.

After this came the Anatomical Physicians — Vesalius, Eustachius, and Fallopius. During the seventeenth century the doctrines of Hippocrates became the prevailing medical philosophy. Harvey discovered the circulation of the blood; Asselli, Rudbeck, and Bartoline explained the absorbent system; Malpighi, Hooke, and others explained the structure and functions of the lungs. Boyle disengaged Chemistry from its mystery. The chemical physicians continued to mix magical ceremonies and astrology with their medicines. The anatomists included in their pharmacopia the Mercury, Antimony and Opium of Paracelsus, and the bleeding, purging, and sweating of the earlier physicians; they only omitted that which was really worth preserving.

Then came the Fermentationists, who believed that certain fermentations in the blood and other fluids were the causes of disease; certain humours were acid, others alkaline, hence disease. Fever was an acidulous disease requiring alkaline remedies. This was advocated by Silvius of Leyden and Willis of England. Sydenham agreed with Willis, but adopted the Hippocratic doctrine, and it is still doubtful whether any more natural doctrine has been found than that expounded by Hippocrates 3,000 years ago.

The Mathematical Physicians who followed used the remedies of the Galenists and chemists.

Then came the Vitalists, who originated with Van Helmont, who originally belonged to the chemical school. The Vitalists, however, are really followers of Hippocrates.

The Solidists, who followed, belonged to the chemical and mathematical schools. In 1671, Glisson published a treatise advocating muscular irritability as a specific property in opposition to the humoral pathology of Hippocrates.

These revolutions in theory had little effect on practice. The prescriptions were alike whatever the hypothesis the physicians adopted. Are we not very much in the same position to-day? What effective system of medicine have we? For Bronchial Catarrh, with a weak heart, the orthodox use Oxygen to help the breathing, and Strychnine and Digitalis injections for the heart, contradictions on the very face of them. The simple and obvious are rejected or not given any thought; the vital power of the patient is further destroyed, and the greater efforts of the vital power to overcome the disease and administered poisons are checked with further injections of Hyoscine or Morphine, so that the end can be said to be peaceful; the end is none the less made sure.

GOLDEN RULES

In Infancy and Childhood

Practise the quiet manner and the gentle voice.

Win the confidence of the children; do not frighten them.

Always tell the child the truth, it imparts confidence.

The infant is peculiarly susceptible to diseases of the digestive tract; the child because it comes in close contact with others, more easily contracts contagious diseases.

Examine the throat in every case of acute fever.

The loss of weight in breast-fed infants, not due to digestive disturbance, may be caused by pregnancy of the mother.

Remember the diarrhœa in infants may be a symptom of any acute disease.

"Milk as Food"

To the Editor, "The Medical Herbalist"

Dear Sir,—With reference to the letters by Mr. Abbott in your March issue, I judge that the "obvious reason" for the "Southport Visitor" not finding space for his communication bearing upon the campaign against T.B. was, that it was not suitable for publication in that journal. A campaign of that character cannot be countered in the way Mr. Abbott tried to do. His letter would do no good, but would have drawn correspondence which would not have flattered anyone.

The other letter contains a reference to Scripture, and for comment on this we may be permitted sufficient space. I shall not say much about the other points he wishes to make.

A friend of Mr. Abbott's once told me he had benefited both by abstaining from and by using meats and dairy products during different periods.

Mr. Abbott, like many others, is stumbled by Scripture, and says that the portion he named is not to be taken as having a literal meaning.

He might just as well have said that he did not agree with Marre Israel in faithfully stating that "the Scriptures are the true guide in all the important matters of life."

However, the portion referred to definitely means what is written. Fifteen times from Exodus 3 to Ezekiel 20 reference is made to God's definite promise to a stiff necked people (Israel) concerning the fruitfulness of the land that He would bring them into the benefit of if they would obey Him.

Deut. xxxi. 20 answers the unbelieving: "When I shall have brought them into the land which I sware unto their fathers, that floweth with milk and honey; and they shall have eaten and filled themselves, and waxen fat; then will they turn unto other gods, and serve them . . ." These portions of Holy Scripture were written concerning the blessing to be had through the obedience of Israel. Jer. xxxi. 23, 24, says: "They came in, and possessed it; but they obeyed not Thy voice, neither walked in Thy law, . . . the city is given into the hands of the Chaldeans."

We are introduced to a highly fertile land which was so abundantly fruitful as to be figuratively described as "flowing" with milk and honey. The people were "waxen fat," and I anticipate they were as healthy on milk, honey and flesh as a normal law-abiding Jew is reputed to be. Then, as their disobedience increased, they indulged and suffered the diseases of the Gentiles—whom they desired so often to imitate.

The application of the words in question is clearly that the Jews in that land would find an abundance of milk and honey (and flesh) for food.

I uphold the use of milk. Its influence on the stomach and the nerves of many sufferers is pronounced. That is saying little as to its virtues.

I blame the Veterinary Profession more than any other for their failure to do anything worth while to arouse the farmers to the dangers and the urgent necessity of keeping disease free animals and supplying pure milk. The question as to how to obtain a clean supply and what to do in its absence I cannot go into.

I am not versed in the keeping of bees, but I always understood that honey was drawn from Nature (the flowers), and that the keeper having in due season "robbed the hives" of most of the honey, the bees are provided with a substitute in the form of our commercial sugar in order to provide winter food. If that is so, we do not get the denatured product hinted at by Mr. Abbott, but, honey as true in name and quality as was ever produced by the industry of the bee.

I have nothing but appreciation for the article on Milk by Marre Israel, and hope these lines will help to show that the Jews did consume milk, flesh and honey, and to settle the minds of many that the Divine permission (given after the fall of man) for flesh to be eaten has not been withdrawn (Lev. xi. 3). A.B.-Y.Z.

Diseases of Women and Children—Cont.

SARAH A. WEBB, M.D. (U.S.A.).

The gaseous distension of the abdomen is a serious complication of diseases of pleura and lungs, usually the result of over-feeding.

An acute paroxysmal abdominal pain from flatulent colic is common in infancy. It occurs especially in breast-fed infants, and may be apparently very severe. Prostration, however, rarely follows the attack.

An infant should hold its head up in three or four months, be able to sit up unsupported at six or seven months, and should be able to stand, with slight support, at nine or ten months.

Remember that the skin and mucous membrane of the newly-born infant are very susceptible to infection and irritants, so do not wash or rub the skin too much, and be careful that bathing does not convey an infection from one part of the skin to another.

Circumcision is best performed after three weeks. Do not perform this operation if jaundice is present.

Light, plenty of fresh air, and plenty of water to drink are very important for babies. Stuffy rooms and too much clothing predispose to "colds."

Do not allow the sucking of a "pacifier" or of the thumb. It is a bad habit, and often causes deformity of the teeth or jaws.

If the child's stomach gets out of order, stop the milk and give water only, or albumen water.

APPENDIX

Infant's Food.—It is relished by the infant, readily appropriated, does not distress the digestion, may be given warm or cold, as seems best, and the child thrives on it from the first. Whole-wheat bread contains to a very large extent the elements for cell growth that are required by the infant. It is prepared by steeping two or three slices in hot water for half-an-hour. The bread should be properly prepared and selected. Biscuits or crackers are not to be used. After being properly boiled, this should be strained through a thin cotton cloth, and the mass thoroughly compressed until the largest possible amount of nutrition of the bread is in the liquid. To perhaps half a pint of this—ten ounces—a teaspoonful, or even two teaspoonsful, of the sugar of milk may be added. For young infants the amount should be carefully adjusted, and it should be fed warm from an ordinary feeding bottle. When properly prepared, it has the appearance of mother's milk. Children fed on this food are known to be strong, vigorous, and healthy.

Slippery Elm Food for Infants and Invalids.—Cut an ounce of Slippery Elm Bark (Ulmus Fulva) obliquely into small pieces about the thickness of a match. Pour on 1¼ pints of boiling water; let it stand an hour or more in a warm place, and the liquor will become mucilaginous. Add half a cup of milk to the same quantity of liquor. A little stick of Cinnamon may be added when infusing in cases of vomiting or diarrhœa. For a pleasant drink, leave out the milk and add a slice of lemon.

Caraway Water.—Place 2 tablespoonsful of crushed caraway seed in a small muslin bag, and put this in a pint of water. Boil down to half a pint. Put 2 teaspoonsful into the baby's bottle. It will remove colic, and is quite harmless.

Albumen Water or Egg Water for Young Infants.—Beat the white of an egg into one pint of ice-cold water. Do not shake. Flavour to taste.

Coddled Egg.—Place a fresh egg in the shell in boiling water, and immediately remove from the fire. Let the egg remain in the water, which is gradually cooling, for 8 minutes, when the white should be of the consistency of jelly. For a delicate digestion, only the white, which can easily be separated from the yolk, should be given.

"The Stormy Life of England's Most Famous Herbalist

"Long-nosed Nick Culpeper, as he pored over books already well-fingered, in his dingy rooms at Cambridge, did more than learn Greek and Latin. He learned what the medical writers of antiquity had to teach about healing.

"Thus, when the thoughtful Nick left Cambridge to become apprenticed to a London apothecary, he was already a man of some learning in his sphere.

"He had, too, formed ideas—political and otherwise—that he was to hold on to through abuse and poverty and battle.

Puritan

"Nick was a dyed-in-the-wool Puritan, fiery, in his support of the Roundhead cause, for all that he had been brought up in a quiet country parsonage among the wood and bracken-covered hills and fields of Surrey.

"And he concluded that 'such as study Astrology are the only men I know that are fit to study Physick, Physick without Astrology being like a lamp without Oil.'

"In the days when the conflicting ideals of Englishmen were boiling into the passions that swept the land with civil war, Nicholas set up for himself as an astrologer and physician in Spitafields.

"War drums echoed through those old narrow streets of top-heavy houses that the Great Fire was to bring crashing down in blazing ruin a generation later.

" 'Prentices left their sobbing sweethearts and marched out to conquer cavalier forces; and in those days, it is believed, Nick left his pills and phials and books and fought for his beliefs. He was badly wounded in the chest.

'Soon, however, he was back from the war, healed again and becoming widely known as a healer in London.

"His repute was spread far beyond the circle of those who actually knew him when, in 1649—the year a masked executioner struck off King Charles's head in Whitehall—he brought out a book.

"Nick called the book 'A Physical Directory, or a Translation of the London Dispensatory.'

Attacked

"This work was, in fact, a translation of the Pharmacopœa, of the College of Physicians, and the members of that worthy body were outraged that Nick should have had the impertinence to publish a translation without their permission and authority.

"A royalist writer saw fit to attack Culpeper in a way that showed more political bias than enthusiasm for the diffusion of knowledge. This writer said that the book had been 'done (very filthily) into English.'

> "Then he declared that Culpeper, 'by two years' drunken labour hath Gallimawfred the apothecaries' book into nonsense, mixing every receipt therein with some scruples, at least, of rebellion or atheisme, besides the danger of poisoning men's bodies.
>
> 'And (to supply his drunkenness and leachery with a drunken reward with a thirty-shilling reward) endeavoured to bring into obloquy the famous societies of apothecaries and chyrugeons.'

"This and other unfair abuse which was heaped on Culpeper did not affect the popularity of his work, for two new editions were brought out in the next five years.

Popular

"Culpeper also brought out a work called: 'The English Physician Enlarged With Three Hundred and Sixty-Nine MEDICINES made of English herbs That were not in any IMPRESSION until THIS.'

"The 'English Physician' was enormously popular; from generation to generation the cumbersome printing presses of the seventeenth and eighteenth centuries turned out edition after edition.

"On numberless bookcases in numberless English homes Nick's book stood as fountain of knowledge to be applied to when any of the family were ill.

"In the edition before me, on the flyleaf, has been written 'A Recipt for the itch. White Elebore root steept in milk 6 days then rub it well into every joint. . . . Henry Courtoy His Book London 1825.' And long after 1825, people referred to Nick's book: to this day many regard it as the framework of herbal knowledge, and Kipling wrote one of the 'Puck Stories'—'A Doctor of Medicine'—about him.

Swindled

"For all that, Nick had a continual struggle to keep his wife and seven children in anything like comfort. His books brought him little money, and he was (he said) swindled out of his inheritance.

"Nick was, too, more humane than worldly-wise, for the poor man who knocked at his door ever received the best of his knowledge of medicine free of charge.

"By the time he reached his middle thirties, Nick was in the grip of consumption—perhaps the aftermath of the wound he had got in the ranks of the Roundheads. At 38, worn out, he was dead."

The Right Thing at the Right Time

MARRE ISRAEL

"To everything there is a season." Not only should we seek to do and say the right thing at the right time, but we should eat and drink in season also. As the earth brings forth good things month by month, so should the housekeeper, like the wise and faithful servant, who his lord did make ruler over his household, to give meat (nurture) in season, assign to those in her care, their supplies at the proper time. (Matthew xxiv. 45).

When a herb is a food as well as a medicinal remedy, it is safe to say that if the full and proper use is made of the herb in the kitchen, it will not be required in the sickroom.

Sage in May

Sage is antiseptic, strengthens the nerves, quickens the senses and memory, and promotes longevity. Although any etymological connection between the words is not apparent from the root-words given, yet there does seem to be a close connection between Sage, the herb, sage, a wise man, and sagacity, the quality of acute mental discernment. A man is what he eats, and whether a man becomes a sage by eating it, or whether he eats sage because he is one, it makes no difference.

Here is a good way to use a little in your salad. Lettuce, two or three ripe, black olives, a sprinkling of onion powder, and half a teaspoonful of sage. This can be served also in the form of a salad sandwich, and many other varieties of vegetables can be used with pleasing results.

He that would live for aye,
Must eat sage in May."

"Why should a man die, who has sage growing in his garden?"—(Maxim of School of Salerno).

"Salvia salva" — "Sage will save."—(Old Proverbs).

RHEUMATISM, GOUT, ETC.

Meadowsweet	½	ounce
Buckbean	½	"
Yarrow	½	"
Broom	½	"
Sassafras Bark	¼	"
Prickly Ash Berries	¼	"
Celery Seeds	¼	"
Ginger Root	½	"
Sennas Leaves	as required	
Spanish Licorice	½	ounce

Pour on above one quart of boiling water, stand in the oven for 20 minutes, then strain through a fine cloth. Dose: Adults, half teacupful, children, half to one wineglassful every three or four hours after meals.

CHRONIC RHEUMATISM

By F. Worthington, M.N.A.M.H.

Chronic Rheumatism commonly manifests itself about or after middle life, although it may occur in the young, developing slower and lasting longer in some forms than that of Acute Rheumatism.

In some cases it may completely spoil all the enjoyment of life, leaving its victim helpless, and they very seldom make a complete recovery.

Chronic Rheumatism attacks the muscles (Muscular) and joints (Articular), and their membranes (Synovial), having various names according to the parts affected.

Muscular Rheumatism (Myalgia) is a chronic inflammation and congested state of the fibrous tissues, which are in many structures of the body, such as the muscles (myositis and fibrositis), tendons (tenonitis and tenosynovitis), ligaments (ligamentitis), aponeurosis (aponeurositis; the fibrous interlaced sheath into which the muscles are inserted), the periosteum (periostitis; the fibrous membrane covering the bones), and the neurilemma (neurilemmatitis; the fibrous membrane or sheath surrounding the nerves).

SYMPTOMS

The first sign of this disease is pain in the fingers and toes, later involving the larger joints, knees, shoulders, and hip. At first, this pain is not increased upon movements; it is worst during the night and first thing in the morning, and upon the approach of changeable weather, especially before and during storms, usually subsiding afterwards. Fever is absent, and there is no redness and swelling of the joint, but as the disease gets fully established, the joints become larger with a fluid (coagulable lymph) forming in the tendons, ligaments, and muscles surrounding the joint, causing a thickening to the parts, which will pit upon pressure.

CAUSES

The chief causes may be from some toxæmic matter circulating in the body, which is formed in certain diseases, such as septic throat, septic blood diseases, septic typhoid, dysentery, tuberculosis, gonorrhœa, syphilis, and other diseases where there is that injurious poisonous matter retained in the blood stream.

TREATMENT

The patient should go to bed as soon as the pains appear, in a well ventilated room to keep the body in an even temperature; care should be taken to prevent any draughts by means of a screen round the bed. A hot-water bottle should be placed at the feet, and the parts affected should be well washed with soap and hot water, dried, and Methyl Salicylate Ointment (which can be got from good herbal stores) gently applied; cover the parts with flannel—this should be repeated three times a day.

MEDICINE

Get from any Herbalist of repute the following:—

Yarrow	¾	ounce
Meadowsweet	¾	"
Clivers	½	"
Broom	½	"
Bittersweet	½	"
Sassafras Bark	¼	"
Prickly Ash Berries	¼	"
Celery Seeds	¼	"
Spanish Licorice	½	"
Ginger Root	¼	"
Senna Leaves	As required	

To the above pour on one quart of boiling water, stand in the oven for 20 minutes, then strain through a fine cloth.

Dose: Adults, half to one teacupful; children, half to one wineglassful (hot) every four hours.

See to the diet.

Diseases of Women and Children—Cont.

SARAH A. WEBB, M.D. (U.S.A.)

Linseed (Flaxseed) Tea.—Take 1 oz. of whole linseed, juice of 2 lemons, 2 small sticks of Liquorice Root, crushed, and 1 heaped teaspoonful of sugar. Pour on these, 2 pints of boiling water and stand in a hot place for 3 or 4 hours. Strain.

Chicken Broth.—Chop fine a small chicken and boil in 1 quart of water for one hour, adding a blade of mace and parsley, also some rice and a crust of bread. Skim from time to time, and strain.

Beef Juice.—Select round steak free from fat. Chop into pieces less than inch square, and put in a double boiler (no water with the meat). Place on a slow fire where the water will simmer (not boil) for 3 hours. Press out the juice, and season.

Mutton Juice.—Cooked as above, is also very nutritious.

Linseed (Flaxseed) Lemonade.—Pour 1 quart of boiling water over four teaspoonfuls of whole Linseed, and steep 3 hours. Strain: sweeten to taste, and add the juice of 2 lemons. If too thick, add a little more water. This is excellent for fevers and colds.

Baths and Compresses

Mustard Bath.—Add 2 teaspoonfuls of mustard to 1 gallon of water. For very small infants it is better to put the mustard in a piece of thin muslin and let it remain in the bath, gently squeezing it from time to time.

Salt Bath.—Dissolve 4 heaped tablespoonfuls of common sea salt to each gallon of water. A plunge in such a bath, followed by a brisk rubbing, has a decidedly tonic effect.

Bran Bath.—Put 1-lb. or more of bran in a muslin bag, and boil in water for 15 minutes. Squeeze occasionally and add this water to a bath until it has a milky appearance.

Warm Compress.—Fold a piece of cloth into several thicknesses, dipping it in tepid water, and placing it on the affected part. Cover with oil silk. Hold the compress in place by a bandage. This is good for a Sore Throat and Inflammation.

Hot Fomentations. — Are made

as above, only cloth must be put in very hot water and wrung out.

Cold Compress.—This is made in the same way, only cloth must be put in cold water and wrung out, changing it often, not allowing it to become warm, and not covering it with oiled silk. This is good for Sprains, and Inflammations.

Infant's Cordial, for expelling wind or for use in cases of Gripes. —Take 1 ounce of concentrated Dill Water. 4 ounces of distilled Aniseed Water, 3 ounces distilled Best Jamaica Ginger Water. Mix, and give from half to one teaspoonful when required, to infants from 1 to 2 days old, increasing dose according to age up to a tablespoonful for adults.

Health Brevities

WHY is it the average individual will be exceedingly careful in buying a suit of clothing, even checking the fibres of its material to see if it is wool or shoddy, and yet will blindly accept a tablet or the contents of a bottle without a thought as to their respective merits? He will see that only the purest milk and the finest food is put on his table, and yet allows an inocculation or serum to be injected into his bloodstream without any questioning.—*Dr. Wm. H. Fought.*

* * *

BURDOCK has a very soothing effect on mucous surfaces, in the respiratory, digestive and urinary tract. It is a true renal depurant and where we desire to increase the solid contents of the urine, there are few better remedies that infusions decoctions or tinctures made from the seeds and roots of this herb.—*John Fearn.*

* * *

NECESSARY drainage in the human body refers to the removal of wornout substances, and other things that must be carried out of the body. Things that may be poison if they are not moved with rapidity toward a body outlet. Here again life force must move these substances through the tubes toward and to points of elimination, and if life force is obstructed the work cannot be done correctly, and sickness to the extent of failure is sure to follow. — *Dr. Willard Carver.*

* * *

IT seems more than odd that a so-called learned profession of scientifically trained persons should find itself constantly in the role of opposition to progress and advancement. Over the centuries the profession of medicine has placed itself in that position, both on matters within its own field as well as on developments in other departments of human progress.—*Dr. Lyndon E. Lee.*

* * *

The only key to the bleak and barren soul of medical art is economics. If you have this key—in the form of a new serum, a new pink pill, a propagandist idea that will drive people into doctor's offices, the door will open to you. If you have an idea that in any manner encroaches upon the domain of this profession, you are taboo and that is final.—*Cash Asher.*

BLOOD PRESSURE

By J. MILTON, N.D., M.N.A.M.H.

In attempting to cure an ailment, it is necessary to first ascertain the cause. Blood Pressure is too freely spoken of as a disease in itself. With this idea in mind, neither patient nor doctor can hope for a cure. It is not a disease in itself, but a symptom of some abnormal condition in the system. Hardened arteries, hypertension of the arteries, kidney trouble or a general toxic condition will be found to be the real disease and cause of high pressure. This condition is always brought about by wrong feeding. Invariably it will be found that the sufferer is a big starch and protein eater, and scarcely ever takes raw salads or fresh fruits. This wrong combination of foods brings on the toxic condition resulting in hardened arteries. These become thickened, probably lined with deposits of lime. The heart must then contract with greater vigour to keep the various parts of the body supplied with blood through these narrow channels.

Mineral drugs, herbal medicines or "blood pressure" tablets cannot cure this condition. It is obvious that the cause must first be attacked. The intake of wrong foods (the cause) must be stopped.

Before detailing treatment, there is another fallacy that must be exposed. It is the unctuous idea that the normal blood pressure is the age of the person plus 100. That is an entirely wrong statement. The blood pressure of an adult is 120 to 130. If it is above 140, then sound health is not the lot of such a person.

In many fruit-growing districts, particularly around Cambridgeshire, there are to be found many men and women of over 80 and 90 years of age. Test them for blood pressure, and very few will be found over 140. Yet, in our towns, there are hundreds of over-eating businessmen of less than 40 years of age, with a blood pressure of over 150.

As to treatment: this is best taken under supervision. From the facts given, it is perfectly obvious that a complete rest from all food is indicated. Three days' fast can be done at home without supervision, but if a longer fast is necessary, then expert supervision is imperative.

During these three days, the patient should take two tablespoonfuls of orange juice every two hours during the day. The body should be sponged down with tepid water each day, and the bowels should be washed out each evening with a quart of water at body heat.

Following the three days on fruit juice, the diet afterwards should be as follows:

On rising in the morning, a glass of water, slowly sipped.

Breakfast of fresh fruit only. Of these, oranges and grape fruit are easily the best.

Mid-day meal: Salads selected from watercress, lettuce, celery, young cabbage, tomatoes, followed by wholemeal biscuits and butter.

Evening meal: Vegetables of

non-starchy nature conservatively cooked. A little steamed fish (except salmon), or a lightly poached egg. Fresh fruits, particularly apples.

No salt or soda must be used in cooking nor taken with food. This is of vital importance.

A drink of Dandelion Coffee or Maté Tea (without sugar) is permissible a half hour before evening meal. Water can be taken **ad lib.** except at meal times. This applies also to the days of fasting.

Fresh air and easy walking exercises are also essential, but in case of very high pressure with persistent dizziness, no exercise must be taken. The patient in such a case must rest and remain perfectly quiet, and no visitors or other disturbing elements be allowed.

Where it is not possible to undertake a long fast, the procedure outlined, i.e., the short fast, should be repeated every twenty-one days. During the fast, no food or medicine should be taken whatever, and smoking is absolutely prohibited.

During the period when food is being taken, the following herbal prescription will be found an additional useful "food."

Lime Flowers, Balm, Avena Satura and Motherwort of each half an ounce. Boil in three pints of water down to two pints. Strain when cold, and take a wineglassful four times a day except on the days of fasting.

If a sufferer wishes to benefit, it is necessary to follow the whole of the treatment outlined. Many want to choose the "bits" that are easy to follow, such as taking the medicine, but not doing a fast, or still continuing to smoke, or having breakfast and taking fruit at teatime. Such a partial method is worse than useless. Sufferers from blood pressure **must** first help themselves. Curb their appetites, and rebuild their health on rational lines.

Herbal Aids to Beauty

How to Remove Freckles

If you are one of those people who are subject to these unsightly blemishes on the skin, when summer comes, well here is the remedy for them.

You will obtain Fresh Elder Blossoms, take half a cupful of these and add cold water until they are covered over, clear or filtered rain water, or distilled water is best; if this is not obtainable then boil ordinary tap water for one hour then let it get cold. After covering well over with water (say three-parts of a cupful) allow them to stand over night, then strain the liquid off and use this to bathe the freckles morning and night.

Health Brevities

SAY "No" to that extra cup of coffee! "No" to that cigarette you are mechanically offered and mechanically accept without really wanting it; say "No" to yourself from time to time and to most other people all the time. If somebody asks if perhaps you aren't a little bit "touched," say "No" with emphasis, and find comfort in the fact that besides sparing your body from abuse, you will at last have attained a positive side to your character, that is, the possession of a positive "No."—*Health Digest.*

JUNIPER

By HUBEERT B. FIGG, F.F.Sc., F.I.C.A., M.P.S.

Synonyms. — Juniperi Fructus; Juniper Berry.

Juniper consists of the ripe fruits of Juniperus communis and belongs to the Linnaean class and order, Dioecia Polyandria and to

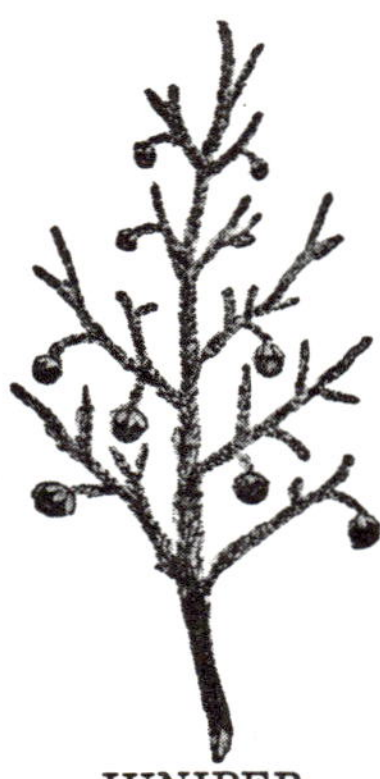

JUNIPER

the Natural Order, Coniferae or Pinaceae. It is a common indigenous evergreen shrub or small tree growing chiefly on chalky downs, dry hills and banks in temperate Europe, Asia and North America.

It assumes a low spreading form, but sometimes rising erect to the height of eight feet, or under cultivation to twice that altitude.

It is easily known by its minute crowded, spine like leaves, and its peculiar odour when these are bruised. It flowers in Spring (May) and the flowers are succeeded by small roundish berries about 0.5 to 1 centimetre in diameter, deep purplish black, sometimes with a reddish tint, and covered with a greyish waxy bloom, they contain three seeds. The berries require to remain on the trees two years before they are fully ripe.

The berries have a peculiar aromatic terebinthinate odour, and of a corresponding taste, with some sweetness at first but followed by bitterness.

They are imported into this country from the Baltic and the Mediterranean.

Juniper in the Bible. — In "Wooton's Chronicles of Pharmacy" the following reference is made:—

> "The Hebrew word 'roethm,' translated juniper in our Authorised Version, has given much trouble to translators. The Septuagint merely converted the Hebrew word into a Greek one, and the Vulgate followed the Septuagint.
>
> "The allusions to the tree are in I. Kings xix, 4 and 5, where Elijah slept under a Juniper tree; Job xxx. 4 speaks of certain men so poor that they cut up mallows by the bushes and juniper roots for their meat; and Psalm cxx. 4. 'Sharp arrows of the mighty with coals of Juniper.' The tree alluded to was almost certainly the Broom, and it is so rendered in the Revised Version either in the text or in the margin in all the instances.
>
> "The Arabic name of the Broom is 'Ratam,' evidently a descendant of 'Roethem.'
>
> "The Genista roetam is said to be the largest and most con-

spicuous shrub in the deserts of Palestine, and would be readily chosen for its shade by the weary traveller.

"The mallows in the Book of Job are translated 'salt wort' in the Revised Version. Renan gives 'They gather their salads from the bushes.' Salads were regarded as indispensable by the poorest Jews. The coals of Juniper (or Broom) are supposed to have reference to the lasting fire which this wood furnishes, but other translations suggest as the proper reading of the verse. 'The arrows of a warrior are the tongues of the people of the tents of Mizram.' "

Juniper was known to Discorides, by whom its fruit was used as a tonic, expectorant and diuretic.

Juniper Oil.—The Oil, the chief active ingredient of the berries, is obtained by distillation with water, and a similar oil can be obtained from the leaves.

It is very pale greenish, lighter than water, specific gravity 0.862 to 0.890, the gravity increasing with the age of the oil. Soluble when freshly distilled 1 in 4 of 95 per cent alcohol, and becoming less soluble with age.

It has an odour and taste similar to that possessed by the plant. Juniper Oil contains an ester, to which the peculiar juniper-like odour and taste are supposed to be due; but this cannot be the case, as the odour persists after the complete saponification of the small amount of the ester.

The B.P.C. 1934 states: "The characteristic odour of Juniper is due to a substance which has not been identified." The proportion of oil which Juniper Berries afford is variously given as from 0.3 per cent to 2.3 per cent. The usual yield is probably about 1 per cent.

Oil of Juniper Wood.—Oleum Juniperi Ligni, a trade name for Fictitious Juniper Oil supposed to be made from the wood, but is generally a mixture of Juniper Oil and Turpentine.

The adulteration of Oil of Juniper with Turpentine can easily be detected. The Specific Gravity of the mixture being less than that of the unadulterated Oil of Juniper.

Foreign Juniper Oil (Hungarian Oil), which contains a larger proportion of the lighter constituents, has a less pronounced Juniper colour and flavour.

Commercial Oil of Juniper (so-called), a third quality, is obtained as a by-product in the manufacture of an alcoholic liquor (Borowicks) and of a Juniper extract, for which there is considerable demand.

Juniper Oil should be preserved in well-stoppered, completely filled, amber-coloured bottles, in a cool place, protected from light.

Action and Uses.—Juniper, its berries, and its oil are stimulant, carminative and diuretic. It also acts as an urinary antiseptic, but it should not be given where there is renal disease. In large doses it is said to irritate the urinary organs; its irritant properties during excretion cause reflex contractions of the uterus, and the drug has been used as an emenagogue.

The oil is held by some to be an excellent diuretic, and to act also like copaivae in arresting mucous discharges, especially from the uretha.

The oil is used as a carminative

in flatulence and colic, and also in the treatment of lumbago.

Juniper is contained in the spirituous liquor called "Hollands," one of its best forms as a diuretic. One well-known Herbal Authority writes:—"I have sometimes found five minims of the oil with a fluid drachm of spirit of nitrous aether given thrice a day, in any common vehicle, produce diuresis in dropsy where other means had failed.

PREPARATIONS

The following are well-known and well-tried preparations of Juniper:—

Spiritus Juniperi B.P.C.:

Oil of Juniper 1 in 10 in alcohol 90 per cent.
Dose 5 to 20 minims.
This spirit was included in the British Pharmacopœia, 1914.

Spiritus Juniper Compositus:

Oil of Juniper...........	8
Oil of Caraway.........	1
Oil of Fennel...........	1
Alcohol 99 per cent......	1400
Water to	2000

Dose 2½ drachms.

Vinum Diureticum (P. Helv.):

Juniper	15
Squil..................	10
Orange Peel	10
Absinthe	5
Sweet Flag	5
Dry Southern Wine.....	1000

Dose ¼ to 1 ounce

Species Juniper. Juniper Tea:

Anise Seed	1
Licorice Root	1
Juniper Berries	8

(Norwegian Pharmacopœia).

Juniper Juice. Juniper-Berry Syrup.

Syrup Juniperi:

Juniper Berries (freshly bruised)	8 ounces
Water (hot)	31 "

Mix, stir frequently during 12 hours, express and evaporate the liquid to a thin extract.

(German Pharmacopœia.)

Herbal Aids to Beauty

For Sun Burn

Perhaps this summer you will go sunbathing and become tanned the lovely brown that your friends will admire so much; but they will not admire the very painful effects of sunbathing caused by being exposed too long with a tender white skin that has been covered up all the winter. In case you get sunburnt by too much exposure (it is extremely painful indeed) the following will prove a blessing to you and it may be obtained from your nearest Herbalist: Glycerine, ¼ oz., Distilled Witch Hazel ½ oz. and Olive Oil, ½ oz., mixed together and applied as required.

CYSTITIS

By FRANK WORTHINGTON, M.N.A.M.H.

Cystitis is an inflamed condition of the urinary bladder, which is a very unpleasant and painful complaint, and generally attacks a person in two stages— acute and chronic.

Acute Cystitis is inflammation of the inner mucous membrane of the bladder, and may attack a person of any age, generally commencing with a cold, shivery feeling all over the body, quickly followed by fever. The pulse becomes hard, sharp and quick, and the patient has a desire to frequently urinate, tenesmus (to strain), and some irritation will be experienced.

There will also be more or less throbbing and a burning sensation over the region of the bladder and pubes (or pubic bone), which is very much increased by pressure, or when the urine is retained for a while.

A dull aching pain is felt, which may extend downwards into the testicles and the gland (or head) of the penis of a male patient, and down as far as the thighs. The latter is experienced in both males and females.

The pain will also extend upwards into the ureters and kidneys, affecting the back (loins and sacrum). The urine passed is scanty, of a high specific gravity, acid in reaction, and being very acrid (acid), it causes bad shooting and burning pains in the neck of the bladder when passing it, and in some cases, the pain and difficulty is so bad, that it can only be passed when in a kneeling position.

The urine has a dark, heavy sediment of an offensive smell, especially on standing for a while, and upon a urinary test will find to be composed of blood, pus, mucous and mucous shreds, albumin, with urates and perhaps crystals of triple phosphates.

CHRONIC CYSTITIS

Chronic Cystitis (or catarrhal) is a condition of chronic inflammation of the mucous membrane walls of the bladder, later involving to a greater or lesser extent the submucosa tissue, and the muscular structure of the bladder. It may follow sooner or later after an attack of an acute form, coming on insidiously (slowly), and is very often met with in elderly persons.

The first onset of this condition is usually a dull aching pain in the abdomen, and over the region of the bladder for a time, with a feeling to strain and a desire to pass urine, which sometimes dribbles away. When it has been passed, there is little or no change at first, except for a slow, increasing quantity of mucous, and a strong odour of ammonia, but later as the condition gets more established, there can be seen a heavy, thick sediment containing blood pus, albumin, mucous and much epithelium tissue, and crystals of triple phosphates, and is alkaline in reaction.

The difficulty and pain has been slowly increasing, until the patient, in extreme cases, or where ulceration has occurred, is in agony each time they try to pass urine. This causes the patient to become very weak and prostrated by the effort. Very often a catheter has to be used. The general constitution of the body becomes affected, failure of appetite and digestion, headache and constipation is present, and the skin is dry and harsh, and eruptions may form, caused by the imperfect general elimination of the waste matter from the body. The patient at this stage becomes very irritable and impatient.

Causes, which are many, may be from sudden exposure of the body to severe cold or draughts, when the excretory glands of the skin are in active process, causing that action to be checked. The waste (or poison) is driven back into the system.

Drinking large quantities of cold water when the body is perspiring has the same action.

Long exposure to cold, causing a loss of body heat, thus setting up a chilled condition of the body, is another.

Neglected colds and fevers, a fall or a blow over the abdomen or the pubic bone, or holding the urine too long when there is a desire, but no opportunity, to pass it at such a time, or by some irritation in the bowels, due to intestinal worms, diarrhœa, constipation (the latter thus causing a distention of the walls of the bladder) and stretching its wall, are some causes.

Cystitis may also follow labour in women, from the pressure or injury from the passage of the fœtal head, or by some infection, such as the lack of cleanliness and care in using the catheter, or leucorrhœa (whites) in women, or gonorrhœal infection both in males and females.

It may be the result of abuse of Nature's laws, or from some organic disease condition, as gout, rheumatism, etc., or from some local inflammation or irritation, as enlarged prostate gland, piles, stones, gravel, tumors, cancer, stricture, etc., etc.

TREATMENT

At the first sign of this trouble, the patient should have a hot sitz bath, and if constipated, an injection to the bowels.

They should then go to bed, and the body kept in a mild perspiration with hot water bottles.

Methyl Salicylate (fort) ointment should be gently rubbed over the bladder, afterwards cloths applied which have been dipped in hot water. These hot applications should be kept up for a few days or so, to remove the congestion and inflammation.

MEDICINE

Get from any Herbalist of repute the following:—

Clivers Herb	¾	ounce
Uva Ursi Leaves	¾	"
Marshmallow Herb	½	"
Dog Grass Root	½	"
Sanicle Herb	½	"
Ginger Root	¼	"

Senna Leaves as required.

Pour on them one quart of boiling water, stand in the oven for 20 minutes, then strain through a fine cloth.

Dose: Adults, ½ to ¾ teacupful; Children, ½ to ¾ wineglassful (hot) every 3 or 4 hours.

See to the diet, avoid starchy foods and meats, coffee, cocoa, and alcoholic liquors.

Vegetables, such as asparagus,

carrots, turnips, onions, and others should be taken freely.

Should you require any advice on Nature's remedies, etc., consult a Herbal Practioner.

Editorial

When philosophical arguments were at their height a few years ago, a phrase which was often repeated at Lectures, made reference to a comparison between the macrocosm and the microcosm. In plain language this meant that the outer or greater world was reflected by the inner world of man.

This was recalled to our mind when we accepted a kind invitation to the Annual Dinner of the London and Home Counties Branch of the Association, on Thursday the 16th of September. In a sense we were there "incognito," except to a few, and we may say in passing that if a copy of the excellent photograph of those present is scrutinized for our frontal features they will be disappointed. Which, we think, is fortunate for us!

Next month we hope to give a full account of the occasion with extracts from the very sensible after dinner speeches, which were undoubtedly given from the heart by the speakers concerned. We were deeply impressed by their sincerity.

Our purpose now is to record our impressions of the guests—hence our allusion to the macrocosm—we hoped to see epitomized as it were our public; and in this we were not disappointed.

Good-fellowship was apparent from the onset—everyone present seemed bent on increasing the comfort and happiness of those nearest them, so that very soon we were a jolly party indeed. At our own table there was much spontaneous laughter which was due in no small measure to the gaiety of one member who must be very healthy, or rather agile, judging from the Branch President's account of his prowess in climbing stairs!

We noticed also that there were no lack of advice on matters herbal. Not that we mean to infer the talking of "shop," rather to emphasis the free giving of therapeutic aids to all and sundry. One lady present even presumed to.... but we are digressing and another thing is perhaps we were not meant to hear, so we will be silent.

Now it would not be possible for all readers of the Medical Herbalist to be present at such a function though any would be very welcome, not only at the London Branch but also at similar functions which occur also in the provinces. But—as we have frequently mentioned in these columns—more and more people are becoming attracted to Medical Herbalism, because they realize that **herbs can cure,** not only in Great Britain but throughout the World.

Some however feel themselves isolated and it is indicative of the great purpose of this magazine in serving the public, that we are enabled to put in touch correspondents who, though almost neighbours, have written to us a thousand miles or more away, for information regarding the names and addresses of those nearest them interested in herbal matters. To those of you who are in a similar position and have hesitated as new readers to write to us, we would like to assure you that we are here to help. With this end in view, any reader who would like to get into contact with residents in his or her village, town or country, may send their address, which will be published in our columns so to achieve the purpose desired.

There is no reason why not that readers, especially in countries far away, should enjoy social gatherings such as that we have mentioned in London. The getting together feeling is fine—the interchange of ideas wonderful—producing enthusiasm which in turn begets more adherents to the theory and practice of Medical Herbalism.

The Approach Of Winter

Judging from the recent weather, it will not be long before winter is upon us with its damp and cold, and the wise ones will have on hand a supply of herbs in order to combat the ailments peculiar to the season.

Chills, Colds and Coughs are of course the most prevalent and for those complaints the herbalist has many remedies which are proved and tested. Peppermint and Elder—blossom taken as in a tea is best for "chills" and no household should be without a small stock. These two herbs every year are brought to the notice of people who have not hitherto tried herbs, with the good result of not only performing a cure but also creating another fresh addition to our supporters.

Catarrh is another troublesome complaint and for this is recommended, Garlic, Horehound, Maidenhair, or certain botanic snuffs made up from Golden Seal, Bayberry and Wild Cherry Bark.

The frequency of the Cough is annoying and should be fought by the avoidance of draughts and the reduction of foods of an excessive starchy nature. Here again herbs are in great demand, Marshmallow, Elecampane, Linseed, Marjoram, Coltsfoot, Lungwort to mention but a few, are excellent.

A visit to a Qualified Herbalist now should be made by every prudent housewife as many herbs are obtainable which can be added to the household's medical chest for readiness against the attack of winter's army of microbes. We say have herbs on hand as they are so efficacious when given at the onset of disease. Many a chill has been avoided overnight by the prompt use of Yarrow or Elder and Peppermint. And before setting off in the damp, depressing mornings to business a cup of that old, old favourite Composition Powder will be the finest value in "insurance" ever.

The elder folks all look forward to the ravages of the forthcoming season with dread—it is such a trying time for those with troublesome difficulties in breathing. Let them go forthwith to their local Herbal Practitioner for advice and live through the season in comfort. The skill is there, the herbs are there, the rest is up to you in freeing the vital force within you, thus putting up the barriers against the invasion of disease.

ANSWERS TO READERS ENQUIRIES

By MEDICON

Question.—I have had some wonderful information from the pages of "The Medical Herbalist" in the past, for which I thank you. If you would kindly let me know how to make Chickweed Ointment (also Marshmallow Ointment, if space permits), I should be more than grateful. Is there any publication dealing with the making of ointments from herbs, and where obtainable? Trusting you will forgive me for asking so many questions in my first letter to you, with the best of all good wishes for "The Medical Herbalist," Yours very sincerely—(R. McP., Hull).

Answer. — Marshmallow Ointment can be made in the following way: Take Marshmallow Leaves 2 ozs.; Slippery Elm Bark, cut small, 2 ozs.; Beeswax, 4 ozs.; Lard, 4 ozs.; Heat together in a warm oven for half an hour, strain through a coarse cloth, and stir until cold.

Chickweed Ointment is made in the same way, substituting the Chickweed Herb for the Marshmallow Leaves.

If you are not intending to use large quantities of the ointments, I would advise you to purchase ready-made Marshmallow Ointment and Chickweed Ointment from your qualified Herbalist, since it is more difficult to make it for oneself than one would imagine.

Q.—Would you please advise me what medicine to give for nervous twitchings in a child of ten. She seems in fairly good health, and is quite all right for months at a time, then the twitchings start again. (Len, Barnsley).

A.—First of all I would advise you to watch the motions closely in case the child has worms. This is only a precaution, since I am of the opinion that the twitchings are due to nothing more than a touch of overstrain of the nerves. Children are apt to be excitable and also to expand a tremendous amount of nervous energy. The muscles are left in a very tired condition, and when relaxed, as in sleep, they sometimes jump. There is a medical explanation of this, but it is too technical to expound here, but I can assure you that it is not serious. However, here is a prescription which will soothe the nervous system:—

F.E. Scullcap ....3 drachms
F.E. Valerian ......3 "
F.E. Mistletoe ......3 "
F.E. Hops ....3 "
F.E. Licorice ....2 "

Add water to 6 ounces. Give two teaspoonsful in water before each meal.

Q.—This lady complains of pains throughout the body, and limbs cold and stiff. She is nervous and depressed, and cannot control micturition at times. (M. McKeown, Femanagh).

A.—In a case such as this it is extremely difficult to diagnose the complaint without seeing the patient. However, there seems no doubt that the nerves are out of hand, so much so, that all the symptoms may be due to nervous debility. Consequently, the remedy must be directed to the nervous system as a whole and not to each individual symptom.

Here is a prescription which should prove effective. Take of Scullcap, Motherwort, Black Cohosh, Valerian and Wood Betony: ½ ounce each. Boil in three pints of water down to two pints. Take a wineglassful four times daily after meals. As far as your diet is concerned, avoid all rich and greasy foods, and be very sparing with condiments, especially salt. Meat must only be taken three times weekly. A green vegetable salad should be taken once daily with Olive Oil as a dressing. Any kind of fruit is good excepting bananas.

Q.—I am completely run down, so would you let me know what herbs to combine so as to make a good general tonic. (John Caw, Co. Down).

A.—Take half an ounce each of Gentian, Calumba Root, Chamomile Herb, Poplar Bark and Pervian Bark. Pour two pints of boiling water on and let it stand for two hours in a covered vessel, then strain. The dose is a wineglassful four times a day.

* * *

Would you please advise me what to take for persistent head colds with sneezing, eyes running, lassitude, etc. It lasts about three days, but keeps re-occurring every two or three weeks. Would you give recipe in fluid extracts as it is easier to take, and also please tell me what would be good for an inhalant.—(Mrs. Brampton).

Your trouble is no doubt a form of chronic catarrh which leaves you open to repeated colds in the changing weather. However, this preparation is what you require:—

Receipt.

F.E. Boneset.
F.E. Yarrow.
F.E. Wood Sage.
F.E. Echinacia, of each ½ ounce.

Add water to 6 ounces. Take two teaspoonfuls in warm water before meals.

The best inhalant is Eucalyptus, but you may get more relief by burning Wood Sage, letting the smoke enter the respiratory passages.

* * *

Lives in Australia, 250 miles way up in the bush, has lack of appetite, sudden stabbing pains in right and left sides of chest. Vomits mucous on rising in morning. Pains in back at times, difficulty in sleeping owing to frequent micturition.—(Fred., Australia).

The collection of symptoms which you mention suggest to me that the trouble is probably Neurasthenia. Most of the sufferings complained of might aptly be set down as sensations, this being typical of the ailment mentioned. There has probably been a good deal of mental strain which has produced a condition of lack of nerve force. This will produce a number of "feelings" which cause the patient to complain of numerous ills.

The right method of treatment is to ignore the individual symptoms and to concentrate on getting the central nervous system built up. This will take a long time but once the results start to come the symptoms will gradually disappear.

I would advise the following herbs. Take of Scullcap, Mistletoe, Hops and Vervain, one ounce of each. Infuse the lot in four pints of boiling water for thirty minutes. Strain and take one wineglassful, four times daily. Stimulating protein foods, such as meat, cheese and eggs, should be avoided, also rich pastries and greasy dishes.

Let the diet consist chiefly of vegetables, salads and fruits, also plenty of milk. Two pints of water should be drunk daily to wash the alimentary canal and the kidneys. Perseverence will be necessary to effect a cure but the results will amply justify the efforts expended.

* * *

A friend writing from India mentions in his letter of a tree called there Kavita, the fruit, leaves and gum of which are used medicinally. Can you give me any further information?—(R. N. K., Richmond).

This tree is **Feronia elephantum** more commonly known as the Elephant-tree. The leaves are aromatic, carminative and astringent. They are used with other decoctions in dyspepsia. The ripe fruit is astringent, digestive and tonic and is a useful remedy in salivation, sore throat and in strengthening the gums. The gum is used sometimes as a substitute for Gum Arabic and is useful to relieve tenesmus in bowel affections.

* * *

To H. A. Tritton: As a preventative against Infantile Paralysis avoid cereals, white bread, sugar and cheap candy. These foodstuffs are apt to cause an acid condition of the blood and lessen the resisting power of the system. Some of the causes of this disease are, exhaustive nervous system, wrong diet, clogged bowels, checked kidneys and the circulation loaded with morbid matter. The first thing to do on treating a case is to give the child an enema of lukewarm water suitable to the age of the child. At the same time give repeated doses of hot water internally with occasionaly fresh fruit juice. Nursing is most important, keep the bowels open and build up with the nourishing slippery elm food.

* * *

To Mrs. L. Burns: Would rather prefer lemon-juice in tea to your suggested use of honey; brown sugar should be used for other purposes. Exposure to cold, dampness and fatigue in addition to impure blood will help to cause lumbago and neuritis; a change of diet will be of great help to you. There is nothing to worry at your age if you have slightly creaking joints you should try one of the blood mixtures given elsewhere in the pages of this issue. The berries of the Mountain Ash have no medicinal properties but a jelly is made from them for culinary purposes. This has a slightly tonic effect when the jelly is made from a good recipe but such is not readily accessible at the time of writing. You will find a recipe for Hay Fever in this issue. Lemons are good for you and the number you mention is not excessive. Salad-dressing? well it depends on its constituents and that you have omitted to mention.

* * *

To R. C. Trenle: Archangel, emmenagogue, Ginseng, tonic and stimulant. Golden-heal, tonic, stomachic. Kola, nervine, diuretic and tonic. Peppermint, stomachic, sudorific and stimulant. Damiana, aphrodisiac. Scullcap, nervine. Mistletoe, anti-spasmodic. Hydrastis, same as Golden-seal.

* * *

To Waino Kotila: An application to the skin, which is most valuable is Grindelia. When poisoned by the plant you mention, it acts promptly and satisfactorily. Tincture of Lobelia can also be used as a local application.

Advance of Medical Science

Extract from The Leeche Booke, 1937.—To Guarde against the DIPHTHERIA PLAGUE: Take of beef broth onne pounde and cooke it till it seethe, coole and adde the germes from the membrane in the throate of onne laide low with the Plague. The germes multiplie and their venome is to be extracted by devious rites—and you may then have gotte the TOXIN.

Nowe take onne horse of noble birth and pricke it well. Into the prickes pour the toxin till it shall make the horse vomite and sweate and shiver. When the horse shall recover to the fulle, after dayes, it shall be pricked again and more noxious toxin applyed. So shall this be repeated till the horse be not affected by the poisone.

Nexte the greate veine in the horse's neck must severed be, and the liffe bloode that streams therefrom gathered in pots and pannes till it shall settle into bloode and water. This water does containe the cure, the Antitoxin, and is mixed with the beef-broth poisone.

Take many stronge and healthie childer and into prickes three put this filthie concoctione. If they succombe not unto the fever or to death, they shalle be immune from the Plague.

Note.—The above recipe is a correct outline of the methods employed in producing the toxin-antitoxin mixtures so widely recommended by Medical Officers for the immunization of children. These, and similar processes used in the production of other sera and vaccines, put to shame the recipes of the Leech Books of the dark ages—and they are accepted by a credulous medical fraternity as the peoples of the middle ages accepted the charlatanry and quackery of the Leech doctors.

Though these foolish and dangerous fashions in medicine continue to rise—and fall—the fact remains that a healthy body is the surest safeguard against any form of disease.

MAGIC OF HERBS or BELIEFS AND UNBELIEFS.

By JOHN PASKE

By one of those chances, which somehow rarely occur, I had become interested, and a kind of Medical Botanist, in the true cause of Herbalism.

But I soon found that the knowledge of curative plants and their uses was far below the standard, even in the cases of many so-called Herbalists, while their Medical Botany was not always reliable.

The average Herbalist in this country takes a pride in being ultra-tolerant, over-doing a beneficence, which tends to harm.

It involves a policy akin to weakness, and but for the inherent pluck of some more enlightened Herbalists, we should not be where we are to-day.

We find to-day there are two schools of thought; those who believe in healing with medical knowledge, and those who claim to have the gift of healing.

The knowledge of the first-named leave substantial records behind them, while in the other case, nothing is left behind. The subject of medicinal herbs is an extensive one, with a scientific library of its own. An immense number of plants are used in medicine, many of which are of no curative value, owing to similar common names being given to different plants. A great many cases came to my notice in recent years, showing that a study in the correct naming of herbs is a very important part in the successful treatment of one's patients.

We find an extraordinary and confusing variety of common names in different parts of the country, which goes to prove that the botanical name makes it the only standard of identity. Botanical terminology and the arrangement of natural orders vary a great deal in different countries, making it much more difficult to study.

A few typical examples are Erigeron Canadensis and Pulcaria Dysentrica, which are both called Fleabane, the former being a tonic and diuretic while the latter is used in cases of dysentery, as its name implies.

Tamus communis and Bryonia dioica are both called Mandrake; both are also called Bryony for no apparent reason.

Celandine is also applied to too many plants of a different Natural Order, such as Ranunculus Ficaria, and Cheledonium majus.

Skunk Cabbage is also given to Lysichitum americana and Symplocarpus fœtidus, plants entirely different to each other.

While Lungwort is applied to Sticta Pulmonaria and Pulmonaria officinalis, the former being a moss, the latter is a Boraginaceæ. Lungwort (Pulmonaria officinalis) owes its name and reputation to the white spots on the leaves, which were thought to be the "signature," showing that it would cure infirmities and ulcers of the lungs, but the power to do good is no longer believed in it.

Thus it will be seen that in order to become a Medical Herbalist, one must not only study the correct identification of plants, but know something of their therapeutical action and methods of administration.

In the old days of Herbalism, so many herbs were used and found good for so many disorders, that one wonders that the patients ever died till one examines the precriptions and methods employed, and then one is more astonished that any ever recovered at all. Probably, there are some Herbalists today who will hold on to anything so long as the magic of the herbs plays its part.

To-day, there is an unfortunate tendency among the poor to desert herbs for any quackery they may chance to see advertised to cure nearly all diseases subject to mankind. In the olden days it was well known that Elderflowers were most highly valued, and used in cases of colds and ointments; Marshmallow for inflammation; Marigold Tea a remedy for measles; Camomile as a mouth wash for disinfecting the mucous membrane, and to stimulate the stomach; Rosemary for making the hair grow; Watercress as a great blood tonic, therefore, good for rheumatism; Raspberry, Agrimony and Barberry Bark for consumptive people; the Greater Celandine good for the eyes; while Hops long had the reputation of inducing sleep; Gentian as the most valuable stomachic, Valeriana for nerves; and Dill Seeds have been used for hundreds of years.

Herbal remedies have attracted writers since the earliest times, many believing in the supernatural agencies brought forward to account for uncomprehended phenomena. For instance, Basil was thought to cause sympathy between two people; Rampion was likely to make a child quarrelsome; while Periwinkle will cause love.

Plants were also credited with strong friendship and enmities amongst themselves. Others held views about their sympathetic and antipathies, which was attributed to individual likes and dislikes. From this, it will be seen that particular plants have power to produce certain dispositions in the mind of man and power over his moral qualities.

Dill seeds were able to hinder witches of their will, and used in spells against them, and many believed that by carrying a bag full near the heart would keep them free from "spells." It was also believed that St. John's Wort would drive away evil spirits; Clover enable the wearer to avert infection; and Garlic would keep away unwanted company.

The Nightmare flower, which is found in Argentina, was supposed to contain a drug which causes nightmare, and was employed by some to whoever they wished to torment.

Among plants that have supposed magic power are the Mugwort, which, if laid in the soles of the boots, will keep the feet from tiring. Wreaths of Camomile hung up in a house on St. John's Day, will defend it against thunder. Wild Thyme laid near milk will prevent it being "turned" by thunder. The root of Tarragon held between the teeth will cure toothache and pains in the head. To transplant Parsley is very unlucky, while if Rhubarb is let go to seed, it will bring death to the family before the year is out. This is still believed in many parts of the country. It is supposed to bring bad luck if Holly is brought into the house before Christmas, but if flower seeds are sown on Palm Sunday, they will come out double.

Elder-blossom is specially connected with magic in all parts of the world, such as if a child is placed in a cradle of Elder wood, no peace will result. He who stands under Elder trees will be protected from lightning, while others believe that Elder will prevent fever, drive away spirits, and a twig carried in the pockets a preventive from rheumatism.

A stake of Elder will last longer than a bag of iron the same size. The Elderberries also hold much magical powers.

For ages past herbs and animals appear linked together, as it seems certain that plants must benefit or affect their well-being. Sheep seek the Dandelion; dogs, Couchgrass; lambs, the Lamb's Lettuce; cats, the Catmint; rats, the Great Valeriana, which was thought to be the plant employed by the Pied Piper to attract its victims. The weasel loves Rue; nightingale, the Hop which is supposed to make them sing; the cuckoo connected with Orchis and Plantain; while the swallow restores the sight of her young by the juice of Celandine, that is why in some parts the Celandine is called Swallow Wort. The hawk is attracted to the Hawkweed with equal success; linnets to Eyebright; woodpeckers to the Peony; and jays to Bay leaves.

It is said that snakes love Fennel; frogs, Cinquefoil; toads, Sage; and lizards, Calamintha.

At one time people blessed their cattle with certain herbs, while many are deadly poisonous to them.

Rest Harrow was held to have marvelous properties if used on tired horses or oxen.

Houndstongue was believed to be the tongue of barking dogs.

In many parts of the country today we find herbs taken with the belief that colour and names have some bearing on their curative values, such as Herb Robert for blood disorders, Marigold for jaundice, and Viper's Bugloss for snake bite.

To-day, when everything is so confusing, little notice is taken of the old folklore of herbs, and their uses, or peep into the depths of minds of the old country folk.

In this respect we lose a great deal, but one must feel grateful that to-day Herbalism is gradually being founded on a scientific basis, to rank with all that is highest in life.

Health Brevities

IN my opinion, it is a social error to criticize the honest effort of any one trying to right their condition. Many a seeker after health via the food route has become discouraged and turned aside from his purpose by the thoughtless ridicule of so-called friends. Being on a diet means nothing more than changing from one group of foods to another, learning to like a greater number of foods, training the body to tolerate foods that our run-down condition would not permit before. Being on a diet does not mean that the first and foremost idea is to reduce. — *Florence Stephenson Hadley.*

LIFE IS NOT CHEMICAL BUT VITAL

By *VITALIST*

TRUTH IN THERAPEUTICS

Poison. People who do not know, often say a little poison does not hurt anyone, but we know different!

We know that a poison is still a poison whether given in small doses or large fatal doses; quantity does not alter quality.

The vitality and tissues of the body always resists and tries to expel all detrimental and poisonous substances from the body, hence vomiting and sweating in many cases naturally occurs in poisoning cases.

On the other hand, vitality accepts and assimulates medicines, because its inherent instinct enables it to differentiate between helpful and harmful substances.

Poisons, exert a chemico-dynamic action upon cell structures, and their virulence is expended almost entirely upon the structure of the nerve cells, and mainly on the nerve centres as these possess less vital resistance than the general bodily tissues.

True Medicine and False

True medicines are possessed of sanative properties which are in a potential and passive attitude in their inherent and logical relation with the vital force, and cannot therefore act in the dynamic or chemic sense of force or energy, either on living matter or cell structure, but true medicine like beneficial foods, furnishes reparative and restorative materials to living matter, by means of which it may maintain its vital integrity; medicines impart or exert a wholesome and helpful influence in aid of the resistive, eliminative and restorative efforts, and results of Vital Force in a disease-state of the organism or any part thereof.

(a) A poison is dynamically active.
(b) A medicine is passive, yet possessed of influence.
(c) A poison is destructive.
(d) Medicines are restorative in their influence.
(e) Poisons are destroyers.
(f) Medicines are builders and constructives.
(g) Vitality and Cell life rejects and resists poisons.
(h) Vitality accepts and assimulates medicines.
(i) Poisons attack living cell structures.
(j) True medicines sanatively influence the living matter of the cell units, by affording helpful material for its assimulation.
(k) Poisons are Pathologic.
(l) Medicines are Physiologic.

The doctors know that small doses of poison given in grains or small parts of grains are less liable to disturb the vital force and cause it to put up a large show of resistance to expel the poison; they also know that the human body tries to adapt itself to changes, or, that it will tolerate poisons to a degree, that is when the nerve cells eventually tire of a long continued resistive effort to expel a poison, it then tries to make the best of it, or tries to adapt itself to the presence of the poison, just as a man may smoke tobacco for years before he finds it is affecting his health, he does not get the satisfaction out of the small amount of tobacco that he commenced with as a beginner, and he find that the desire grows, and that he can smoke more and more, apparently, without it having the effect that it used to, and the same with the drinker of alcoholic beverages, what really happens is the adaption and toleration to the presence of a poison in the body.

The chemical doctors know that this occurs with poisonous chemicals used as medicine, so all goes well for a time, but it is found that the quantity of the deadly drug must be increased to the patient from time to time as the ever resistive instincts of the living matter gains strength from constant suppression.

Take Morphia for an example, to any patient to whom it has been given, should morphia be withheld from them entirely, or even the doses diminished, this long suppressed resistive energy of the central nerve cells breaks forth like a long accumulated energy of a volcano into a storm of resistance that renders the poor victim of the morphia habit frantic with craving for the drug; if a healthy person takes the so-called medicinal dose for a period and then discontinues it, he is racked with the most unbearable pain in every part of his body.

Small doses of poison may be surely lodged in the system without causing immediate death, but the damage done is slow and insidious and not immediately seen or the results felt, but little by little, and as sure as fate, the organs and nerves are weakened and debilitated and many healthy cells of various organs and nerves die as a result; so a person may not feel the loss straight away of a few dozen nerve, liver, kidney or blood cells, but time tells its woeful tale.

Proof of Destructive Poison

Professor Redding—a Physiomedical Herbalist in America—conducted a series of experiments on a microscopic slide with living blood cells kept alive with a suitable menstrum, and treated with various poisonous and non-poisonous substances used in medicine. Under the influence of Cayenne (one of the finest herbal stimulants known), these blood corpuscles attained a vigour and energy never before witnessed; and at the end of one hour all seemed still endowed with new life and animation, whilst at the end of two hours they seemed no less happy, and gradually returning to their normal state. Professor Redding also made experiments with Strychnine, Arsenic and Mercury, and this is what he says:—

> "Treating fresh blood corpuscles on the slide, we found that 1-700,000 part of a grain of Strychnine almost instantly transformed this living matter into non-living fat globules, and that hundreds of living moving bioplasts suddenly and rapidly suspended all vital action from the destructive influence of less than 1-40,000 part of a grain of

Morphia and thus remained a dead and smeary mass."

Other non-poisonous herbs and poisonous chemicals were tried with the same disastrous results from the chemicals, and beneficial results from the herbal remedies; this is the acid test and we should not need to say more to prove our contention.

Strychnine

Commonly used today in many chemical medicines and advertised pick-me-ups on the market, it is a most deadly poison—prussic acid excepted. It is given by the regular profession for nervous diseases in small doses as a stimulant. It is a nerve motor irritant, acting on the neurons of the cerebral portion of the brain. It produces motor and sensory in-co-ordination, also acting on the medulla and the spinal cord, from which reflex impressions are made on the motor areas of the cerebral cortex. They cause under its influence, violent and in-co-ordinate explosions of motor-nerve energy, resulting in symptom complexes called convulsions, motor agitans (shaking palsy), and tetanic contractions of the spinal nerves. Large doses causes an agonising death by spasm whereby the whole body becomes rigid, the eyes fixed with a horrible look of fear and frenzy, and final exhaustion and death by destruction of the nerve centres.

Statements by Medical Men

Dr. Bostock (Author of the "History of Medicine"):—

"Every dose of medicine given is a blind experiment upon the vitality of the patient."

Dr. Schweninger (Physician to Prince Bismarck):—

"People want to be cheated. They fancy no cure to be possible without medicines. We physicians have been talking this apothecary stuff into them till they believe it."

The famous Russian physician, D. W. Weressaj, speaking in his book, "The Confessions of Physicians," of his experience in public hospitals, says:—

"Never leave a patient without medicine, we are told; prescribe something, anyhow, so that the patient may see that something is done for him. And when a diagnosis is wholly impossible, search for one that is, dose the patient with certain medicines, trying one after the other.

"If he responds to the first, the third, or the twelfth treatment, then, he is afflicted with the malady for which this treatment is good, and after that it is plain sailing!"

M. Malgendie (The celebrated French Physiologist):—

"I hesitate not to declare, no matter how sorely I should wound our vanity, that so gross is our ignorance of the real nature of the physiological disorder called disease that it would, perhaps, be better to do nothing, and resign the complaint into the hands of Nature, than to act as we are frequently compelled to do, without knowing the why and wherefor of our conduct, at the obvious risk of hastening the end of the patient. Gentlemen, medicine is great humbug. I know it is called science. Doctors are nearly empirics when they are not charlatans."

In the next issue I will deal with the much used Bromine used in medicine today.

SOME BRITISH WILD PLANTS AND THEIR USES

By W. CROMPTON, M.N.M.A.H.

COMFREY

Symphytum Officianalis. N.O. Boraginaceæ

Synonyms. — Knitbone, Consound, Common Comfrey Gum Plant, Boneset, Slippery Root, Consolida, Black Root, Yalluc (Saxon), Ass Ear.

Habitat.—Europe, Western Siberia, abundant throughout England, by the river banks, in moist and watery places.

Description. — Root perennial, thick, tapering, branchy, fibrous, brownish, black outward, white within; stems, succulent, erect firm, branched, rough, with strong hairs, angular somewhat membraneous at the angles; height 2 feet. Leaves, large, alternate, acute, darkish green, rough and covered with short hairs, lower ones egg-shaped, on foot stalks, upper ones almost stalkless, ovate-lanceolate or tapering to each end, very decurrent, being attached to the stem much below their point of insertion, thus forming a wing-like continuation of the stem. Flowers in cluster on short stalks, drooping, usually all turned towards the same side; colour yellowish white or purple. Carollas, bell-shaped, calyx deeply cleft, narrow and lace-shaped, spreading.

Part Used.—The whole plant, leaves and root.

Chemical Contents.—Allantoin, a large amount of mucilage, also a trace of starch, and tannin.

Medicinal Properties.—Comfrey is gently stimulating, and toning to the mucous membrane, particularly of the respiratory organs. It is demulcent and soothing to the irritated conditions following colds, influenza, catarrh, bronchial affections, and pneumonia. In the irritated mucous membrane of the stomach and bowels, symphytum slowly reaches to soothe and heal.

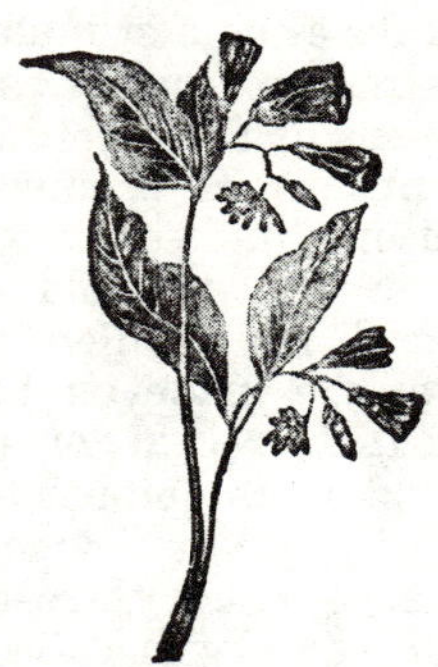

COMFREY

When the veins and arteries are bursted, symphytum is a regular friend that never lets you down.

In hæmorrhage of the lungs and stomach, it will soon set all at rest by its binding, knitting or contracting effects. When given for hæmorrhages it should be combined with astringents. However, when given for ruptures, it may be combined with other mucilaginous media.

Preparation and Uses.—Comfrey Root crushed, 1 oz. Boil in 3 pints of water to 1 pint. Strain. Dose: ¼ to teacupful four times daily.

In case of rupture of the bowels, make and use as follows:—

Comfrey Root crushed 1 ounce
Marshmallow Root
(Althaea Officinalis)..1 "
Mistletoe (Viscum
Album)..1 "
Clown's Woundwort
(Stachys Palustris)..1 "

Simmer in 5 pints of water half hour. Strain. Dose: One small teacupful five times daily. This will give entire satisfaction in all cases suffering from rupture, whatever the cause. It is peculiarly remedial in old ruptures. Perseverance must be sustained, if need be, for a period of two or three months.

The formulæ given as under is a remedy for varicocele:—

Comfrey ....1 ounce
Balmony (Chelone
Glabra)....1 "
Rupturewort (Herniara
Glabra)....1 "

Simmer in 4 pints of water half hour. Sieve. Dose: One wineglassful 5 times daily. This has been well tried, and given great benefit insomuch as there has not been any return of the trouble unless the patient persists in his old habits.

In cases of spitting blood, use the following:—

Comfrey Root crushed .1 ounce
Water Plantain (Alisma
Plantago)....1 "
Mistletoe (Viscum
Album)....1 "
Water Betony (Scrofularia Aquatica)....1 "
Water Avens (Geum
Rivale)....1 ounce

Simmer in five pints of water half hour. Strain. Dose: One wineglassful 4 times daily. This preparation will relieve the most obstinate cases of blood spitting (Hemoptisis). Also the inveterate cases of vomiting blood (hæmorrhages of the lungs and stomach). In nose bleeding, apply also a cold, wet sponge to the back of the neck frequently.

BORAGE

Borage Officinalis. N.O. Boraginaceaæ

Synonyms.—Burrage.

Habitat.—From the Middle and South of Europe to North Africa. Having been naturalised it is found on rubbish and waste ground in this country (England).

Description.—Root long; mostly biennial; fibrous, divided, whitish; stem erect, round, thick, much-branched, covered with stiff hairs, succulent; 1½ to 2 feet high. Leaves alternate, wavy, deep green, covered with long harsh hairs; lower ones obovate or egg-shaped (with broad part of the egg uppermost), with foot stalks; upper ones ovate, nearly stalkless. Flowers terminate, bright blue, star-shaped; it differs from all others of this order by the prominent black anthers; these form a cone and are said to be their beauty spot. The fruit consists of four dark brown nutlets.

Part Used.—Leaves and flowers.

Chemical Contents.—Potassium and calcium combined with mineral salts. The fresh juice contains 30 per cent and the dried herb 3 per cent of nitrate of potash. The stem and leaves supply much salty mucillage; the same, when boiled, deposits nitre and common salt. It is to these qualities and the specially refreshing and invigorating properties which are said to make Borage so wholesome. Due to the presence of nitrate of potash, small sparks are emitted when the dried plant is burned on coals.

Medicinal Properties.—Demulcent, diuretic, emollient, diffusively stimulating and relaxing antispasmodic agent.

Medical Properties. — Borage comforts the heart when saddened with much grief, eases the causes of disturbance in the secretive glands, particularly that of the adrenals, or suprarenal capsules. All the glandular system is gradually reached by the singular action of Borage. It is used to defend the heart in contagious and eruptive fevers. The seed and leaves are said to increase the mothers milk.

Preparation and Uses.—Make as follows:—

Borage .... 1 ounce
Boiling water .... 1 pint

Steep half hour. Strain. Dose: 1 wineglassful 4 times daily between meals.

Make and use the following in case of mind wandering:—

Borage .... 1 ounce
Weed Broadleaf (Plantago Major) .. 1 "
Meadowsweet (Spirea Ulmaria) .. 1 "
Water Avens (Geum Rivale) .. 1 "
Wormwood (Artemesia Absinthium) .. 1 ounce

Simmer in 5 pints water half-hour. Strain. Dose: One wineglassful every three hours.

This will surely relieve neurasthenia, mental oppression, weakness of the central nervous system, and generally rundown conditions following severe illness.

The compound hereunder will make for speedy recovery in eruptive fevers, thus:—

Borage .... 1 ounce
Marshmallow (Althaea Officinalis) .. 1 "
Mugwort (Artemesia Vulgaris) .. 1 "
Masterwort (Imperatorio Obstruthium) .. 1 "
Motherwort (Leonuruus Cardiaca) .. 1 "

Simmer in 5 pints water half-hour. Strain. Dose: One wineglassful three times daily.

This preparation is well suited to make for improvement in measles and all other eruptive diseases.

Use the following in blood poisoning, food poisoning, persistent sickness and vomiting, thus:—

Meadowsweet (Spirea Ulmaria) .. 1 ounce
Plantain (Plantago Major) .. 1 "
Rupturewort (Herniara Glabra) .. 1 "
Polypody of the Oak (Polypodium Vulgare) .. 1 "

Simmer in 5 pints water half-hour. Strain. Dose: One wineglassful three times daily.

The above will give complete service in blood poisoning from whatever cause.

RED CABBAGE

By E. GRUNDY, M.N.A.M.H.

The Red Cabbage, like all other foods, should be spoken of in terms of their food values, or the elements they contain. We have been taught to look upon foods as something palatable and as something which fills the stomach, irrespective of their good or bad effects. With the result that today we have thousands of people suffering from some unknown cause or set of germs. This is not surprising in view of the fact that Orthodoxy thrives in its effort to stamp out the effects not the cause of disease.

The human body is made up of fourteen known elements, and a food should be spoken of in terms of the Vital content which will supply the shortage of those elements necessary to maintain the body in perfect health; i.e., build up, energise and vitalise it.

Man's diet should be constructive, and an intelligent understanding of the different foods and their combinations would demand no other. Besides being palatable, our foods must contain active principles which maintain life; Neuclean, the life principle; Vitamin, the active principle; the Vital mineral elements; the regulating and equalising principles. Unless our food contains one or more of these agents, it cannot be considered as real food, though it does freuently take the place of such.

Articles of diet, both singly and in combinations, classed as food, which although not actually detrimental to health, can be so deficient in the life-giving and sustaining principles that they should not be used; they give the digestive and eliminatory organism extra work, and use up a considerable amount of stored energy which they in no way replace. Hence, the necessity for a thorough understanding of the body's requirements and the correct foods to supply the demand, which is my reason for writing this article on the Red Cabbage, the analysis of which is Potassium 44.5, Calcium 16.3, Sodium 10.0, Sulphur 10.0. Understanding the former, we find the Red Cabbage a wonderful food where-ever the blood stream is impure or any cancerous condition exists; it is also invaluable wherever Calcium is called for, being indicated in the building up of the teeth and boney structure in children, infectious teeth, weakness of the boney structure, weak arteries. Due to its Calcium content, it is also indicated in gastric disturbances, digestion and assimilation of food.

As a Potassium food it is indicated in neurotic tendencies, constipation, cancer, old sores, low vitality, low muscular tone, and lack of recuperative power.

As a Sulphur food it is indicated in diseases of the skin, diseases of the hair, infections, lack of bile secretion, intestinal putrefaction.

WILD FLOWERS OF THE MONTH

By MRS. B. EMMOTT, F.N.A.M.H.

MARCH

I always think of March as the month of smiles, because it is the birth of Spring and the herald of Summer. How pleasant after the dark days of Winter—even though the days may still be cold; they are longer, the light shines forth. The sun is shining, telling of warmer days to come; the trees are budding, the first Spring flowers are beginning to show their heads, and their golden glory, in the shape of the daffodil, which truly is the March flower.

"Daffodils,
That come before the swallow dared, and take
The winds of March with beauty."

The trumpet daffodil is the type known as the English daffodil, and is the one that enriches the Midland meadows in Springtime. The double daffodils belong exclusively to the garden, but to my mind these double flowers do not equal the single ones in gracefulness although the double ones are very attractive. The manner in which the process of doubling is accomplished is really wonderful. There are some flowers that are double within the trumpet only. In this case the organs of reproduction may be supposed to be converted into petals, or their equivalents. Other flowers occur that are double outside the trumpet, which remains intact in the midst of a crowd of golden banners, and others are double throughout like a double rose, the trumpet being completely lost in a confused mass of petals.

If we inquire into the origin of these many petals, we find that we can in theory account for many of them. For example, the outer petals are six in number, the trumpet consists of six lobes united at their edges, there are six stamens, and a stigma of three lobes. Thus in a common single trumpet daffodil there are twenty-one parts. It is almost impossible to find how many parts there are in a double flower, it being so difficult to count them. You may find from sixty to three times as many, a considerable portion of them being just green scales like miniature leaves.

As garden flowers, the finest of the double daffodils are **Telamonius plenus,** the largest golden yellow; **Cernuus plenus,** a lovely white rosette flower; and **Cernuus bicintus,** a very pretty white flower with a double trumpet and two rows of guard petals. Trumpet daffodils will thrive almost anywhere. They are suitable for rockeries and common borders. A certain amount of shade is favourable to their well-doing, but they also love light and air, and to be greatly shaded is unfavourable to their flowering.

In March, when you go on your botanical ramble, one of the first herbs to greet you will be the "Chickweed." See the sheltered hedgebank with a glorious sheet of emerald green sparkling with whitest stars, a sight beautiful to behold, and with this beauty comes

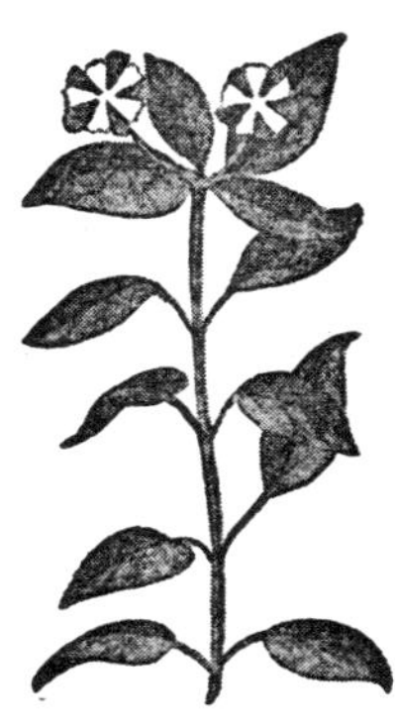

CHICKWEED

usefulness, for Chickweed is indeed a wonderful remedy both internally and externally. Now is the time to mix Chickweed in your salad, it is good for you, as well as for the singing birds. It is time too, to make Chickweed ointment, that will heal all kinds of wounds and ease those inflamed piles, or sooth the burning irritation of erysipelas.

During our rural rambles, in these early days of Spring, we come across the pale primrose lying in deep contrast upon its beautifully formed leaves, whose surfaces appear to have been embossed by deeply-cut dies of elegant workmanship. We usually find them in clusters, in the shade of a grove, or on a sloping mossy bank, overhung by the branches of some lofty tree.

When admiring these lowly flowers, don't forget to look up at the trees, and enjoy their delicate tracery, the interlacing of their slender branches. Observe the downy catkins of the hazel nut, they are the male flowers and always seen in the topmost parts of the tree. The beech, the willow and the birch flowers in precisely the same manner. The male flowers, appear in the Autumn and attain complete development in the Spring, when the female flowers, which are less conspicuous become perfect in form and function.

By all means, admire the primrose, the wood-anemone and the daffodils, but don't miss the beauty and the changing colours and form of our wonderful trees.

* * *

APRIL

"The flowers of April are as numerous as the stars of heaven, and like the Milky Way in heaven they make a glowing girdle round the earth."

April does indeed give to us many flowers, but, it claims as its birthright the modest violet. There are many species of violets and they can be found in almost every Country. At this time of the year they are found abundantly in our woods with their delicate little flowers hidden amid their clustered leaves. What magic power lies in the odour of fresh violets! There are few people to whom even a faint whiff will not bring some picture of the past, some old time recollection, be it sad or gay. Its subtle influence never fails to touch the answering heart cord, which leads the mind a helpless captive, many stories have been and could be told about violets. Truly Wordsworth was right when he wrote:—

"Long as there are Violets.
They will have their place in
story."

Many poets have sung its praises, including Browning and Shakespeare. This is not to be wondered at, for the shy and modest Violet appeals to the human sympathies and emotions to a greater degree than most of our English flowers. It may not be as beautiful as the rose, nor have the daffodil's bright colour, nor the graceful stature of the columbine, but, could it boast no other dower, this "sweet shy hermit of the shade" with its matchless perfume, would still be crowned the loved Queen of Spring. Shakespeare's poor crazed Ophelia, found flowers

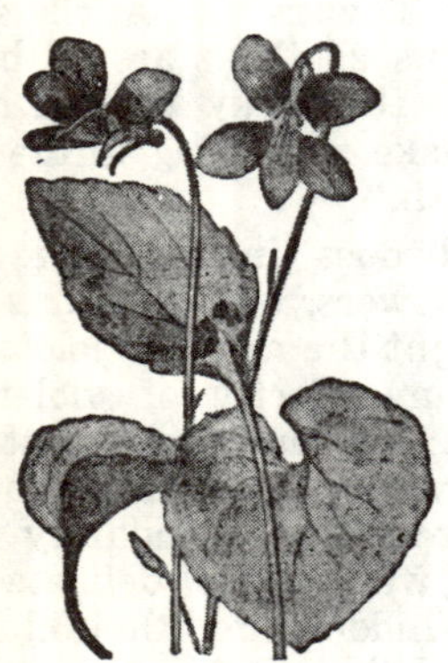

VIOLET

in plenty, for King, Queen, and brother, but for this sweet emblem of innocence there could be no place among her 'posies' now that the stain of wickedness and murder lay upon the court. "I would give you some violets, but they withered all, when my Father died" said Ophelia.

Violets, with their sweet perfume, their lovely colouring and velvet bloom, have oft brought love and comfort to sorrowing hearts, giving their message of love, hope, and encouragement.

Add to this the value of the violets medicinal properties, which for generations has been used by those versed in the healing art. Then indeed do we sing the praise unto God for this little flower, whose fragrance is superior to all that we receive from the rich East. We all know the value of Syrup of Violets, which is made in the following manner:—

Take 1 lb. of fresh petals of violet; add two pints of boiling water; marcerate for 24 hours in a covered glass vessel; pour off the fluid, then strain through fine linen or filtering paper, and with twice the weight of refined sugar made into a Syrup without boiling. The dose is from one to two teaspoonfuls. With the addition of a little Almond oil it forms a useful laxative for infants and young children. Acidulated with a small quantity of lemon juice or raspberry vinegar it may be given with benefit in coughs and sore throats. The Violet with all its virtues with all its usefulness brings the message of modesty.

The Violet droops its soft and
bashful brow,
But from its heart, sweet incense
fills the air.
So rich within—so poor without
are thou,
With modest mein and soul of
virtue rare."

Springtime is a lovely time, not only do we get the golden glory of the daffodil, but, April brings us, along with the violet, the primrose and cowslip.

What is more enchanting when walking through the country, than to come by chance upon a sunny clearing, starred with clustering groups of Spring primroses, there to feel that nature has taken you into her confidence, has given you a message of love, a message of life's return, the promise of a new beginning.

The beautiful primrose is the first flower to come in such profusion to delight the little ones. What nicer picture is there, than a child with a bunch or a basket of these sweet scented blossoms, truly every child loves the delicate fragrance of "The soft starlike primrose drenched in dew."

Along with the primroses comes the cowslip. These little flowers call out. "Rejoice and be glad in the light of my beauty." Forget the cold and frosty dame of winter. Smile in the warmth and sunshine of her daughter Spring. The note that has stirred all things in nature calls out, to you with a promise of hope. Get attuned with nature and health, that wealth and wisdom may be yours. Hope is a living vital thing. The Winter has passed Spring is here.

* * *

JUNE

The June flower is the Queen of Flowers—Her Majesty the Rose. What a variety of roses there are from the wild roses **(Rosa arvensis and Rosa canina)** which grow in our untrimmed hedges, to the beautiful Gloire de Dijon, and the Marechal Niel, which are cultivated in our gardens. There are two grand divisions of roses known as the Summer and the perpetual roses. The former bloom once in Summer, hence their name. Under this class are included what are familiarly called June roses, June moss roses and June climbers, all of which with sundry varieties, are hardy and easy to culture. The perpetual roses are those which flower several times in the season and include Bengal, China, tea-scented, Bourbon and Noisette roses.

In each division according to their habit of growth may be found climbers, intermediate and dwarfs. The climbers throw out long main branches, well supplied with shorter side branches, which produce the flowers, they are different from the others only in the matter of length. The half climbers, reach about one-half, the intermediates one-fourth and the dwarfs one-eighth as high as the climbers.

No matter what kind of rose, the purity of the blossoms, the delightfull texture of their velvet petals with the perpetual incense that arises from their opening lips ever charm and enchant. It is said that Hymen, the god of matrimony, used to wear a crown of roses, and that "his locks dropped perfume." The rose of whatever species, colour or name, holds supremacy in the hearts of the people and never will its glory wane until roses cease to bloom.

All nations have prized the rose. In ancient days ever warriors wore wreaths of its flowers and the Greeks and the Romans strewed petals over the dishes on festive occasions. When Cleopatra invited Anthony to an entertainment, the royal apartments would be covered with roses. In eastern lands the rose is prized above all flowers and in England its message is love, home and beauty.

We all know the value of rose-leaves as an astringent lotion for inflamed or weak eyes. The rose is not alone in its beauty as the flower of June. There are many flowers, indeed, that are plentiful everywhere and in the hedgerow and meadow we find some that belong rather to May than June. The heath lands and rocks are sweetly dotted with the fresh growth of ferns and the rivers and streams are newly fringed with their own peculiar forms of vegetation.

Borage and Comfrey

Among the flowers we may meet with in June is the common Borage, with its splendid blue flowers. The Viper's Bugloss is a rough but robust relative of the Borage, and one of the most elegant of all our wild flowers. It attains a height of two to three feet, the flower spike often measuring a foot in length. The flowers are in a succession of short comb-like tufts, the buds bright pink, the flowers pale blue, or deep blue, and ofttimes richest violet. Truly a glorious assemblage is given to this plant.

Perhaps less beautiful, but more useful than any other member of the borage tribe, is the Comfrey, which is known by its light green hairy leaves, and clusters of white, yellow or pink flowers. Often in the moist places in which you find Comfrey, is to be seen the true Forget-me-not, the Water Scorpion Grass with its beautiful pale blue flowers.

By the water side we find the Buckbean, a charming aquatic with bright green leaves and lovely pink flowers.

It would be strange if in a June ramble we did not somewhere meet with the honeysuckle. The common Woodbine or honeysuckle of the woods is too well known to need description. It is the Woodbine of Shakespeare, and with him the companion of wild rose.

"I know a bank whereon the wild
thyme grows,
Where oxlips and the nodding
violet blows,
Quite over canopied with luscious woodbine,
With sweet musk roses and with
eglantine."

Many of the Yarrows are now in bloom, the Cranesbill attracts our attention during the sunny month of June and by this time the Furze and the Broom are getting their share of our admiration. The grasses too, are flowering, gleaming in the meadows like silver feathers, sparkling amid the herbage of tangled groves with their white, yellow and reddish sprays of beauty. Glorious month of June, with thy flowers so beautiful, and so numerous that all cannot be mentioned, but above all the rose reigns supreme—the Queen of Flowers.

"Of all flowers,
Me thinks a rose is best,
It is the very emblem of a maid,
For when the west wind courts
her gently,
How modestly she blows, and
paints the Sun.
With her chaste blushes."

"THE GARDEN OF THE LORD"

By Rev. T. GWERNOGLE EVANS, M.N.A.M.H. AND *Mr. ALFRED HALL,* M.P.S., F.N.A.M.H.

PLEURISY

This disease is ushered in by the usual symptoms of inflammatory action, such as rigors, headache, etc.; these are succeeded by an acute pain usually in the region of the fifth rib. The pain is sharp and pricking, which is increased upon coughing, or taking a long breath. It may attack one or both sides. The breathing is hurried and painful, the pulse hard and quick, the face flushed and the whole surface dry and hot. Pleurisy consists of inflammation of the lining or membrane of the lung, and soon extends to the substance of the lung. Exposure to cold and dampness is the main cause of this malady, whereby the blood is thrust upon the internal organs in an undue quantity. The main item in treatment should therefore be to stimulate the system and keep up circulation, and thus prevent fluid on the lung.

Treatment.—Apply first a cayenne poultice to the chest for about twenty minutes, and then apply the chest oils and cover the chest with flannel. Repeat the poulticing if the pain still continues and give the following medicine:—

Pleurisy Root	1	ounce
Vervain	1	"
Hyssop	1	"
Yarrow	1	"
Ipecacuahana Root	1/4	"

Boil in 4 pints of water and simmer down to 1 pint. Strain, and add 2 drams of Essence of Cayenne and 8 ounces Honey. Give one tablespoonful every three hours, and regulate the bowels with liver pills. In the case where the inflammation extends to the substance of the lung, treatment as recommended for Inflammation of the Lung.

PNEUMONIA—OR INFLAMMATION OF THE LUNG

By Dr. W. H. Webb, from "The Herb Doctor," February, 1927:—"The best combination I have found to clear the lungs in Pneumonia is the following:—

Pleurisy Root Powder	1	ounce
Mallow Leaves	1	"
Boneset Herb	1/2	"

Infuse the Mallow and Boneset in 1½ pints of boiling water, and the Pleurisy Root in a separate jug with the same quantity of boiling water. Stir well and stand covered until the Pleurisy Root Powder is well settled. Then mix the two teas in wineglass or half-teacup doses, and give frequently, warm, say every fifteen minutes or so. Add a little Cayenne to stimulate when the medicine gets fairly to work, but not until the system gets fairly relaxed. Infusions of Black Horehound, Wild Cherry Bark, sweetened with Honey, are good to tone and nourish the system when the lungs are clear. Slippery Elm Bark as a drink will help wonderfully, especially in the first stages of the complaint. Cut an ounce in small pieces on an angle with the grain, pour on 1¾ pints of boiling water, and when well infused, add a little Lemon juice. During convalescence add a little Cinnamon, and mix with milk; but the infusion with Lemon is best until the lungs are clear. It is about all the food that is needed at this stage. The British Herb Tea is a good general tonic to follow the Horehound and Wild Cherry Bark. It is composed of equal parts of Agrimony, Meadowsweet, Wood Betony, Raspberry Leaves, and Great Burnet. Make a cup of the fresh infusion every time, adding milk and sugar as desired. The tea may be taken at or before meals. Be careful that the patient does not over-eat, as the tissues are now relaxed to bear the strain of heavy work. Calf's-foot Jelly, or sparely buttered toast, with baked apple, and a light-boiled egg, are good foods in convalescence. Don't fail to sponge the body when perspiring with tepid vinegar and water, and rub the chest with good liniment, followed by Chickweed or Mallow Ointment. It will assist expectoration and relieve the breast. See that the room is ventilated, as fresh air is life itself, but protect from draughts. In America, deaths are practically unknown among the Physico-Medical doctors."

POLYPUS

This is a pendulous tumor which most frequently grows in the back of the nose and in the womb. Polypi are of two kinds: the simple and malignant. The former is soft and attached to the mucous membrane and generally arise in clusters, so that when situated in the nose, often project beyond the soft palate and prevent free breathing. Malignant Polypus has a broad base, and is either fibrous or cartilaginous structure, and ulcerated on its surface.

Treatment.—Make the following solution and use with a syringe:—

Fluid Ext. of Celandine....1 oz.
" " " Witchazel ...1 "
" " " Oak Bark ....1 "
" " " Blood Root ..1 "
Tincture of Myrrh.........1 "
" " Lobelia ....1 "

One teaspoonful to be mixed with a gill of lukewarm water, and use with a syringe or douche three or four times a day.

PREGNANCY

During the whole course of pregnancy, the bowels, if not naturally moist and easy, should be kept so by mild laxatives, such as Rhubarb, Infusion of Senna or Syrup of Figs. Once the quickening stage has commenced, 4½ months, we can thoroughly recommend the following tea, which will ensure a safe and comparatively easy time at childbirth. Take:—

Raspberry Leaves .....1 ounce
Black Currant Leaves..1 "
Mugwort Leaves ......1 "
Senna Pods ....1 "
Ginger Root ....1 "

Boil in 2 pints of water for 5 minutes. Strain, and when cool add 1 ounce of Tincture of Gentian. Take a tablespoonful three or four times a day, so long as the bowels are not too free. After birth, this is an excellent tonic and cleanser.

RHEUMATISM

This disease in which there are two states, acute and chronic, are well defined. The chronic is generally the sequel of the acute. The chronic differs from the acute in the absence of general fever in the inflammation of the parts possessing less urgent symptoms, being characterised almost entirely by pain and stiffness, by the swelling, if any, passing from one place to another, which is most common in the acute stage.

The Acute or Inflammatory Rheumatism is known by sharp pains in the joints, muscles, back, knees, ankles and hips, extending over the whole system; loss of strength, shivering, heat, thirst and general discomfiture; there is little sleep, white-coated tongue, dry skin; the bowels are constipated and the pulse hard.

The Chronic is not accompanied with fever, but the swollen joints are very tender to touch and stiff, and when untreated the joints become enlarged and distorted. Dampness and cold are the chief causes, as also the sudden checking of profuse perspiration. Twisted muscles or sprains when neglected soon become rheumatoid.

Treatment. — Turkish baths are indispensable, failing this hot mustard baths, to assist circulation and perspiration. After the bath give Yarrow Tea until a copious sweat is produced and keep the body warm from this point with hot bottles at the feet.

Now give the following mixture:—

Tincture of Guaiacum ½ ounce
" " Gelsemum .2 drams
Fluid Ext. of Yellow Dock....½ ounce
" " " Poke Root 2 drams
" " " Cascara .3 "
Potassium Iodide ......2 "
Decoction of Sarsaparilla to 8 ounces

Give two teaspoonful every four hours in water, and take every night a good dose of Yarrow Tea until the pains cease, or if pain is excessive use the following:—

Oil of Cloves ....2 drams
Oil of Wintergreen ...½ ounce
Oil of Eucalyptus .....½ ounce
Oil of Origanum ......½ ounce
Essential Oil of Camphor to 3 ounces

To be well rubbed into the painful parts 3 or 4 times daily.

RICKETS AND SOFTENING OF BONES

This disease is peculiar to the young, and is first noticed during the teething period, or follows measles, scarlet fever, whooping cough, or some other infantile disease, which induces great constitutional weakness. With this affection, the limbs become bent and twisted and the head appears swollen. The child at first walks with great difficulty, and in most cases the limbs are unable to support the weight of the trunk. The pelvis and chest become deformed and naturally there is derangement of the digestive organs, the knee and hip joints are greatly swollen. In most cases the urine is found to deposit a large amount of white deposit. Diarrhœa also sometimes accompanies Rickets, when Cherry Bark should be given.

Delicately born children or those

with scrofulous tendency are most susceptible to this disease; in all cases sun baths and fresh air, or in other words, open-air, is absolutely essential.

Treatment.—In bad cases where the limbs are so much affected by the softening of the bones, the patient should be in recumbent posture, the head and shoulders supported by some light apparatus.

Sea-salt baths containing mustard are excellent. To prepare, add 1 lb. of Bay Salt and a tablespoonful of mustard to each bath and immerse the body in same for 10 minutes. Massage the legs, etc., while in the cool bath occasionally in order to stimulate the muscle and tendons, and a good rubbing with the towel while drying will also benefit.

The undermentioned mixture is beneficial:—

Liquid Ext. of Malt...	5	ounces
Cod Liver Oil........	5	"
Honey	5	"
Juice of three Lemons		
Ext. of Bone Marrow	5	"

Take a teaspoonful after each meal, continue this treatment for a week, and then give for the next week:—

Infusion of Gentian....	2	ounces
" " Cinchona ..	2	"
" " Calumba ..	2	"
Honey	1	lb.

One teaspoonful three times a day after meals as a tonic. By alternating the medicines the system will be gradually toned up. Diet in this complaint is an important factor, malted foods made of milk, Oatmeal, broths, eggs and fish are excellent, judging the food, of course, according to the age of the child. For 18 months, all the above may be given.

Massaging the legs with Olive Oil is also good.

RINGWORM

There are two distinct kinds, the one occurring in an eruption of small vesicles encircling a portion of healthy skin on any part of the body; the other, and more infectious form, is a pustular eruption of circular form, occurring on the head.

The pustular form is very contagious; the patches are circular when the pustule bursts, the discharge is profuse, the crusts thicken, the hair falls out, and in neglected cases, the whole scalp is sometimes involved. This must not be confused with Alopecia (see article). In the former, the ring and bare patch is a dusky red colour, while in the case of Alopecia, the bare patch is white and white patches emerge into each other, forming a large patch.

Treatment. — Wash the head every other night in a solution of Lysol, Listerine or any such antiseptic fluid, brush the hair when dry to loosen any diseased hair, and paint on the following night and morning:—

Fluid Ext. of Jaborandi	1	dram
" " " Blood Root	1	"
Lysol	1	"
Tincture of Cayenne...	1	"
Glycerine	4	drams

Note.—All brushes, combs, hats, etc., used by the infected person should be thoroughly washed and disinfected, and other children should never be allowed to use these things, otherwise the disease will be carried to them.

WOOD BETONY (Betonica Officinalis)

By the REV. F. B. DENNES

There are contrary opinions as to the knowledge which people possess respecting the identity of Wood Betony, one writer states "It is the best known herb in the vegetable kingdom," another one says, that "Nineteen out of twenty people would not recognize it growing in the midst of other herbs such as Red Dead-nettle, the Stachys and others."

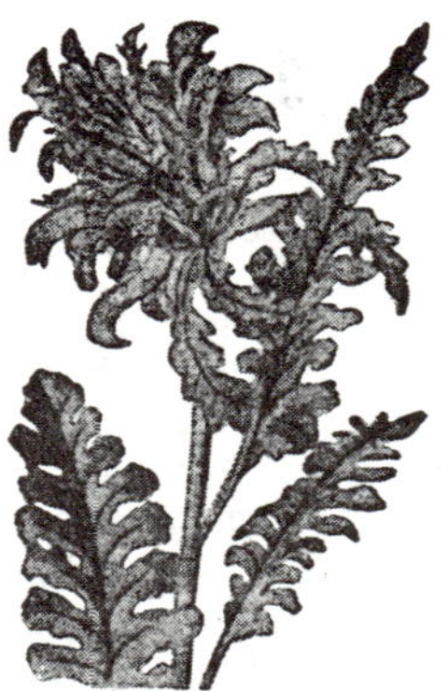

WOOD BETONY

It seems to be very rare these days, in this country. I have never seen it growing wild in Norfolk, Hertfordshire, or Cambridgeshire. A friend of mine told me it could be found growing plentifully in the Kelshal Woods, Herts. that you could reap it there, so when I was on my holiday a few years ago staying in easy distance from these woods, I motorcycled out there and found the Game Keeper and asked permission to go through the woods. He very kindly granted my request and accompanied me through them, but there was no trace of any plant I thought Betony should be like. We then passed out of the woods along into an adjoining field and as we walked on we came across a plant which was very plentiful, the flowers were red, and were placed in whorls around a square stems towards the top, I gathered some of this thinking it might be Betony, upon my return home I sent a sample of it away for identification, and this inquiry proved it was not Betony. The people to whom I sent the specimen sent me a piece of Wood Betony and then I could see it was different from the plants growing in the field, so if Betony was growing in these woods when my friend saw it some years before it had vanished by the time I went, or he had mistaken it for a plant which I think was Wood-basil.

My next adventure was to send away for three plants of Wood-betony to see if they would grow in my garden, which they did, and from the seeds others came until I had eight or nine plants.

Having now seen the plant growing and being sure as to what it was like, when I was out near Kelshal woods again I went with the Game Keeper and had another search but betony was not there.

The herb grows up every year with a number of leaves on long foot stalks, and in the midst of these there arise several stems from one to two feet high, square, with a pair of leaves upon alternate sides.

It is stated—"that two sides of the stem are more deeply hollowed than the other two, these deeper grooves are gutters of the plant leading down to its reservoir, namely, the soil immediately around the root, and they run from the points between the leaves of one pair to the mid-rib of each of the leaves in the pair below it, the surfaces of the leaves collect moisture and tilt so as to send it down the next groove, and so on, and thus the greater part of the rain is gathered into two streams which increase in volume as the base of the plant is reached."

I have examined several of the stems with a magnifying glass, and find the above statement to be correct.

The edges of the leaves are round like a set of teeth, different from most herbs which have often sharp teeth like a saw, the edges of the leaves and the venation at the back of them, and the stalks, have a number of fine hairs upon them. The flowers are a purple red colour arranged in whorls at the top of the stem which together forms short spikes; the shape of the flowers are like a tube, belonging to the two lipped or **Labiatae** family.

If we follow the guidance of history and tradition we must place Betony in the front rank of herbal remedies because of the high esteem in which it was held by our forefathers.

It was considered of such value that a proverb was current which said, "Sell your coat and buy Betony." It was so important to have it in the house. If a person was very virtuous there was a saying abroad. "You are more virtuous than Betony."

It is recorded that the great Roman Emperor, Augustus Caesar, had in his service the Physician, Antonius Musa who valued it as a cure for no less than forty-seven diseases, from the bites of mad dogs to indigestion, from the stings of serpents to the toothache, from a splinter in the thumb to the plague, there was nothing it could not put right, "and it was not the practice of Caesar to keep fools about him," remarks Culpepper. The same old herbalist further endorses the eulogy in the words, "It is a very precious herb for certain, and most fitting to be kept in a man's house."

Turner, a Physician at the end of the seventeenth century, recounts nearly thirty complaints that Betony will cure, and adds, "I shall conclude with the words found in an old manuscript under the virtues of it. 'More than all this have been proved of Betony'."

The late Mr. W. H. Box, of Plymouth, when about seventeen years of age was in the grip of consumption, and in his trouble he heard, as if someone whispered, "There is something in nature that will cure you." At this time he only knew of about six herbs, but nothing of their properties or uses, and he continues thus, "Of the six herbs I knew two were gathered and decocted as directed by me, a wineglass of which I took three times a day. In a fortnight there was a great change for the better, and in ten weeks the cure was complete."

In other parts of his books he tells us that the two which cured him were Wild Sage, and Wood

Betony. He lived to be a great healer of other sufferers.

Betony is considered of equal value for the stomach, indigestion, and belching after food.

John Gerarde says, "It maketh a man have a good stomach and an appetite for meat. It prevaileth against belchings."

He also says, "Betony with white flowers is seldom seen, it was found in a wood in a village called Hampstead near unto a worshipful gentleman's house, one of the clerks of the Queen's Council (called Mr. Wade) from whom I bought some plants and placed them in my garden where they flourished as in their natural place of growing."

Wood Betony is of historical interest and deserves more careful study, and a greater emphasis placed upon its value in the treatment of disease, and if preserved with, greater results would accrue from its use.

Complexion Problems of the Month

By KATHLEEN COVENTRY, M.N.A.M.H.

I came across some interesting reading the other day when examining an old book. The ladies of the time were advised to treat their skins in a way which, I am afraid, would not be very popular nowadays. For blotchy skins this old herbal advised its readers to rub in the juice of Field Scabious (**Scabiosa arvensis**) and wonderful testimony was paid to its value in removing "the foulnesses of the skin."

Another favourite external treatment in the old days was a skin wash of a decoction of Hogs Fennell or Sulphur Wort and here again the virtues were extolled. Another recipe given I tried out with excellent results, and that was, to brush over the teeth with powdered Water Dock; as a dentifrice it strengthens the gums and cleanses the teeth.

Meadowsweet was a great favourite in those days of old and ladies would introduce into their bath a bag containing this herb and afterwards would vigourously rub the skin. It was claimed that this imparted a healthy tone to the skin.

I have been asked for a good anti-wrinkle lotion. A friend of mine who has tried the following says it is good:—

Tincture of Benzoin, 1 Fl. drm.
Essence of Eau de Cologne, ½ Fl. drm.
Glycerine, 1 Fl. drm.

Distilled water to make up to one pint.

Your local herbalist can make this up for you cheaply.

In answer to a correspondent (Mabs, Folkestone):—I do not advise you to use any preparation to stop excessive perspiration under the arms. You had better see a herbalist. The discomfort will certainly be checked harmlessly by washing under the arms with a simple decoction of Holy Thistle. One ounce of the herb to one pint of boiling water.

IS MEDICAL SCIENCE RUINING HUMANITY?

By *JAMES I. BARDSLEY*, D.C., Ph.C., N.D., Ph.N.

A SCATHING INDICTMENT

The heading of this article is so foreign to what you have been reading in your newspapers, that you may gasp with wonder; read again with shock, then draw your conclusion, with red face and bursting blood vessels that I am "crazy." That I should be placed in a straight jacket and locked in a padded cell, where such proclamations will be heard within only four walls and sink into my own ears.

But if you read this article, which can only cover the highlights of the subject, I believe that you will draw your final conclusion to the degree that I am right; and that the medicine men, who create the damaging material which is ruining you, should be placed where you first wished to place me.

FALLACIOUS FAITH IN CHEMICALS

The compounding of chemical formulas are intriguing, and for a good many centuries it was thought that chemistry held the secret of life. For the last two decades, it has proved to be an instrument of death. Tradition and custom chain us to our system of weights and measures in chemistry, when our own experience and judgment prove that all is not well. The old experience of the "blind leading the blind."

When you are ill, your first thought is of the medical doctor, because either it is custom, or you do not know otherwise. You realise inwardly that he fails in so many cases, and nearly in every case you wonder whether you retained your health because of medicine, or in spite of it. But you still cling to the hope that he might strike something that may help, thus you consult him.

MEDICINE DYING—DRUGLESS HEALING RISING

It is realized to-day that there are other sciences, namely, drugless professions, which are doing far more good and accomplishing everything that medicine hopes to accomplish, and curing many diseases which medical science has pronounced incurable; that medical science is being made a fool of in the field of healing.

Now and then we run into a person who condemns these drugless sciences, such as Chiropractic, Naturopathy etc., and we ask them why? The answer forthcoming is: "Our medical doctor said their champions are quacks or charlatans." That they were taking person's good money, and not assisting them in their health. We wonder just what these persons would expect the medical doctor to say about the drugless profession, which has taken over 40 per cent of the United States population away from them. They of course, would not recommend another one to go to them. But this person who is under the influence of his medical doctor, proceeds to repeat that the drugless doctors are quacks. I believe this is the worst form of ignorance. Condemnation without investigation.

Victims Turn to Drugless Healing

But the funny part of all this story is: that this same person, who so loudly shouted condemnations upon the drugless professions, generally ends up in one of their offices, seeking that same health which he expected from the medical profession, and was unable to receive.

I have seen these patients come to a Chiropractic office, white with fear and trembling from head to foot, the fright which had been instilled into them by the medical profession. Forcing themselves to enter where health awaited them. I have seen them burst into hysterical laughter, after their adjustment, after they had seen how simple and easy a way the drugless method was by which to regain their health. They admitted how foolish they had been to be frightened, or to allow themselves to be frightened. However, the medical profession's greatest whip is fear.

The Real Quacks

But enough of that; let us see what medical science (?) is offering them, and why its exponents are allowed to apply the term quack to the drugless professions, when the word is so suitable to themselves.

I could supply you with stories where whole families of children have been wiped out through the use of serums, vaccines and toxins. Three little coffins in a row, in one case, to be buried without redress, sacrificed on the altar of medicine. You never heard of any such results in the drugless fields. I will just start out with a very commonly used drug. I do not know of any person living, and capable of thinking, in any city of the United States and many other cities of the world, who have not heard of it. It is known by the name, aspirin. Eaten like candy, this drug is slowly but surely ruining the humans who are using it. I have preached this for years, but "medical science" shrugs its shoulders and keeps its mouth shut, for the sake of big business. I have seen aspirin drug addicts, and possibly so have you. I have seen women's and men's nervous systems shattered for life through the use of it. Persons heart shattered for life by it; and yet it is advertised that it will not harm the heart.

The Deadly Harm of Aspirin

We now see by the following that after all these years, aspirin is at last being realized as damaging and harmful. The extract from the article which follows here, is taken from the Des Moines Tribune, and reads:—

"Washington, D. C.—The Bayer Co., Inc., of New York, was ordered Wednesday by the Federal Trade Commission to cease 'unfair competitive practices' in the sale of aspirin. The company is prohibited from asserting without proper qualifications, that the product has no harmful after effects, does not depress the heart, and the like. . . ."

This article was kept very quiet,

and the people to-day still do not realize that aspirin will cause great harm, and eventually death. The authorities did not stop the manufacture of this drug, which is just as deadly as any other drug. The dangers of its contests or its continued use are not printed on the box. It is not only allowed by prescription. It is sold on any counter, whether drug, department magazine, candy or cigar store, in all cities of the United States. Some persons eating it by the box daily. Not using it as an emergency, but as a habit. Ignoring nature rather than find the cause which is creating the headache or pain in the system.

The Action of Aspirin

In corroboration of the above, we read the following, by Dr. H. C. Temple, taken from "Good Health Magazine":

"The steady increase in deaths from heart disease since 1900 may in part be due to the free use of drugs derived from coal tar, in the opinion of Dr. H. C. Temple, writing in the Ohio State Medical Journal. He lays special stress on acetysalicylic acid, which has an enormous sale under the trade name of aspirin. It may be obtained not only in drug stores, but at news stands and stationery shops. People use it as a remedy for headaches and pains of all sorts. It belongs to the same group of coal tar derivatives as acetanilid antipyrin, acetophenacidin and other well known heart depressants.

"The physiologic action of any of this general class of drugs is to reduce arterial tension and weaken the contractibility or elasticity of the muscular fibres of the heart. By the continued use of aspirin, the heart muscles become soft and flabby, the heart valves relax and use their power to perform their normal function properly, and by degrees, the blood begins to regurgitate with each heart pulsation back into the blood vessels, thus gradualy resulting in a valvular heart lesion. Once this is established, it is never cured, but continues to grow worse until death results. Yet this drug is advertised as being quite harmless."

My friends; just think of the millions of people using this drug daily. Picture the damaged hearts and other organs and nervous systems this drug is creating; then these same medical doctors want to know why there is so much heart disease to-day. Do they know why? Only too well. With such drugs as above, and vaccines, serums and toxins being pumped into the blood stream by the tons.

They ask you to contribute millions to heart hospitals and heart laboratories yearly, to assist and discover why there is so much heart trouble, and why so many people are dying from it.

This Dr. Temple came out and told them why. But his statements were confined to the Ohio State Medical Journal, which after all, is one of their own organs. Why not come out in the daily papers in large headlines with such statements? The newspapers fear the loss of advertising from the drug manufacturers. The people must die for the lack of knowledge, and big business, big business don't forget, must be preserved, even at the cost of thousands of lives yearly.

CLEAN CULTURE AND HEALTH

EXPERIMENTS OF SAMPSON MORGAN

By JOHN MAXWELL, N.D.

To have clean bodies we must have clean foods. To have clean foods we must have clean soil. To have clean soil we must avoid dressings of unclean fertilizers, manure, blood or so-called tankage from the stock-yards.

Clean soil, combined with fresh air, sunshine and rain, produces vigorous healthy vegetation which insects will not wantonly destroy; healthy plants with good keeping quality; so different from the sappy, extra-stimulated, quality-weakened product which has been forced by artificial stimulation through the use of nitrate of soda or sulphate of ammonia.

Clean soil is not the habitat of weevils, corn borers or other pestilential visitors whose work in life seems to be that of scavengers to clear off the unfit, to destroy vegetation which is below par.

Clean soil is like that which is formed by the alluvial deposits proceeding from the erosions from basic rocks, granite, gneiss and porphry, washed down into the valleys from the mountain sides age after age, rich in all the essential minerals; finely comminuted mineral of such a texture that it can be taken up in solution by water and conveyed to the roots of plants. Clean soil, rich soil, has been built up of this basic material, plus vegetable matter, layer after layer of each, commingled.

There are such deposits at the mouths and deltas of large rivers in many parts of the world, as in the delta of the Nile, the mineral material carried down from the Abyssinian mountains by spring rains, this fine mud overflowing the banks of the Nile, depositing rich fertilizers on the land as the water evaporates, sinks into the soil or is later carried back to the bed of the river. The mouth of the Rio Grande River in the U.S.A. gives a similar illustration.

There is no fertilizer equal to this!

The kind of food we eat has a lot to do with the cleanness or uncleanness of our interior. and the kind of soil in which that food is grown very seriously affects the issue.

SICK SOIL

Sick soil produces sick food and sick food makes sick people.

Much soil is made sick by unnatural treatment; by constant cropping, without replenishing the elements extracted from the soil. Then the use of artificial stimulants instead of using natural basic food. Nitrate of soda, sulphate of ammonia and heavy doses of nitrogen in animal manure cannot be called real aid. Plants thus stimulated have not sound texture, have not good keeping qualities.

The situation was very clearly described by the late Mr. McCrillis, of Boston, as follows:—

"The common use of manure and commercial fertilizers, particularly the nitrate of soda generally employed (or other compounds of nitrogen artificially manufactured) will, it is recognized, produce a rapid growing plant structure, and one is sometimes deceived by the apparent luxuriousness of its foliage and other outward characteristics. The process, however, as we shall attempt to show, is largely a forcing process, and not one which will replenish or restore those mineral elements that are essential to healthy plant structure."

Mr. McCrillis goes on to say: "All or nearly all the commercial fertilizers are developed on the modern nitrogen theory, which is that almost all plants except the legumes, do not get their nitrogen from the air, but must have it in easily soluble form in the soil. This leads to the production of various commercial chemical compounds which contain nitrogen, and which are sold at a relatively high price to the farmers to supply this assumed need. It seems peculiar that the Creator of the Universe, in forming the air, should have made nearly eighty per cent of it out of nitrogen, if it had not been intended that the plant structures through their leaf formation, should in some manner be able to absorb this nitrogen, so necessary to their development, directly from the air. It seems absurd that they must get nitrogen through commercial combinations placed in the soil."

Sampson Morgan

Now let me quote Sampson Morgan, who worked hard as a writer and a practical horticulturist, for more than forty years in the interests of Clean Culture.

I received from his widow some years ago, a life-size picture of an apple which measured, I think, twenty-seven inches in circumference and weighed twenty-six ounces. This was sent to him in London by an orchardist who had attended to his trees in the way and manner suggested by Mr. Morgan, and sent this as a specimen from one tree. This was taken to a meeting of fruit brokers at Covent Garden Market, who unanimously proclaimed it the finest looking apple they had ever seen. Each one desired to possess it, so Sampson Morgan had it put up to auction and it was finally knocked down to one who bid £14. The money was then given to charity and the fortunate broker was happy. It would be interesting to know what he did with the seeds; if improved seedlings were produced from them.

Here is something good from Sampson Morgan's pen:

"In a healthy soil, nitrifying organisms, the good bacteria, which in a sweet, well-drained aerated soil, thrive freely on uncontaminated green material, moisture and bland mineral, alone would rule.

"Sir Almroth Wright, the distinguished bacteriologist, since the advent of Clean Culture, agrees that manures and medicines are unnecessary. But whilst he admits that the fertility of the soil may be maintained without manure, and the health of the body without medicine, and commends by cure for unhealthy conditions in the soil, a clean and natural once-burned earth, yet his cure for unhealthy conditions in the body is an unclean and unnatural one — inoculation with dead animal matter."

"The inoculators imagine that they can render man immune to disease by the unnatural injection of vaccine (pus), diseased animal matter. But pus is filth, and its introduction into the human body must be attended with awful consequences, as the huge increase in new forms of disease proves. In a perfectly healthy body even normal leucocytes could not thrive."

Bacteria and Disease

"Pasteur said that germs cause disease, which they do not. My long continued studies in the dust have convinced me that diseases in soils, plants and men arise from conditions brought about by the introduction of poisons and by imperfect environment; and experiments have satisfied me beyond doubt that this is the natural and correct explanation.

"Bacteria do not originate diseases. Their advent is always preceded by the existence of unclean conditions. The eventual existence of filth in the animal and vegetable kingdoms brought the facteria and micro-organisms of disease, as we know them, upon the scene. Before man and plants discarded the simple life, there was no scope for the presence and activities of the pus cells, and of the bad bacteria, because there were no congenial conditions to entice them and no weak, corrupted internal tissue for them to feed upon."

"Disease is the effort of nature to rid the system of morbid accumulations, and a fast will allow nature to work unhampered in that cleansing process. Then, when appetite returns, let the body be fed on clean foods produced by Clean Culture; let there be a clean wholesome environment, accompanied by clear and clean thinking, with man learning to earn his bread by the sweat of his brow.

"When man began to eat flesh (a filth food) he began to be diseased. When he began to feed animals on manure fed grass (a filth food) he introduced 'pus cells' and micro-organisms of disease into the lower animal kingdom. When he began to grow fruits, vegetables, and grains by the aid of waste animal matter (a filth food), he infected them with similar destructive agents. As the result of these three-fold violations of moral law alone Nature has plagued his structure with purulent diseases, which have in the majority of cases made life a veritable curse.

Poisoned Soils

"In consequence of my Clean Culture teaching, English medical investigators of note took up the study on the Continent, having found, as others had long previously, that the wounds of soldiers who had been used to a meat dietary do not heal anything like so cleanly or quickly as do the wounds of soldiers who have been used to a fruit and vegetable dietary. They also found that the most difficult wounds to heal were those of soldiers who had been used to living upon sewage and manure grown products. I could personally quote scores of cases to prove this which have come under my personal notice. Awful dangers attend the repulsive use of dead and waste animal matters in the growth of foodstuffs. These highly fed and poisoned soils are a menace to the health of the people wherever they exist.

"If clean plant foods through a clean soil produce healthy tissues in roots, fruits and grains, and through the consumption of the latter, healthy tissue in the human body, it naturally follows that the use of unclean plant foods through an unclean soil must produce unhealthy tissue in roots, fruits and grains, and through the consumption of the latter unhealthy tissue in the human body.

" 'Clean Culture,' writes a member of an important Parliamentary Agricultural Committee, 'is the application of the pure food principle to plant as well as animal life,' but it is more. It is the application of the pure food principle to soils also.

"An authority on physical reform writes: 'It goes right to the root of the building of a healthy body. By studying what shall go to build up the foods that shall eventually build our bodies, and by insisting on the necessity of the purity of the food you have got down to the actual foundation of the food question.'

"Though the farmer may turn his sheep into the meadows marred by tall over-luxuriant tufts of coarse grass, the sheep avoid and will not eat them, even after the pasture around them has been grazed quite bare. They know instinctively that the short succulent sugary healthy grasses are the most savoury and richer in nutrients than the tall coarse bladed stuff, which springs up where the foul carbonate-of-ammonia laden manure has been dumped upon the sward."

Natural Fertilisers

Among the agencies for the cure of sick soils, let us use dressings of finely comminuted rock dust from the basic rocks, granite, gneiss and porphry, from marl pits, and for extra dressings, when needed, of finely pulverized limestone, colloidal phosphate rock, iron ore, etc.; grow and plough in cover crops to supply essential humus, not only as a medium in which beneficial bacteria work, but to hold moisture in the soil and prevent its too rapid evaporation. In addition to all of the above, Sampson Morgan recommended the burning of coarse fibrous vegetation; that which would take too long to rot naturally, and use the ashes freely as extra fertilizer. This he called "bonfire ash."

In one article supplied to the "Chemical News" he wrote: "A gentleman in the west of England has written to me in high praise of the new soil science. He says: 'I wish I had known of Clean Culture when I was in the colonies, where I passed the greater part of my life as a planter. I would have had the bush burned in situ, and the ashes conveyed to my sugar fields. When in Barbadoes I was told that the father of Sir Graham Briggs amassed a large fortune in sugar by cutting and burying the bush in his sugar fields. All his neighbours, of course, set him down as a crank. Practically he was carrying out part of Clean Culture teaching. In Cornwall there are potteries where the fuel for the kilns consists entirely of gorse and furze, and the ashes which result from this burning are sold at six pence a bushel. They tell me the effect of the ashes on roses is wonderful.'

"As a matter of fact, I might here mention that the use of these ashes for roses especially was brought about by my advice, and this advice is emphasised in my Fortnightly Review Paper, for June, 1910."

If Sampson Morgan and Luther Burbank had been associated, I think we would have seen marvellous results from the partnership.

Like Burbank, Morgan was an optimist. He said: "I insist that the golden age of soil productivity in Europe, Asia and Africa is not behind, but before us. Clean Culture, Nature's method, is capable of making the miasmatic swamps of the tropics as sweet and healthy as England, and the huge deserts even of Africa fertile beyond description."

The chemist is dealing with proximate principles; he simply gives us drugs, inorganic dope, artificial stimulants; something of an entirely different order to nature's method of working. The bacteria in the soil fit in with dressings which are of a natural order. Just as Bechamp, the renowned French chemist and physicist, discovered minute animalculae which he named microzyma, which had lain dormant for centuries in the chalk hills, but possessed ability to produce ferments in certain media; so we find, in the finely comminuted basic rocks, microzyma; organized elements, which work with the mineral elements in the rocks, and the humus from vegetable matter, to nourish vegetation.

Perfect Food

Such vegetation, grown under favourable conditions, where every mineral need is supplied, has great potency as food for man. Sampson Morgan says in another place: "I have in my experiments with plants and soils demonstrated the positive affinity between perfect food and health, and imperfect food and disease. Since then, Professor Potter, in a paper at a British Association Meeting, endorsed Clean Culture in my words as follows: 'Susceptibility to disease in influenced by manurial treatment in the vegetable kingdom, and high fertilization with nitrogenous manures lowers the power of the plant or organism to resist infection."

"The maintenance of fertility in the soil is due to the unimpeded activity of minute organisms. Their activity depends upon congenial conditions and perfect food. The laws of nature dominate the life of the microbe as well as that of the mammoth.

"Though in some forms of sedimentary, organic and igneous rocks, we have ample materials of undeniable importance for fertilizing purposes, possibly granite, a crystalline rock of considerable beauty, is best for enchancing soil fertility and enriching all crops naturally.

"The disintegrated rock formed the basis of the soil in the beginning, but no more. Soil consists of vegetable and mineral amalgamations, and only with such is it possible to enjoy perfect crops and perfect products.

"According to my Clean Culture teaching, bonfire ash is one of the mightiest factors, in the production of perfectly healthy soils, vegetable and animal cells, beneficent bacteria, grasses, plants, trees, and human beings.

"In experiments, by digesting

powdered felspar, hornblende, and other minerals in water for a week, from a third of one per cent to one per cent of the mineral was dissolved out by the water.

"The ordinary farmer and gardener know little about the dissolving properties of rain water, or understand that the presence of simple particles of the primary rocks in the cultivated soil are necessary to assure the elaboration of healthy supple tissue in the animal organism, or flexibility in flax, in the stem of grain-bearing plants and the branches of fruit trees.

"The postassa in the granite is worth its weight in gold to the English and Irish flax growers, who cannot by any possibility produce that pliancy of thread which is the chief characteristic of flax of the highest commercial quality. It is utterly impossible to grow supple flax of the finest grade with carbonate of ammonia laden manure or forcing chemicals."

"The Garden of the Lord" —Cont.

ST. VITUS' DANCE, OR CHOREA

This is a peculiar kind of convulsion; the convulsive motions generally affect the extremities. The patient loses all voluntary power over the parts, so as to be unable to move them in the desired direction, or restrain the various motions. Different parts of the body, especially the face, are subject to involuntary twitchings, and when the disease is violent the speech becomes affected. This disorder arises from the derangement of the digestive organs; sometimes frights, exposure to cold and repelled eruptions, the editary nerve disorders are frequent causes.

Treatment.—Quietude, rest, open air, pure food are the essentials; avoid anything that will excite the brain or cause general excitement or bring about violent temper. Give the following medicine:—

Scullcap	1	ounce
Mistletoe	1	"
St. John's Wort	1	"
Valerian Root	1	"
Peruvian Bark	1	"
Gentian Root	1	"

Add 5 pints of boiling water and carefully simmer down to 2 pints. Strain. Cut up 3 large oranges and again simmer for 10 minutes with the strained fluid; now add ½ lb. sugar and again strain. Dose: Take a tablespoonful after each meal, for a child 10 to 15 years; also give one Compound Asafœtida and Lobelia pill at bedtime. Should this disease arise as the result of the stoppage of the menses, treat first that affection and follow with the above nervine and tonic.

SCARLET FEVER

This term is employed to denote a disease attended by fever, sore throat, and a red rash on the surface, which rash generally appears between the second and fourth day of illness, first upon the face and neck, and then spreads over the whole body, terminating between the seventh and tenth days. The rash has very much the appearance of the shell of a boiled lobster. The eyes are red and swollen, as also the tonsils, and the breath is offensive. Oppressed breathing, partial diarrhœa, deafness, and great prostration prevail almost from the beginning of the disease. Not unoften is there delirium at nights.

Treatment.—If there is soreness of the throat and much mucous or bronchial effects, give a dose of Syrup of Lobelia every four hours, according to age. Give a hot bath for a short while, and quickly dry and place patient in a warm bed. Give a dose of Syrup of Figs, and follow with:—

Pleurisy Root	½	ounce
Vervain	½	"
Ground Ivy	½	"
Red Sage	½	"
Centaury	½	"

Boil in 2 pints of water and simmer down to 1 pint. Sweeten with sugar, honey or treacle if found necessary. Give, according to age, a tablespoonful three times daily. If the bowels are kept moderately opened and an even temperature of the room maintained, there is no fear of dangerous results.

SMALL POX—VARIOLA

The highest state of impurity of the blood, which our bodies are capable of attaining is evidenced in this disease, yet under proper treatment there need be no anxiety. The disease is ushered in by a cold stage, thirst, drowsiness, loss of appetite, coldness of the body, sore throat, headache, pains in back and loins. In children convulsions sometimes take place previous to the eruptions, which generally appear about the fourth day. At first the spots are similar to flea bites and come on the neck, breast and face. As the disease advances these spots become larger and contain at first a white and then yellow matter; about the eighth day the spots or pustules begin to suppurate and the fever is more pronounced; the face is red and much swollen. About the tenth day the face and neck subside, after which the pustules discharge their contents and then become dry; they fall off in crusts, leaving the skin brownish in colour, but ultimately is restored to its former state.

Treatment. — Assist Nature to drive out the putrefaction and keep the determining powers to the surface. Bathe the patient in warm water and have hot-water bottles to the feet. Drink the following tea:—

Wood Sage	1	ounce
Pitcher Plant	1	"
Vervain	1	"
Marigold Flowers	½	"
Saffron	1	"
Peppermint	1	"

Add to 3 pints of boiling water and simmer down to 1 pint. Strain, and add 1 ounce of Bayberry Powder. Give a teaspoonful every 4 hours. An injection of decoction of Eucalyptus Leaves is the best method of dealing with any constipation. As soon as the pustules begin to scab and itch, apply a little Olive over the surface; this will not only keep the scab soft but will prevent the ghastly looking poc mark. Diet, etc., follow principles laid down as in all other fevers.

Note.—As a preventative against Small Pox, make an infusion of 1 ounce Pitcher Plant and 1 ounce Ground Ivy in 2 pints of boiling water and simmer down to 1 pint. Take a tablespoonful every 6 hours.

SYRUPS

As these contain the properties of the herbs in a palatable form, they are pleasant for both young and old and are taken readily.

BLOOD PURIFIER AND DECLINE SYRUP

Simmer slowly 3 ounces of Sarsaparilla, 1 ounce each of Yellow Dock, Burdock, Guaiacum, Wood Sanicle, and Poke Root in 4 quarts of water. Simmer down to 1 quart; then strain and press out the herbs. Re-boil the herbs in a quart of water and simmer down to 1 pint; again strain and add to the first liquid. Add 3 lbs. of sugar and boil slowly for 10 minutes; allow to cool and take off the scum. Now add 3 drams of Potassium Iodide, 1 ounce of Tincture of Queen's Delight, 1 ounce of Spirits of Wine, and 1 ounce of Fluid Extract of Sassafras, and shake. It is an excellent blood purifier, and in this lies the secret of its success in rheumatism, scurvy, boils, abscesses, ulcers, eczema and skin diseases. Dose: One tablespoonful three or four times a day.

COUGH SYRUP

Take 1 ounce each of Horehound, Elecampane, Cherry Bark, Coltsfoot and Thyme, all finely cut, and simmer in 4 quarts of water down to 1 quart. Strain and press out the herbs. Dissolve 1 lb. of sugar in the liquid, and then add 1 lb. of honey, 1 ounce of Ipecacuanha Wine, 1 ounce of Vinegar of Squills, and 2 drams of Tincture of Aniseed. Dose: Adults, a dessertspoonful three times a day; children, from ½ to 1 teaspoonful, according to age.

We find this a splendid remedy for all coughs, croup, whooping cough, consumption, bronchitis and all affections of the lungs.

COUGH SYRUP (CHILDREN'S)

Syrup of Tolu	1 ounce
Syrup of Red Poppy ...	1 "
Oxymel of Squills.....	1 "
Glycerine	1 "
Ipecacuanha Wine	4 drams
Aniseed Water	6 ounces

For children under one year, give half a teaspoonful three times daily. From 7 on to 14 years, one teaspoonful. Mothers will find this safer and better than Paregoric; it acts quickly where the breathing is difficult.

SYRUP OF LOBELIA

Boil 2 ounces of Lobelia herb in 2 pints of water and simmer down to 1 pint. Strain and by gentle heat dissolve 2 lbs. of refined sugar. Dose: 5 to 20 drops. Useful in coughs, but note, taken in large doses it will act as an emetic.

SYRUP OF RASPBERRY

Slowly boil for half an hour in a covered vessel 1 pound of Raspberries in a pint of Malt Vinegar. Press and strain, and in the clear liquid dissolve by the aid of heat 1 lb. of sugar, ½ lb. of honey, 4 ounces of glycerine, and 2 ounces of Syrup of Lobelia. Take a teaspoonful four times daily. This is an excellent remedy for asthma, croup, whooping cough, and dry and hard tickling coughs. If 5 drops of Fluid Extract of Pleurisy Root and 1 drop of Essence of Cayenne be added to each dose of Raspberry Syrup, it makes a splendid mixture for inflammation of the lungs.

SYRUP OF SQUILLS

Dissolve 2 lbs. of sugar in a gill of water by gently heating; when cool, add a pint of Vinegar of Squills. Dose: One teaspoonful. This is a useful syrup for coughs and colds, especially in conjunction with other herbs. Taken with Yarrow Tea, it is an excellent remedy for catarrh or cold in the head.

SYRUP OF TOLU

Make the simple syrup as in Syrup of Squills, and add to every 10 ounces of syrup 4 drams of Tincture of Tolu, and shake. Dose: Half to one teaspoonful. Useful for coughs and bronchitis in children; it is generally given with other medicaments.

Recommended Herbal Remedies

Nervous Conditions

Mistletoe . . . . 1/4 ounce
Scullcap . . . . 1/4 ounce
Valerian . . . . 1/2 ounce
Tansy . . . . 1/2 ounce

Simmer in two pints of water down to one pint, strain and bottle. Dose—a wineglassful three times a day.

* * *

Kidney Haemorrhage

F.E. Cranesbill . . . . 2 drams
F.E. Bistort . . . . 2 drams
F.E. Witch Hazel . . . . . 2 drams
F.E. Bayberry Bark . . 2 drams
F.E. Comfrey Root . . . 2 drams
Tinct. Gentian Root. . . . 4 drams

Made up with water to fill a 12-ounce bottle. Dose a teaspoonful every hour, until the haemorrhage ceases and then every three hours.

* * *

Boils

Yellow Dock Root. . . . . 2 ounces
Red Dock Root. . . . . . . 1 ounce
Brooklime . . . . 1 ounce
Nettle . . . . 1 ounce

* * *

Cancer of the Breast

F.E. Phytolacca . . . . . . 2 ounces
F.E. Gentian . . . . 1 ounce
F.E. Dandelion . . . . 1 ounce

Mixed with some simple syrup up to one pint. Dose—a teaspoonful after each meal.

* * *

Inflammation of the Uterus

Powdered Slippery-elm Bark. . . . 2 ounces
Powdered Marshmallow Root. . . . 2 ounces
Powdered Comfrey Root. . . . 2 ounces
Powdered Composition 1/2 ounce
Powdered Sugar . . . . . . 6 ounces

Mix this thoroughly and for a dose take two teaspoonfuls and place in a cup. Fill half way up with boiling water and stir well, then fill up with hot milk. A very nourishing and soothing drink.

* * *

Flatus

Dandelion Root . . . . 1 ounce
Parsley Root . . . . 1 ounce
Mountain Flax . . . . 1 ounce

Boil in two pints of water for abount twenty minutes, take a wineglassful as required.

A BOTANICAL RAMBLE

By MRS. B. EMMOTT, M.N.A.M.H.

On Sunday, September 5th, members and friends of the Lancashire Branch of the National Association of Medical Herbalists, met at Clitheroe for a botanical ramble.

Leaving the Station by the County Lane, we passed through meadowland and Pastureland, where cows were grazing peacefully. Many and varied were the old-fashioned stiles we passed through; rough and rocky a portion of the way; but we all enjoyed it, even the Elder Berries, who, although not so nimble as the younger ones, got through their difficulties very well. Soon we were on the banks of the Ribble, passing through a glorious valley, where God's Messengers' "the flowers," greeted us, and those who had ears to hear, heard the message: "We are they, whom He had sent for your use, for meat and Medicine."

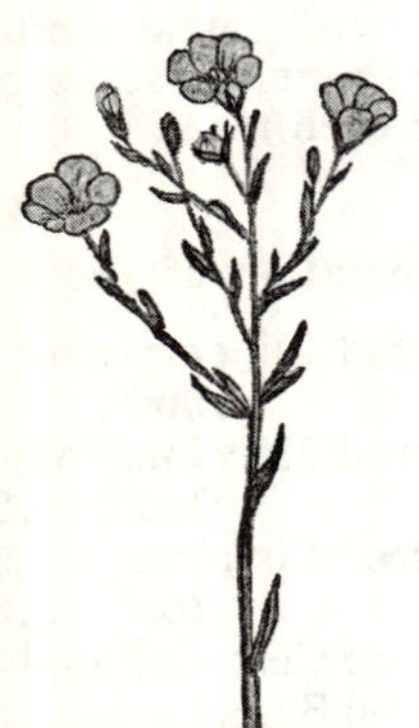

MOUNTAIN FLAX

Small beautiful flowers, each bringing its own message. The delicate Eyebright with its pure white flower, streaked with purple, was crying out "Here I am, Why don't you gather me? I will brighten your eyes. A cup of tea a day, made from my leaves, and a lotion made from me, will make your eyes as pure and clear as my own small flower."

We met the Water Figwort, with its heart-shaped flower, in its close panicle. The figwort may not be as beautiful as some flowering plants, but it is certainly tall and attractive, and as most Herbalists know, it is a very useful plant, its alterative properties making it of great value in all cutaneous eruptions. Its leaves are as soothing in their healing when applied, as poultices in cases of abscesses and wounds. In the year 1628, at the siege of Rochelle, during a season of famine, the soldiers of the garrison supported themselves by eating the roots of the plant, and applied the leaves to their wounds, which it speedily healed. That is why in France it is still spoken of as "Herbe de Siege."

I think every member got a specimen Prunella—the herb that ought to be in every home. Its dense short spikes, of purple flowers, came peeping at us everywhere, and it seemed to be calling out: "Healall, Healall." Its very name tells how useful it is, and ought to be in every Herbal Medicine Chest. Its action is astringent, it is most useful as a gargle in relaxed—sore throat.

It is a woman's herb and is useful in all female weaknesses, leucorrhoea, etc. Many cases are recorded by old herbalists in which wounds inflicted by sickles, scythes and other sharp instruments, were healed by its use.

Another small and lovely flower—of whose usefulness enough cannot be said—greeted us with a sunny smile. The Ladies Mantle, so called from its leaf being in the form of a cloak, truly the foliage of the plant is more attractive than its small but pretty flowers. Its usefulness is in its astringent properties, and may be given for excessive menstruation, dysentery and all haemorrhages. It is also most valuable in diabetes.

We had many specimens including our friend Yarrow. One member found a sample of Mountain-flax so useful for its laxative properties. Mountain-flax has a long established reputation amongst the old Welsh country-folk as a cure for rheumatism.

Amongst my specimens was a small purple-red flower. One of our members who gave it to me, said: "Your favourite." Just my favourite. Not for its pretty flower, nor its sweet fragrance, but for its great help to mankind, has the Clover become my favourite. Alterative and sedative, we know its soothing action on the bronchial membrane, we know its excellent power as a syrup for whooping cough, but, what is more, we know the ease that can be obtained from this little flower when man is suffering from that most dreaded of all diseases—cancer.

On our ramble we visited Mr. and Mrs. Moorey, who kindly provided refreshments. Then on to Hey's Farm Guest House, where we got a lovely view of the Ribble Valley.

Recommended Herbal Remedies

Prostatitis

Tinct. Sabal serrulata.

Dose ten drops in a wineglassful of water once in three hours

or

Tinct. Aesculus hippo.

Dose—Add thirty drops to four ounces of water. Take one teaspoonful once in two hours.

* * *

Eczema

F.E. Yellow Dock .....1 ounce
F.E. Mountain Grape ..1 ounce
F.E. Burdock Seed....½ ounce

Made up with a simple syrup to eight ounces. Dose—two teaspoonfuls three times a day before meals.

Common Wayside Herbs

The Borage Family

This family of rough-leaved plants contains many herbs of excellent value which will cure the minor ailments that occur in every household.

If we take as an example such a familiar member of this group as the Forget-me-not (though of no medicinal value) the main characteristics will be seen whereby it can be distinguished.

It will be observed that the leaves are of a fleshy texture, and covered with stiff short hairs which grows older; also the leaves are placed alternately on the stem.

The flowers are arranged in a very curious manner, as the stalk which bears them is coiled up at the tip so that the youngest flowers are almost hidden. But as the flow-are more pronounced as the plant ers expand the stalk gradually un-coils so that they appear to grow from one side only; this is not so,

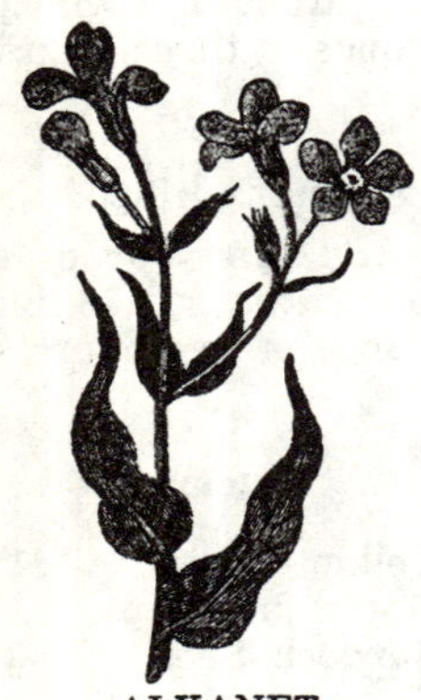

ALKANET

however, they are only turned that way. This "twisting" character is one which will enable you to recognize a plant as belonging to the Borage family.

Some of the plants which are useful as herbal remedies are, Borage, Houndstongue, Alkanet, Viper's Bugloss and Comfrey—all of which are quite harmless.

The most useful one is Comfrey which is to be found growing wild in damp places and is fairly common. In height it is about two feet with coarse stems with either yellowish-white or purple flowers. The leaves are large, with very noticable veins, tapering at the base and running down into the stem as will be seen in the illustration.

Comfrey is an official plant in the National Botanic Pharmocopoeia, so that you can be assured of its purity when obtained from a qualified Medical Herbalist. It is useful for complaints of the lungs and can be applied in the form of a fomentation to all inflammatory conditions of muscles. In years past this latter use gave Comfrey the popular name of knit-bone.

No finer remedy exists than this for ulcerated conditions. A decoction is made from the root by boiling one ounce in a quart of water down to a pint, and a wineglassful taken as a dose three times a day. Better results are obtained when combined with other alternatives, which your Herbalist will be able to provide and make up in fluid extract form. An up-to-date practioner will have on hand at all times a stock of fluid extracts which many prefer for use instead of making a decoction or infusion, as the case may be, from the crude herb.

Comfrey is also of value to those unfortunates, the dyspeptics, and in such cases a decoction should be made with milk, with larger doses than usual. Catarrhal troubles can be cured too, by gargling and spraying in addition to taking the decoction.

In that excellent work "Herbal Simples" by the late Dr. W. T. Fernie, is the following anecdote: "Mr. Cockayne relates that the locksman at Teddington informed him how the bone of his little finger being broken, was grinding and grunching so sadly for two months, that sometimes he felt quite wrong in his head. One day he saw a doctor go by, and told him about his distress. The doctor said: 'You see that Comfrey growing there? Take a piece of its root, and clamp it, and put it about your finger, and wrap it up.' The man did so, and in four days his finger was well."

Auto-Intoxication

OUR success in healing the sick depends more upon the careful looking-after and preventing of the self-poisoning of our patient, than upon any other thing we can do.

We all had thrust upon us repeatedly in practice, the demand of the patient that we purge him or keep the bowels open freely, and as soon as we do that the patient says that his head is better. It matters not where the intoxication is in the body, because the bowels are the important channel for removal from the system of obnoxious matter.

Auto-intoxication is defined as a toxemia caused by substances introduced into the body by tainted foods or microbes and toxins generated within, from the introduction of substances laden with microbes.

There is a law of nature that forbids inertia or a dormant state —inactivity. If the tissues and organs of the body do not properly perform their work they will necessarily die or become foul and in this state the secretions will form toxins which are intensely poisonous to the remainder of the body. Therefore, it should be a cardinal doctrine to keep up an active state of various organs of the body for purpose or renewal of secretions.

Modern Herbal Remedies

On one or two occasions we have reprinted some of the old-fashioned remedies with the object in view of creating interest and perhaps research. Now we have been requested to print a few standard recipes which can be made up by a qualified Medical Herbalist

Blood Mixture

Liq. Sarsae Jam ......4 drams
F.E. Burdock root .....2 drams
F.E. Dandelion root ...2 drams
F.E. Peruvian bark ...2 drams
F.E. Sassafras bark ...2 drams
F.E. Poke root ....2 drams
10 drops Sac. Ust.

This is made up with sufficient distilled water to fill a 12-oz. bottle and a tablespoonful taken after meals.

* * *

Pimply Skin

F.E. Echinacea ....3 drams
F.E. Yellow Dock ....3 drams
F.E. Burdock ....3 drams
F.E. Blue Flag ....3 drams
F.E. Queen's Delight ..3 drams

Distilled water is added to make up an 8-oz. bottle and a tablespoonful taken three times a day.

* * *

Nephritis

F.E. Populus Tremuloides 1 oz.
F.E. Juniperis Communis..1 oz.
F.E. Barosma Grenata ...½ oz.
Mucilage of Gum Acacia...2 oz.

Mixed well together and take a teaspoonful every two hours in half a cupful of an infusion of Meadowsweet.

THE YOUNG PEOPLE'S PAGE

By MISS H. M. BRETT, M.N.A.M.H.

A few weeks ago, many members belonging to the London Branch of our Association enjoyed a delightful expedition to Kew Gardens. Kew Gardens are amongst the most celebrated botanical gardens in the world. When one walks through the gardens and observes numbers of people all taking a delight in the beautiful surrounding, one is impressed that the British Nation is undoubtedly a nature-loving people.

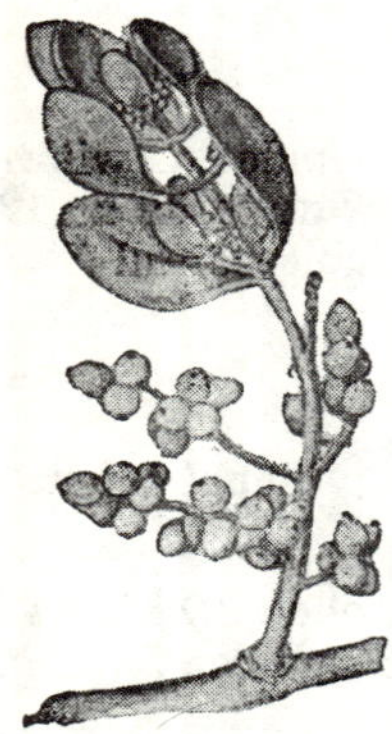

THE MISTLETOE

We had the privilege of seeing many plants which do not belong to this country and trees such as the banana and the rubber tree. Those which interested us most were, of course, in the Herb-garden; those of medicinal value, which, by their use, we are familiar. It was evident with some plants, that they had completed part of their work of the year, which brings us to a very important part in the life of a plant.

We know the Floral Kingdom consists of different groups or families into which the various plants are classed. At this time of the year, most of the plants, and we have been considering the wild flowering plants, will have completed their year's work, part of which is the production of a seed or seeds for future plants.

Although there is a big difference in the various groups, yet the only parts necessary for the formation of the future plants are contained in the flower. The flower, therefore is the most important part of the plant for the production of the seeds as well as being the most ornamental. The flower opens out when it has received fit nourishment from the root and leaves. Most flowers consist of a green outer part called the calyx, which is usually of several leaves, called sepals. The sepals form a protective outer covering for the flower when it is in bud.

When the bud expands, the petals open out forming the corolla. The petals enclose the stamens, which produce a fine dust called pollen; and right in the centre of the flower is the pistil. The development of the fruit takes place after the pistil has received the pollen from the stamens. The bees aid nature a great deal by taking the pollen from one flower to another, in search for nectar to make honey. The wind, too, helps to take the pollen from flower to flower. This process is known as pollination for the development of the seeds. When the seeds are ripe, the plants adopt many ways to get them scattered. Some are blown by the wind, as in the poppy, in which the seeds lie loose at the bottom of the fruit, known as the poppy-head. When the wind blows it bends the flower-stalk and jerks the fruit open and allows the seeds to escape. Other seeds blown by the wind are the dandelion, thistle and groundsel. The wind carries them along and deposits them in all kinds of places. Some seeds are known as winged seeds, and trees as the ash, the sycamore, elm and birch have these. Some plants have a habit of shooting out their seeds. The broom and the gorse do so, their seeds are contained in a pod and when the sun is warm, the pods dry and crack open, letting go the seeds with a "pop."

There are two types of fruits; the dry and the fleshy. The dry fruits consist of the nuts; we have all seen the hazel nuts growing on hedgerow. The fleshy fruits are divided again into two types, known as the berry and the drupe. The berry is fleshy throughout as in the gooseberry, the currant, the elder and the tomato. The drupe is that type of fruit, the inner part of which is hard and stony. It contains a nut enclosed in the pulp, as in the plum, cherry, almond and peach. The raspberry and the blackberry are really composed of compound fruits, which are themselves composed of small drupes. The strawberry differs from other fruits. Its seeds are taken to the outer surface and are called achenes.

The mistletoe gets its seeds distributed in another way. It is a parasite; that is, a plant which grows on another plant, instead of getting its own nourishment from the soil. The berries contain a sticky substance, and when the birds eat these berries, the seeds often stick to the bird's beak, who rubs them off on to the branch of a tree. The seedling is thus from the first attached to the tree on which it lives.

We have thus seen, that one great purpose of the Floral Kingdom, is the production of seeds for new plants. There is another great purpose especially with the medicinal plants. They contain active principles, which are sometimes in the roots, sometimes in the leaves and other parts of the plant. Next month, we shall see how Nature supplies us with a wonderful store of Herbal Remedies in her own laboratory.

* * *

At this time of the year, the trees are almost leafless. If we look closely at them, we shall find, that while this year's foliage has completed its task and fallen, yet the tree has provided itself with next year's buds. They will be found to occur in the axil of the leaf-stem. The leaves, we shall learn, make food for the tree.

The air consists of certain gases; the chief gases being nitrogen and oxygen. Other gases occur in very small quantities amongst them is the gas, carbon dioxide. This gas although in such small quantities, is very necessary for the formation of the starch in the leaves. The green colouring matter in the leaves, is due to a mixture of pigments known as CHLOROPHYLL, which is of great importance to the nutrition of the plant. It is the chlorophyll in the presence of light, which forms the starch in the leaves from the carbon dioxide in the air, breathed in through the tiny pores known as STOMATA, on the under side of the leaves. The chlorophyll is able to separate the carbon from the carbon dioxide and build it up into starch and sugar, and at the same time give off oxygen. The air we breathe out contains carbon dioxide (CO/2), and yet it is in the air around us in very small quantities, that is because it readily dissolves in water and why the air, after the rain, is much purer. As plants use this CO/2, for food, nature maintains a balance. The gas which is waste to us, is food for plants and trees. We know that without plants and trees, no animals could exist. The plants purify the air and give up oxygen, and so fulfill one great purpose of their existence.

Parts of a Plant

The chief parts of a plant are the root, stem, leaves, flowers and seeds. The root penetrates the soil, and by the aid of the root-hairs, is able to absorb the soluble food. All food must be in a liquid state before it can be absorbed. The water in the ground dissolves the mineral salts which is taken in by the root-hairs. In some plants the root is the storehouse for certain foods; especially in the root vegetables and bulbs. In some medicinal plants as the dandelion, the marshmallow, the burdock and many others. All parts of the dandelion can be used, but in medicine it is the root that is used for its tonic effects. Most people know of Dr. Thompson's famous Dandelion Coffee. He was one of our Herbal Pioneers.

When the root is required, it is gathered after the leaves have perished. The proper time to gather any part of a plant, is at the stage of full maturity or development of the part to be used. If the whole plant is to be used, it must be gathered when the leaves and flowers are at their best. We know that

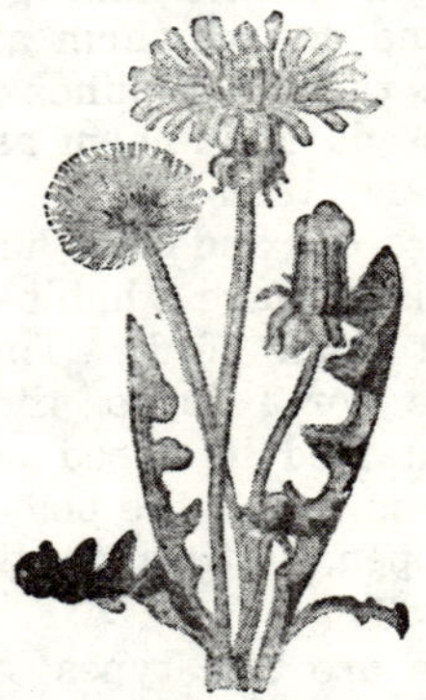

DANDELION

the more freshly gathered are our herbs, the better are the results. There is a right time for everything, especially for the gathering of medicinal plants. Last month we learnt that the function of the flower is principally for the production of seeds. Some flowers contain valuable oils, and other medicinal properties. When the flowers are required, they must be gathered when they are just fully opened and the seeds must be collected when they are ripe.

The stem conducts the liquid food from the root to the leaves and at a certain time; just before the flowers appear, the leaves of medicinal plants contain valuable properties. Such plants as the plantain, horehound, comfrey to mention a few.

Some of the flowers used in medicine are chamomile, hops, red clover, elder flower and many others. The plants mentioned are those which grow in our countryside and which you should be able to recognise. Many of our medicinal herbs however, come from other lands.

* * *

Why Plants Breathe

If we look at any leaf, we shall find it contains numerous veins or channels known as the vascular system through which food substances made in the leaf by the breathing process, travels into the stem. We know the leaves breathe in for the plant. When the plant is living, the sap is always rising from the root. Sometimes the roots absorb more moisture than the plant requires. Then the leaves breathe it out. That is why there are often tiny drops of moisture on leaves, especially in the morning. This breathing out of the superfluous moisture by the leaves ensures a continual flow of sap from the root. In this way the plant is kept alive. In the autumn the fullgrown leaves have finished their work.

The tree wastes nothing which is of value to it so when the leaves have completed their work, the tree makes a layer of thick substance at the base of the leaf through which the sap cannot pass. The leaf then changes colour and falls off, leaving a scar which the tree has already healed over. This is shown very clearly in the horse-chestnut, where also can be seen the tiny holes or the vascular system through which the sap passed. Nature seems to waste nothing. The leaves bud and open in the spring, work all the summer breathing for and feeding the tree. In the autumn they fall and decay and make food which the roots absorb and so the seasons progress each fulfilling its task.

Modern Herbal Remedies

Tape Worm

F.E. Wormwood ....2 drams
F.E. Tansy ....2 drams
F.E. Am. Mandrake ....1 dram
Oil of Male Fern.......1 dram
Oil of Tansy..........24 drops

Make up with distilled water to fill a 6-oz. bottle. Take one tablespoonful night and morning.

* * *

Hay Fever

F.E. Boneset ....2 drams
F.E. Yarrow ....2 drams
F.E. Vervain ....2 drams
F.E. Hyssop ....2 drams
F.E. Bogbean ....2 drams
F.E. American Valerian 4 drams

Make up with distilled water to 12 oz. and take a tablespoonful every three hours.

* * *

Menorrhagia

Witch Hazel Powder.....½ oz.
Bayberry Powder ....½ oz.
Bur-marigold Herb ......½ oz.
Ginger Powder ....¼ oz.

Mix these together and make an infusion by pouring on two pints of boiling water; strain off, and drink half a teacupful every half hour.

MELVIN POWERS SELF-IMPROVEMENT LIBRARY

COOKERY & HERBS

___CULPEPER'S HERBAL REMEDIES *Dr. Nicholas Culpeper*	3.00
___FAST GOURMET COOKBOOK *Poppy Cannon*	2.50
___GINSENG The Myth & The Truth *Joseph P. Hou*	3.00
___HEALING POWER OF HERBS *May Bethel*	3.00
___HEALING POWER OF NATURAL FOODS *May Bethel*	3.00
___HERB HANDBOOK *Dawn MacLeod*	3.00
___HERBS FOR COOKING AND HEALING *Dr. Donald Law*	2.00
___HERBS FOR HEALTH—How to Grow & Use Them *Louise Evans Doole*	3.00
___HOME GARDEN COOKBOOK—Delicious Natural Food Recipes *Ken Kraft*	3.00
___MEDICAL HERBALIST *edited by Dr. J. R. Yemm*	3.00
___NATURAL FOOD COOKBOOK *Dr. Harry C. Bond*	3.00
___NATURE'S MEDICINES *Richard Lucas*	3.00
___VEGETABLE GARDENING FOR BEGINNERS *Hugh Wiberg*	2.00
___VEGETABLES FOR TODAY'S GARDENS *R. Milton Carleton*	2.00
___VEGETARIAN COOKERY *Janet Walker*	4.00
___VEGETARIAN COOKING MADE EASY & DELECTABLE *Veronica Vezza*	3.00
___VEGETARIAN DELIGHTS—A Happy Cookbook for Health *K. R. Mehta*	2.00
___VEGETARIAN GOURMET COOKBOOK *Joyce McKinnel*	3.00

GAMBLING & POKER

___ADVANCED POKER STRATEGY & WINNING PLAY *A. D. Livingston*	3.00
___HOW NOT TO LOSE AT POKER *Jeffrey Lloyd Castle*	3.00
___HOW TO WIN AT DICE GAMES *Skip Frey*	3.00
___HOW TO WIN AT POKER *Terence Reese & Anthony T. Watkins*	3.00
___SECRETS OF WINNING POKER *George S. Coffin*	3.00
___WINNING AT CRAPS *Dr. Lloyd T. Commins*	3.00
___WINNING AT GIN *Chester Wander & Cy Rice*	3.00
___WINNING AT POKER—An Expert's Guide *John Archer*	3.00
___WINNING AT 21—An Expert's Guide *John Archer*	4.00
___WINNING POKER SYSTEMS *Norman Zadeh*	3.00

HEALTH

___BEE POLLEN *Lynda Lyngheim & Jack Scagnetti*	3.00
___DR. LINDNER'S SPECIAL WEIGHT CONTROL METHOD *P. G. Lindner, M.D.*	1.50
___HELP YOURSELF TO BETTER SIGHT *Margaret Darst Corbett*	3.00
___HOW TO IMPROVE YOUR VISION *Dr. Robert A. Kraskin*	3.00
___HOW YOU CAN STOP SMOKING PERMANENTLY *Ernest Caldwell*	3.00
___MIND OVER PLATTER *Peter G. Lindner, M.D.*	3.00
___NATURE'S WAY TO NUTRITION & VIBRANT HEALTH *Robert J. Scrutton*	3.00
___NEW CARBOHYDRATE DIET COUNTER *Patti Lopez-Pereira*	1.50
___QUICK & EASY EXERCISES FOR FACIAL BEAUTY *Judy Smith-deal*	2.00
___QUICK & EASY EXERCISES FOR FIGURE BEAUTY *Judy Smith-deal*	2.00
___REFLEXOLOGY *Dr. Maybelle Segal*	3.00
___REFLEXOLOGY FOR GOOD HEALTH *Anna Kaye & Don C. Matchan*	3.00
___YOU CAN LEARN TO RELAX *Dr. Samuel Gutwirth*	3.00
___YOUR ALLERGY—What To Do About It *Allan Knight, M.D.*	3.00

HOBBIES

___BEACHCOMBING FOR BEGINNERS *Norman Hickin*	2.00
___BLACKSTONE'S MODERN CARD TRICKS *Harry Blackstone*	3.00
___BLACKSTONE'S SECRETS OF MAGIC *Harry Blackstone*	3.00
___COIN COLLECTING FOR BEGINNERS *Burton Hobson & Fred Reinfeld*	3.00
___ENTERTAINING WITH ESP *Tony 'Doc' Shiels*	2.00
___400 FASCINATING MAGIC TRICKS YOU CAN DO *Howard Thurston*	3.00
___HOW I TURN JUNK INTO FUN AND PROFIT *Sari*	3.00
___HOW TO WRITE A HIT SONG & SELL IT *Tommy Boyce*	7.00
___JUGGLING MADE EASY *Rudolf Dittrich*	2.00
___MAGIC MADE EASY *Byron Wels*	2.00
___STAMP COLLECTING FOR BEGINNERS *Burton Hobson*	2.00

HORSE PLAYERS' WINNING GUIDES

___BETTING HORSES TO WIN *Les Conklin*	3.00
___ELIMINATE THE LOSERS *Bob McKnight*	3.00

____HOW TO PICK WINNING HORSES *Bob McKnight* 3.00
____HOW TO WIN AT THE RACES *Sam (The Genius) Lewin* 3.00
____HOW YOU CAN BEAT THE RACES *Jack Kavanagh* 3.00
____MAKING MONEY AT THE RACES *David Barr* 3.00
____PAYDAY AT THE RACES *Les Conklin* 3.00
____SMART HANDICAPPING MADE EASY *William Bauman* 3.00
____SUCCESS AT THE HARNESS RACES *Barry Meadow* 3.00
____WINNING AT THE HARNESS RACES—An Expert's Guide *Nick Cammarano* 3.00

HUMOR

____HOW TO BE A COMEDIAN FOR FUN & PROFIT *King & Laufer* 2.00
____HOW TO FLATTEN YOUR TUSH *Coach Marge Reardon* 2.00
____JOKE TELLER'S HANDBOOK *Bob Orben* 3.00
____JOKES FOR ALL OCCASIONS *Al Schock* 3.00
____2000 NEW LAUGHS FOR SPEAKERS *Bob Orben* 3.00
____2,500 JOKES TO START 'EM LAUGHING *Bob Orben* 3.00

HYPNOTISM

____ADVANCED TECHNIQUES OF HYPNOSIS *Melvin Powers* 2.00
____BRAINWASHING AND THE CULTS *Paul A. Verdier, Ph.D.* 3.00
____CHILDBIRTH WITH HYPNOSIS *William S. Kroger, M.D.* 3.00
____HOW TO SOLVE Your Sex Problems with Self-Hypnosis *Frank S. Caprio, M.D.* 3.00
____HOW TO STOP SMOKING THRU SELF-HYPNOSIS *Leslie M. LeCron* 3.00
____HOW TO USE AUTO-SUGGESTION EFFECTIVELY *John Duckworth* 3.00
____HOW YOU CAN BOWL BETTER USING SELF-HYPNOSIS *Jack Heise* 3.00
____HOW YOU CAN PLAY BETTER GOLF USING SELF-HYPNOSIS *Jack Heise* 3.00
____HYPNOSIS AND SELF-HYPNOSIS *Bernard Hollander, M.D.* 3.00
____HYPNOTISM *(Originally published in 1893) Carl Sextus* 5.00
____HYPNOTISM & PSYCHIC PHENOMENA *Simeon Edmunds* 4.00
____HYPNOTISM MADE EASY *Dr. Ralph Winn* 3.00
____HYPNOTISM MADE PRACTICAL *Louis Orton* 3.00
____HYPNOTISM REVEALED *Melvin Powers* 2.00
____HYPNOTISM TODAY *Leslie LeCron and Jean Bordeaux, Ph.D.* 5.00
____MODERN HYPNOSIS *Lesley Kuhn & Salvatore Russo, Ph.D.* 5.00
____NEW CONCEPTS OF HYPNOSIS *Bernard C. Gindes, M.D.* 5.00
____NEW SELF-HYPNOSIS *Paul Adams* 4.00
____POST-HYPNOTIC INSTRUCTIONS—Suggestions for Therapy *Arnold Furst* 3.00
____PRACTICAL GUIDE TO SELF-HYPNOSIS *Melvin Powers* 3.00
____PRACTICAL HYPNOTISM *Philip Magonet, M.D.* 3.00
____SECRETS OF HYPNOTISM *S. J. Van Pelt, M.D.* 3.00
____SELF-HYPNOSIS A Conditioned-Response Technique *Laurance Sparks* 5.00
____SELF-HYPNOSIS Its Theory, Technique & Application *Melvin Powers* 3.0
____THERAPY THROUGH HYPNOSIS *edited by Raphael H. Rhodes* 4.0

JUDAICA

____HOW TO LIVE A RICHER & FULLER LIFE *Rabbi Edgar F. Magnin* 2.0
____MODERN ISRAEL *Lily Edelman* 2.0
____SERVICE OF THE HEART *Evelyn Garfiel, Ph.D.* 4.0
____STORY OF ISRAEL IN COINS *Jean & Maurice Gould* 2.0
____STORY OF ISRAEL IN STAMPS *Maxim & Gabriel Shamir* 1.0

JUST FOR WOMEN

____COSMOPOLITAN'S GUIDE TO MARVELOUS MEN Fwd. by *Helen Gurley Brown* 3.0
____COSMOPOLITAN'S HANG-UP HANDBOOK Foreword by *Helen Gurley Brown* 4.0
____COSMOPOLITAN'S LOVE BOOK—A Guide to Ecstasy in Bed 4.0
____COSMOPOLITAN'S NEW ETIQUETTE GUIDE Fwd. by *Helen Gurley Brown* 4.0
____I AM A COMPLEAT WOMAN *Doris Hagopian & Karen O'Connor Sweeney* 3.0
____JUST FOR WOMEN—A Guide to the Female Body *Richard E. Sand, M.D.* 4.0
____NEW APPROACHES TO SEX IN MARRIAGE *John E. Eichenlaub, M.D.* 3.0
____SEXUALLY ADEQUATE FEMALE *Frank S. Caprio, M.D.* 3.0
____YOUR FIRST YEAR OF MARRIAGE *Dr. Tom McGinnis* 3.0

MARRIAGE, SEX & PARENTHOOD

____ABILITY TO LOVE *Dr. Allan Fromme* 5.0
____ENCYCLOPEDIA OF MODERN SEX & LOVE TECHNIQUES *Macandrew* 5.0
____GUIDE TO SUCCESSFUL MARRIAGE *Drs. Albert Ellis & Robert Harper* 5.0

_____HOW TO RAISE AN EMOTIONALLY HEALTHY, HAPPY CHILD *A. Ellis* 3.00
_____IMPOTENCE & FRIGIDITY *Edwin W. Hirsch, M.D.* 3.00
_____SEX WITHOUT GUILT *Albert Ellis, Ph.D.* 3.00
_____SEXUALLY ADEQUATE MALE *Frank S. Caprio, M.D.* 3.00

MELVIN POWERS' MAIL ORDER LIBRARY

_____HOW TO GET RICH IN MAIL ORDER *Melvin Powers* 10.00
_____HOW TO WRITE A GOOD ADVERTISEMENT *Victor O. Schwab* 15.00
_____WORLD WIDE MAIL ORDER SHOPPER'S GUIDE *Eugene V. Moller* 5.00

METAPHYSICS & OCCULT

_____BOOK OF TALISMANS, AMULETS & ZODIACAL GEMS *William Pavitt* 4.00
_____CONCENTRATION—A Guide to Mental Mastery *Mouni Sadhu* 3.00
_____CRITIQUES OF GOD *Edited by Peter Angeles* 7.00
_____DREAMS & OMENS REVEALED *Fred Gettings* 3.00
_____EXTRA-TERRESTRIAL INTELLIGENCE—The First Encounter 6.00
_____FORTUNE TELLING WITH CARDS *P. Foli* 3.00
_____HANDWRITING ANALYSIS MADE EASY *John Marley* 3.00
_____HANDWRITING TELLS *Nadya Olyanova* 5.00
_____HOW TO UNDERSTAND YOUR DREAMS *Geoffrey A. Dudley* 3.00
_____ILLUSTRATED YOGA *William Zorn* 3.00
_____IN DAYS OF GREAT PEACE *Mouni Sadhu* 3.00
_____KING SOLOMON'S TEMPLE IN THE MASONIC TRADITION *Alex Horne* 5.00
_____LSD—THE AGE OF MIND *Bernard Roseman* 2.00
_____MAGICIAN—His training and work *W. E. Butler* 3.00
_____MEDITATION *Mouni Sadhu* 5.00
_____MODERN NUMEROLOGY *Morris C. Goodman* 3.00
_____NUMEROLOGY—ITS FACTS AND SECRETS *Ariel Yvon Taylor* 3.00
_____NUMEROLOGY MADE EASY *W. Mykian* 3.00
_____PALMISTRY MADE EASY *Fred Gettings* 3.00
_____PALMISTRY MADE PRACTICAL *Elizabeth Daniels Squire* 3.00
_____PALMISTRY SECRETS REVEALED *Henry Frith* 3.00
_____PROPHECY IN OUR TIME *Martin Ebon* 2.50
_____PSYCHOLOGY OF HANDWRITING *Nadya Olyanova* 3.00
_____SUPERSTITION—Are you superstitious? *Eric Maple* 2.00
_____TAROT *Mouni Sadhu* 6.00
_____TAROT OF THE BOHEMIANS *Papus* 5.00
_____WAYS TO SELF-REALIZATION *Mouni Sadhu* 3.00
_____WHAT YOUR HANDWRITING REVEALS *Albert E. Hughes* 2.00
_____WITCHCRAFT, MAGIC & OCCULTISM—A Fascinating History *W. B. Crow* 5.00
_____WITCHCRAFT—THE SIXTH SENSE *Justine Glass* 4.00
_____WORLD OF PSYCHIC RESEARCH *Hereward Carrington* 2.00

SELF-HELP & INSPIRATIONAL

_____DAILY POWER FOR JOYFUL LIVING *Dr. Donald Curtis* 3.00
_____DYNAMIC THINKING *Melvin Powers* 2.00
_____EXUBERANCE—Your Guide to Happiness & Fulfillment *Dr. Paul Kurtz* 3.00
_____GREATEST POWER IN THE UNIVERSE *U. S. Andersen* 5.00
_____GROW RICH WHILE YOU SLEEP *Ben Sweetland* 3.00
_____GROWTH THROUGH REASON *Albert Ellis, Ph.D.* 4.00
_____GUIDE TO DEVELOPING YOUR POTENTIAL *Herbert A. Otto, Ph.D.* 3.00
_____GUIDE TO LIVING IN BALANCE *Frank S. Caprio, M.D.* 2.00
_____HELPING YOURSELF WITH APPLIED PSYCHOLOGY *R. Henderson* 2.00
_____HELPING YOURSELF WITH PSYCHIATRY *Frank S. Caprio, M.D.* 2.00
_____HOW TO ATTRACT GOOD LUCK *A. H. Z. Carr* 4.00
_____HOW TO CONTROL YOUR DESTINY *Norvell* 3.00
_____HOW TO DEVELOP A WINNING PERSONALITY *Martin Panzer* 3.00
_____HOW TO DEVELOP AN EXCEPTIONAL MEMORY *Young & Gibson* 4.00
_____HOW TO OVERCOME YOUR FEARS *M. P. Leahy, M.D.* 3.00
_____HOW YOU CAN HAVE CONFIDENCE AND POWER *Les Giblin* 3.00
_____HUMAN PROBLEMS & HOW TO SOLVE THEM *Dr. Donald Curtis* 3.00
_____I CAN *Ben Sweetland* 4.00
_____I WILL *Ben Sweetland* 3.00
_____LEFT-HANDED PEOPLE *Michael Barsley* 4.00